Solubility and Related Properties

DRUGS AND THE PHARMACEUTICAL SCIENCES

A Series of Textbooks and Monographs

Edited by
James Swarbrick
School of Pharmacy
University of North Carolina
Chapel Hill, North Carolina

Other Volumes in Preparation

Solubility and Related Properties

Kenneth C. James

Welsh School of Pharmacy
University of Wales Institute
of Science and Technology
Cardiff, Wales

MARCEL DEKKER, INC.   New York and Basel

Library of Congress Cataloging-in-Publication Data

James, Kenneth C., [date]
    Solubility and related properties.

    (Drugs and the pharmaceutical sciences ; v. 28)
    Includes index.
    1. Solutions (Pharmacy) 2. Drugs—Solubility.
3. Solubilization. I. Title. II. Series.
RS201.S6J29   1986   615'.19   86-4418
ISBN 0-8247-7484-1

MARCEL DEKKER, INC.
270 Madison Avenue, New York, New York 10016

Current printing (last digit):
10 9 8 7 6 5 4 3 2 1

PRINTED IN THE UNITED STATES OF AMERICA

Preface

There are several excellent books on solubility but, because their approach is theoretical, they deal exclusively with molecules with low polarity. There is rarely much practical interest in such systems, but the work that has been published on more complicated systems usually involves an element of empiricism and is therefore not applicable to theoretical treatment. This book is written with the practical aspects of solubility in mind so that it is appropriate to extend the scope to polar, interacting, and conducting systems. Despite the practical emphasis, the theoretical background of the properties of solutions has not been neglected and particular attention has been paid to explaining and deriving concepts that are normally taken for granted. Rather tedious proofs of equations therefore appear in some of the early chapters, and there are examples throughout the text showing how theory can be used in practical situations.

The book has two basic aims. The first is to enable the reader to select the most suitable solvent for the purpose he has in mind. This is necessary in the formulation of liquid pharmaceuticals, for which there is still a demand, even though drugs are almost always taken in the form of tablets and capsules. The very old, the very young, and many otherwise normal patients are incapable of swallowing tablets or capsules, and must be provided with liquid oral forms of dosage. The unconscious patient is unable to swallow at all and must receive his drugs by injection. Similarly, drugs that are metabolized or destroyed by digestive enzymes when taken orally must be administered parenterally. Intramuscular and subcutaneous injections are usually solutions, and intravenous injections must be entirely liquid. Enteral feeding preparations have similar requirements.

Solubility is equally important with colors. Dyes are used in solution but pigments are used in suspension; dyers are interested in solvents and painters in "nonsolvents." Whether or not a color dissolves will control the properties of the product. For example, nail varnishes, which are solutions, give a clear glossy finish while the suspensions give a pastel effect. Sometimes colors exist in both forms in the same base, as in lipsticks, in which the bromo acid is dissolved and the pigment is not.

Sometimes the most efficient solvents are unsuitable (they may be toxic) and less efficient solvents must be considered. In these circumstances one must be able to predict approximate solubilities, in order to select the most suitable solvent. This is the second basic aim of the book, namely, to provide information from which the reader can estimate solubilities that have not been determined experimentally. The answers obtained are not always accurate, but they do give an idea of where the solubility lies and can suggest whether or not a particular line of investigation should be attempted.

Lipophilic solvents are required for lipid drugs that are to be administered in soft gelatin capsules, suppositories, topical preparations, or injections. In these circumstances the most efficient, nontoxic solvent may still not be the best for the purpose in mind. Bioavailability from suppositories, percutaneous absorption from topical preparations, and duration of biological activity following intramuscular injection are all dependent on the degree of saturation of the drug in the solvent. Therefore, an ability to predict solubility is important in order to select the solvent giving the appropriate biological response.

Estimated solubilities are usually adequate for correlations with other physical properties, as in linear free-energy relationships (LFER). Quantitative structure-activity relationships (QSAR), used in medicinal chemistry, form the most important pharmaceutical application of linear free-energy relationships. These involve correlations between biological activities and various physical properties, and are used to predict the potencies of known, untested compounds, and to suggest new compounds of possible pharmacological interest. The octanol-water partition coefficient is one of the more important of these physical properties. A chapter is devoted to partition law and methods of predicting partition coefficients.

Sometimes the structure of a solute is modified to increase its aqueous solubility, such as the conversion of hydrocortisone, which is insoluble in water, to hydrocortisone hemisuccinate, which is soluble in aqueous alkali. Alternatively, the structure may be changed to render a water-soluble drug insoluble. Thus, benzylpenicillin is very soluble in water but is unstable in aqueous solution. The procaine salt of benzylpenicillin is soluble in 200 parts of water, and suitably formulated aqueous suspensions retain 90% of their potency after 1 year at ambient temperature. Similar considerations apply to plastics: Chemical modification can render a polymer that is soluble in water and suitable as a film former in hair setting agents to one that requires an organic solvent to dissolve, is water-resistant, and is suitable for use in hair spray. In contrast, cellulose, which is insoluble in water, can be rendered water-soluble by esterification and becomes an efficient adhesive and suspending agent.

Pharmaceutical solutions are not always simple and frequently contain more than one solute, sometimes with widely different solubility characteristics. Solvent mixtures are required in these situations, necessitating a knowledge not only of the behavior of the solutes in solution, but also of the miscibility of the solvents. Even when the individual solutes are soluble in the same solvents, they sometimes interfere with each other when mixed. There are laws, equations, and other devices that help us to understand these complicated systems.

Should the reader wish to determine solubilities, activities, or partition coefficients experimentally, the methods and their pitfalls are described within. Methods of predicting physical properties related to solubility, such as molar volume, parachor, and heat of vaporization, are also described.

Authors of research papers involving solubility appear to be reluctant to convert to SI units. It has been attempted in this text to use SI units as far as possible, but it has not always been practicable, particularly when the topic is associated with solubility parameters, whose units involve the old calorie unit. In a similar way, natural logarithms have been used wherever possible, since they are just as easy to use as logarithms to the base 10 in this age of the electronic calculator. However, where the original papers used logarithms to the base 10, and it was considered that conversion to the natural form would cause confusion, logarithms to the base 10 have been retained.

Kenneth C. James

Contents

1

Solutions and Solubility

I. INTRODUCTION

The essential opening to any discussion is to establish exactly
what is going to be discussed. It is therefore necessary to define
the subject under discussion, namely the term *solubility*, which is
what this book is all about. Closely associated with solubility is
the solution.

A *solution* is a molecular dispersion of a solute in a solvent.
There can be more than one solute, and the solvent can consist
of more than one substance. To be precise, a mixed solvent is
itself a solution; for example, a solution of benzoic acid in 95% v/v
ethanol should really be regarded as a solution of benzoic acid and
water as solutes, in ethanol as solvent, but for most purposes it is
convenient to look upon ethanol-water and similar mixtures as solvents
in their own right. With some systems, such as solutions of solids
in liquids, the identities of solute and solvent are unambiguous, but
with solutions of liquids in liquids, the choice of which is solute and
which is solvent is often optional. It is normally assumed that the
liquid in excess is the solvent, but this is arbitrary.

A solution is capable of continuous variation in composition,
within limits. This distinguishes it from a chemical compound, which
is a molecular dispersion, but is not capable of continuous variation.
The lower limit is the philosophical point at which the solution is so
dilute, it must be regarded as pure solvent, and the upper limit occurs when the solvent is incapable of dissolving any more solute,
and a new phase consisting of undissolved solute appears in the
system. The solution in equilibrium with undissolved solute is a
saturated solution, and the concentration of the saturated solution
is the solubility of the solute in that solvent. The presence of excess solute is necessary to avoid supersaturation.

Solubilities vary with temperature, and when the solute is volatile, also with pressure. These two properties must therefore be
specified to make any solubility statement meaningful.

The subject matter of this book will be confined to consideration of molecular dispersions, including those in which the solute,
by virtue of its high molecular weight, comes within the colloidal
range (e.g., proteins and polymers). The contributions of

solute-solute, solute-solvent, and solvent-solvent interactions to solubility are discussed, but solvophobic colloids and solubilized systems are considered to be outside the scope of this book.

II. METHODS OF EXPRESSING CONCENTRATION AND SOLUBILITY

Before carrying out a solubility determination, it is necessary to decide how the result is to be expressed. The better known methods will be described generally and coupled with methods of expressing concentration.

A. Parts

In pharmacy, solubilities have traditionally been expressed by *parts*; for example, chloroform is said to be soluble in 200 parts of water at 20°C. This means that at 20°C, chloroform requires the addition of 200 times its volume of water before it will dissolve completely and produce a saturated solution. This statement is independent of the units in which the liquids are measured, provided that the same units are used for both, and therefore provides a simple, unambiguous method of expressing the solubilities of mobile liquids in mobile liquids. With materials that are not readily measured by volume, the system can no longer be considered in unambiguous terms. Castor oil, for example, is too viscous to be measured accurately by volume, and in common with other viscous liquids, is traditionally measured by weight. Thus when it is stated that at 20°C castor oil is soluble in 2 parts of ethanol, it is implied that the castor oil has been measured by weight. However, ethanol, being a mobile liquid, is traditionally measured by volume, and since ethanol has a density of 790 kg m^{-3} at 20°C, a solubility of 1 kg in 2 dm^3 (2 liters) of ethanol corresponds to 1 kg in 2 × 0.79 = 1.6 kg of ethanol. A large error is therefore possible if the wrong units are assumed. The problem is avoided by laying down universal rules, as follows:

1. Mobile liquids are measured by volume.
2. Gases, solids, and viscous liquids are measured by weight.

This scheme should be followed when expressing solubilities by parts, but to avoid any confusion, it is recommended that the units be stated (e.g., 1 kg of castor oil is soluble in 2 dm^3 of ethanol at 20°C). Solubilities expressed by parts are rarely meant to be precise and are normally quoted only as a guide for the preparation of solutions.

B. Percentage

Percentage concentration is expressed as the quantity of solute
which is dissolved in 100 equivalent units of solution. Logically,
therefore, a solubility expressed as a percentage implies the percentage concentration of the saturated solution. The choice of
units follows the scheme given above; for example, solids in liquids
are traditionally expressed as weight of solute in total volume of
solution. Percentage weight in volume, measured in grams per
100 ml, is more concisely termed *gramarity*, or can be expressed
in the abbreviated form % w/v. *Milligramarity* refers to concentration expressed as milligrams per 100 ml. The units grams per
liter (dm^3) and milligrams per milliliter are also commonly used.
Corresponding expressions are percentage weight in weight (% w/w),
or *gramality*; percentage volume in volume (% v/v); and percentage
volume in weight (% v/w). The particular expression employed can
be inferred by the nature of the solute and solvent, but it is
nevertheless desirable to declare on every occasion exactly which
units are employed. Solutions of gases in liquids are traditionally
expressed as weight in weight.

C. Molarity and Molality

Molarity is concentration expressed as molecular weight in grams of
solute in 1 dm^3 (1 liter) of solution and is usually written, mol
$liter^{-1}$ or mol dm^{-3}. *Molality* is the number of moles of solute in
1 kg of solution and is symbolized m. Molality is independent of
temperature; molarity is not.

D. Mole Fraction

Mole fraction concentration is the number of moles of the component
of interest divided by the total number of moles in the solution. If
the number of moles of solvent is n_1 and the number of moles of
solute is n_2, then

$$\text{Mole fraction of solvent} = X_1 = \frac{n_1}{n_1 + n_2}$$

and

$$\text{Mole fraction of solute} = X_2 = \frac{n_2}{n_1 + n_2}$$

Also,

$$X_1 + X_2 = 1$$

The suffix 1 is always used to designate solvent, and 2 to designate solute.

E. Volume Fraction

The *volume fraction* of a solvent (ϕ_1) in a solution is defined as the volume of solvent in the solution divided by the total volume of solution. It is therefore expressed as

$$\text{Volume fraction of solvent} = \phi_1 = \frac{n_1 V_1}{n_1 V_1 + n_2 V_2}$$

where V_1 and V_2 are molar volumes of solvent and solute, respectively. Similarly,

$$\text{Volume fraction of solute} = \phi_2 = \frac{n_2 V_2}{n_1 V_1 + n_2 V_2}$$

Also,

$$\phi_1 + \phi_2 = 1$$

For a precise definition of molar volume, intermolecular volume should be taken into account, but this is usually ignored. Also, since the coefficients of expansion of solute and solvent are invariably different, volume fraction will vary with temperature. This effect is usually neglected.

F. Interconversion of Units

The following examples are given to illustrate conversion from one method of expressing concentration to another.

Example

Suppose that 2.776 g of a saturated solution of a nonvolatile solid in a volatile solvent is evaporated to dryness and leaves a residue of 0.057 g. The density of the saturated solution is 1507 kg m^{-3} and the molecular weights of solute and solvent are 122 and 199, respectively.

Solution: (a)   The solute is soluble in

$$\frac{2.776 - 0.057}{0.057} = 48 \text{ parts of solvent by weight}$$

(b)   The gramality of the saturated solution is

$$\frac{0.057 \times 100}{2.776} = 2.05 \text{ % w/w}$$

(c)   The gramarity of the saturated solution is

$$\frac{0.057 \times 100 \times 1507}{2.776 \times 1000} = 3.09 \text{ % w/v}$$

(d)   The molality of the saturated solution is

$$\frac{0.057 \times 1000}{2.776 \times 122} = 0.168 \text{ mol kg}^{-1} \text{ (m)}$$

(e)   The molarity of the saturated solution is

$$\frac{0.057 \times 1000 \times 1507}{2.776 \times 122 \times 1000} = 0.254 \text{ mol dm}^{-3}$$

(f)   The mole fraction solubility of the solute is

$$X_2 = \frac{0.057/122}{(2.776 - 0.057)/199 + (0.057/122)} = 0.0331$$

Example

n-Butanol is soluble in 45 parts of water at 20°C. Calculate (a) the mole fraction solubility, and (b) the volume fraction solubility, given that:

	Density at 20°C ($kg \ m^{-3}$)	Mol. wt.	Molar volume (cc)
Butanol	810	74	92
Water	1000	18	18

Solution: 1 ml is soluble in 45 ml of water. Therefore,

$$1 \text{ g is soluble in } \frac{45 \times 1000 \times 1000}{810 \times 1000} = 55.6 \text{ g of water}$$

Therefore:

(a) Mole fraction solubility $= X_2 = \dfrac{1/74}{1/74 + 55.6/18} = 4.36 \times 10^{-3}$

(b) Volume fraction solubility $= \phi_2 = \dfrac{92/74}{92/74 + (55.6 \times 18/18)}$

$$= 2.19 \times 10^{-2}$$

III. ELECTROLYTE SOLUTIONS

A. Activity and Activity Coefficient

The most characteristic feature of aqueous electrolyte solutions is their ability to conduct electricity. This property is called *conductance* and is expressed quantitatively as the specific conductance (κ), defined in cgs units as the reciprocal of the resistance in ohms set up between the opposite sides of a 1-cm cube of the solution. Specific conductance provides a means of comparing one solution with another but gives no indication of the charge-transporting abilities of the individual ions. The equivalent conductance (Λ), defined by

$$\Lambda = \frac{1000 \, \kappa}{M} \tag{1.1}$$

serves this function. The greater the equivalent conductance the greater the efficiency of the ions in transporting electricity. M is concentration in mol dm^{-3}. Λ is inversely proportional to concentration, so a plot of Λ against 1/M should give a straight line of slope 1000 κ, but in practice two types of plot are obtained, neither of which is rectilinear over the whole concentration range. Typical examples are shown in Fig. 1.1. The lower plot is characteristic of weak electrolytes; equivalent conductance increases curvilinearly to a constant limiting value, the limiting conductance (Λ_0), at high dilution. The principal reason for this behavior is that weak electrolytes, as the name suggests, are only partially ionized in strong and moderately strong solutions, most of the molecules in solution remaining in the nonionized state, but as the solution is diluted, more molecules dissociate, until the equivalent conductance reaches Λ_0, when the solute is completely ionized.

Equivalent Conductance

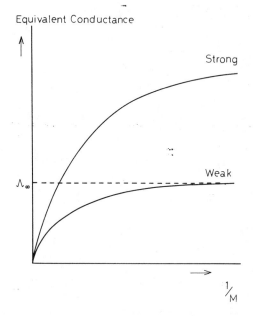

FIGURE 1.1 Equivalent conductances of strong and weak electrolytes.

Limiting conductance has two useful features:

1. Because it applies to very dilute solutions, it can be as-
    sumed that weak electrolytes are fully dissociated.
2. It can be calculated by summing the contributions of in-
    dividual ions. These contributions are called *mobilities*
    (λ) and are standard for specific ions at specific tempera-
    tures. Some examples are shown in Table 1.1. Thus for
    hydrogen chloride at 25°C,

$$\Lambda_0(HCl) = \lambda_{H^+} + \lambda_{Cl^-} = 349.8 + 76.4 = 426.2 \text{ ohm}^{-1}$$

The fraction of the solute molecules that are ionized at a given
concentration is called the *degree of dissociation* (α), and can be
calculated from

$$\alpha = \frac{\Lambda}{\Lambda_0} \tag{1.2}$$

An indication of the degree of dissociation can be obtained from
osmotic pressure (Π) through

$$\Pi = iRTM \qquad (1.3)$$

and

$$\alpha = \frac{1-i}{1-n} \qquad (1.4)$$

where R is the gas constant, T the temperature, M is molarity, and i the van't Hoff factor. n represents the number of ions per molecule; for example, for acetic acid, n = 2. Degrees of dissociation obtained by this route agree well with those obtained from conductance measurements.

A similar interpretation could be applied to the strong electrolyte plot in Fig. 1.1, but is not valid because strong electrolytes are known to be completely dissociated at all concentrations, and also because the results obtained with Eqs. (1.2) and (1.4) do not agree.

It will be shown in Chapter 5 that nonelectrolyte solutions of liquids in liquids rarely obey Raoult's law precisely, and that in most situations concentration must be multiplied by an activity coefficient (f) before meaningful vapor pressures can be calculated. A similar interpretation applies to the strong electrolyte plot in Fig. 1.1. The behavior of a given ion in solution is influenced by the presence of ions of opposite charge. Each ion will be surrounded by an atmosphere of oppositely charged ions, which will decrease the mobility of the ion. The process is called the umbrella effect, for obvious reasons. Ions will be brought into closer contact in concentrated solutions, and hence the mobility of the ion will become increasingly more affected as concentration increases.

Although the concept of activity coefficients of electrolytes was originally derived from conductance measurements, its application

TABLE 1.1 Ionic Mobilities of Some Common Ions in Water at 25°C

Cation	ohm^{-1}	Anion	ohm^{-1}
H^+	349.8	OH^-	198.3
Na^+	50.1	Cl^-	76.4
K^+	73.5	Br^-	78.1
Ag^+	61.9	I^-	76.8
$(1/2) \ Mg^{2+}$	53.0	NO_3^-	71.5
$(1/2) \ Ca^{2+}$	59.5	$(1/2) \ SO_4^{2-}$	80.0

Source: Ref. 1.

actually extends to any situation in which the active mass of an electrolyte is considered. Active masses are usually taken to be equal to concentrations. This is approximately true for dilute solutions, but in more concentrated systems, concentration must be multiplied by the activity coefficient to give the activity (a), which is the precise measure of active mass.

The magnitude of the activity coefficient depends on the units of concentration to which it applies. The most important activity coefficients are the practical or molar activity coefficients (f_M), based on molar concentrations and applied in the form

$$a_M = f_M M \qquad\qquad (1.5)$$

in which M represents molar concentration, and the rational or mole fraction activity coefficients (f_X), based on mole fraction concentration, and applied in the form

$$a_X = f_X X \qquad\qquad (1.6)$$

where X represents mole fraction concentration. The molal activity coefficient (f_m), defined by

$$a_m = f_m m \qquad\qquad (1.7)$$

is based on molal concentration. The coefficients differ less with increasing dilution, and below 0.01 M can be considered equal.

Like all thermodynamic properties, activity coefficients must be defined relative to a standard state. For electrolyte solutions the standard state for the solvent is the pure liquid, and for the solute it is the infinitely dilute solution. As the solute concentration approaches zero, the activity coefficient approaches unity and the activity approximates to the concentration.

The activity coefficient of an electrolyte is a composite value, embracing the cation(s) and the anion(s), and varies from one electrolyte to another. It is dependent on the concentration of all the ions in the solution, rather than only those of the solute of interest. Furthermore, the way in which the activity coefficient varies with the concentration of ions in solution differs from one electrolyte to another. Examples are shown in Fig. 1.2. Total ionic concentration is assessed as the ionic strength (I), defined by

$$I = 0.5(M_A z_A^2 + M_B z_B^2 + M_C z_C^2 + \cdots + M_N z_N^2) \qquad\qquad (1.8)$$

Activity Coefficient

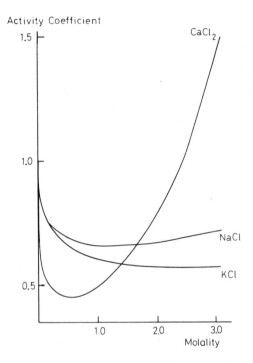

FIGURE 1.2 Activity coefficients of some strong electrolytes.

where z is ionic charge and A, B, and so on, represent the various ions in solution.

Debye and Hückel calculated the electrostatic free energy required to charge a neutral particle to the potential of an ion in its oppositely charged ionic atmosphere. This was equated to RT ln f_M, giving

$$\ln f_M = -4.198 \times 10^6 \, \frac{z^2}{(\varepsilon T)^{3/2}} \, \sqrt{I} \qquad (1.9)$$

Substitution for the dielectric constant (ε) and T for water as solvent at 25°C gives

$$\log f_M = -0.51 z_+ z_- \sqrt{I} \qquad (1.10)$$

z is split up into z_+ and z_- because under practical conditions two oppositely charged ions must be considered. Equation (1.10) is

called the Debye-Hückel limiting law, limiting because it applies only
to very dilute solutions. It holds reasonably well up to I = 0.01.
Beyond this, the activity coefficient decreases more slowly with increasing concentration. The scope can be extended to about I =
0.25 by correcting for the sizes of the ions. This takes the form
of two parameters: A, which is the distance of approach of the
ions and approximately equal to 10^{-9} m, and B, which is derived theoretically and is approximately equal to 10^9 m^{-1}. These are inserted
into Eq. (1.10) to give

$$\log f_M = \frac{-0.51z_+z_-\ \sqrt{I}}{1 + AB\ \sqrt{I}} \qquad (1.11)$$

which, since AB = 1, leads to

$$\log f_M = \frac{-0.51z_+z_-\ \sqrt{I}}{1 + \sqrt{I}} \qquad (1.12)$$

In more concentrated solutions the ions will increase the dielectric constant of the medium in their immediate vicinity. This causes
a decrease in interionic forces, and the activity coefficient becomes
greater than would otherwise be the case. This is corrected by adding a term proportional to root ionic strength,

$$\log f_M = \frac{-0.51z_+z_-\ \sqrt{I}}{1 + \sqrt{I}} + CI \qquad (1.13)$$

C is calculated from experimental results. An estimate of C is
given by [2]

$$C = 0.1(z_+z_-) \qquad (1.14)$$

Example

Calculate the ionic strength at 25°C of an aqueous solution containing 0.4% w/v of sodium sulfate decahydrate and 0.3% w/v of potassium chloride. What are the activity coefficients of the two salts in
the solution?

Solution:

$Na_2SO_4 \cdot 10H_2O$: molecular weight = 322.2; therefore,

$$\text{Molarity} = \frac{0.4 \times 10}{322.2} = 1.24 \times 10^{-2}$$

KCl: molecular weight = 74.5; therefore,

$$\text{Molarity} = \frac{0.3 \times 10}{74.5} = 4.03 \times 10^{-2}$$

$$I = 0.5(M_{Na}z_{Na}^2 + M_{SO_4^{2-}}z_{SO_4^{2-}}^2 + M_{K^+}z_{K^+}^2 + M_{Cl^-}z_{Cl^-}^2)$$

$$= 0.5(2 \times 1.24 \times 10^{-2} \times 1^2 + 1.24 \times 10^{-2} \times 2^2 + 4.03 \times 10^{-2}$$

$$\times 1^2 + 4.02 \times 10^{-2} \times 1^2)$$

$$= 0.5(2.48 \times 10^{-2} + 4.96 \times 10^{-2} + 4.03 \times 10^{-2} + 4.03 \times 10^{-2})$$

$$= 7.75 \times 10^{-2}$$

This is greater than 0.01 and less than 0.25, so Eq. (1.12) applies.
$Na_2SO_4 \cdot 10H_2O$

$$\log f_M = \frac{-0.51 \times 1 \times 2 \sqrt{7.75 \times 10^{-2}}}{1 + \sqrt{7.75 \times 10^{-2}}}$$

$$= -2.22 \times 10^{-1}$$

Therefore,

$$f_M = 0.600$$

KCl

$$\log f_M = \frac{-0.51 \times 1 \times 1 \sqrt{7.75 \times 10^{-2}}}{1 + \sqrt{7.75 \times 10^{-2}}}$$

$$= -1.11 \times 10^{-1}$$

Therefore

$$f_M = 0.774$$

Example

Calculate the approximate activity coefficient of sodium chloride in a 0.5 M solution in water at 25°C.

Solution

$$C = 0.1(z_+ z_-) = 0.1$$

$$\log f_M = \frac{-0.51 z_+ z_- \sqrt{I}}{1 + \sqrt{I}} + CI$$

$$= \frac{-0.51 \times \sqrt{0.5}}{1 + \sqrt{0.5}} + 0.1 \times 0.5$$

$$= -0.2112 + 0.05 = -0.1612$$

Therefore,

$$f_M = 0.690 \quad (\text{lit.} = 0.681) \; [2]$$

B. Interrelationships Between Activity Coefficients

Molar activity (a_M) is related to free energy through

$$\Delta \overline{G} = \Delta G_M^\circ + RT \ln a_M \tag{1.15}$$

where $\Delta \overline{G}$ is the partial molar free energy or chemical potential and ΔG_M° is the standard free energy, both on the molar scale. A similar relationship applies to mole fraction activity; that is

$$\Delta \overline{G} = \Delta G_X^\circ + RT \ln a_X \tag{1.16}$$

Since both equations relate to free energy, the right-hand sides of the two equations can be equated, and on rearrangement give

$$\Delta G_M^\circ + RT \ln M + RT \ln f_M = \Delta G_X^\circ + RT \ln X \tag{1.17}$$
$$+ RT \ln f_X$$

A molar solution is equivalent to M_2 moles in $(1000\rho - M_2 W_2)/W_1$ moles of solvent, where ρ is density of the solution in g cm^{-3} and W_1 and W_2 are molecular weights; therefore,

$$X_2 = \frac{M_2}{(1000\rho - M_2W_2)/W_1 + M_2} = \frac{M_2W_1}{1000\rho + M_2(W_1 - W_2)}$$

or

$$\ln \frac{X_2}{M_2} = \ln \frac{W_1}{1000\rho + M_2(W_1 - W_2)} \tag{1.18}$$

Rearrangement of Eq. (1.17) for solute gives

$$\ln f_{M,2} = \ln f_{X,2} + \ln \frac{X_2}{M_2} + \frac{\Delta G^\circ_{X,2} - \Delta G^\circ_{M,2}}{RT} \tag{1.19}$$

As $M_2 \rightarrow 0$, $\ln f_{M,2} \rightarrow \ln f_{X,2}$; therefore, substitution in Eq. (1.19) gives

$$\ln \frac{M_2}{X_2} = \frac{\Delta G^\circ_{X,2} - \Delta G^\circ_{M,2}}{RT} \tag{1.20}$$

Also as $M_2 \rightarrow 0$,

$$X_2 \rightarrow \frac{M_2W_1}{1000\rho_1} \tag{1.21}$$

So that substitution from Eqs. (1.18), (1.20), and (1.21) in Eq. (1.19) gives

$$\ln f_{M,2} = \ln f_{X,2} + \ln \frac{W_1}{1000\rho + M_2(W_1 - W_2)} \tag{1.22}$$

$$+ \ln \frac{1000M_2\rho_1}{M_2W_1}$$

which simplifies to

$$f_{X,2} = f_{M,2} \frac{\rho + 0.001M_2(W_1 - W_2)}{\rho_1} \tag{1.23}$$

where ρ_1 is the density of the solvent.

For electrolyte solutions, Eq. (1.23) becomes

$$f_{X,2} = f_{M,2} \frac{\rho + 0.001M_2(nW_1 - W_2)}{\rho_1} \tag{1.24}$$

in which n represents the number of ions into which each molecule of solute dissociates.

Similar equations can be derived, as follows:

$$f_{X,2} = f_{m,2} (1 + 0.001nm_2W_1) \tag{1.25}$$

$$f_{m,2} = f_{M,2} \frac{\rho + 0.001 M_2W_2}{\rho_1} \tag{1.26}$$

The equations apply when there is more than one solute, by substituting Σ nm for nm, Σ nM for nM, and Σ M for M; Σ represents the sum of the terms for all solutes.

IV. DETERMINATION OF ACTIVITY COEFFICIENTS

A. From Solubilities

The chemical potential ($\Delta \overline{G}_{M,2}$) of a nonelectrolyte in solution is given by the van't Hoff equation,

$$\Delta \overline{G}_{M,2} = \Delta G^{\circ}_{M,2} + RT \ln M_2 f_{M,2} \tag{1.27}$$

where $\Delta G^{\circ}_{M,2}$ is the standard free energy, M_2 the molar concentration of the nonelectrolyte, and $f_{M,2}$ its practical activity coefficient. Saturated solutions are, by definition, in equilibrium with the pure solute, under which circumstances Eq. (1.27) can be written in the form

$$\Delta \overline{G}_{solute} = \Delta G^{\circ}_{M,2} + RT \ln M_{s,2} f_{M,2} \tag{1.28}$$

in which $M_{s,2}$ represents the solubility and $\Delta \overline{G}_{solute}$ is the free energy of the pure solute. If the solubility ($M'_{s,2}$) is determined in the presence of a quantity of dissolved electrolyte, the chemical potential of the nonelectrolyte in the new solution will be given by

$$\Delta \overline{G}_{solute} = \Delta G^{\circ}_{M,2} + RT \ln M'_{s,2} f'_{M,2} \tag{1.29}$$

where $f'_{M,2}$ is the activity coefficient of the solute in the presence of the electrolyte. Equating Eq. (1.28) with Eq. (1.29) then leads to

$$\frac{M_{s,2}}{M'_{s,2}} = \frac{f'_{M,2}}{f_{M,2}} \tag{1.30}$$

Activity coefficients can be determined from Eq. (1.30) by measuring solubilities in a range of concentrations of inert electrolyte and plotting the logarithm of $M_{s,2}/M'_{s,2}$ against the square root of ionic strength ($\sqrt{I}$). A straight line should be obtained. The intercept at $\sqrt{I} = 0$ represents the conditions at zero ionic strength when $M_{s,2} = M'_{s,2}$, and ln $(M_{s,2}/M'_{s,2})$ should be zero. The correction is applied by subtracting the intercept value from all the points and calculating a new regression equation, from which activity coefficients can be calculated. The procedure could be applied to the determination of activity coefficients of electrolytes.

Example

The solubilities of potassium bromate in a series of solutions of sodium chloride in water are given below. Construct an equation for calculating practical activity coefficients of potassium bromate at specific ionic strengths. The molecular weight of potassium bromate is 167.

NaCl (M)	0.00	0.25	0.50	0.75	1.00	1.50
KBrO ($g\ dm^{-3}$)	78.8	82.9	87.2	90.4	93.9	99.0

Solution:

When [NaCl] = 0, [$KBrO_3$] = 78.8/167 = 0.472 M (= M_0).

$$I = 0.5(M_{K^+}z_{K^+}^2 + M_{BrO_3^-}z_{BrO_3^-}^2)$$

$$= 0.5(0.472 \times 1^2 + 0.472 \times 1^2)$$

$$= 0.472$$

$$\sqrt{I} = 0.687$$

When [NaCl] = 0.25, [$KBrO_3$] = 82.9/167 = 0.496 M.

$$I = 0.5(M_{K^+}z_{K^+}^2 + M_{BrO_3^-}z_{BrO_3^-}^2 + M_{Na^+}z_{Na^+}^2$$

$$+ M_{Cl^-}z_{Cl^-}^2)$$

$$= 0.5(0.496 + 0.496 + 0.25 + 0.25) = 0.746$$

$$\sqrt{I} = 0.864$$

$$\log \frac{M}{M_0} = \log \frac{0.496}{0.472} = \log 1.051 = 0.0215$$

These and the remaining results are summarized in the following table.

KBrO$_3$(M)	0.472	0.496	0.522	0.541	0.562	0.593
log M/M$_0$	0.0000	0.0215	0.0439	0.0585	0.0760	0.0991
$\sqrt{I}$	0.687	0.864	1.011	1.136	1.250	1.447

A plot of $\sqrt{I}$ against log M/M$_0$ is shown in Fig. 1.3 and is rectilinear. Linear regression analysis will therefore provide an equation from which activities may be calculated. Linear regression analysis, also known as least squares analysis, is a mathematical procedure for calculating such relationships and is built into most electronic calculators. The basic methodology will be shown in this example, but for subsequent calculations it will be assumed that the reader will have the necessary hardware. Any reader who does not have such a facility is referred to this example for the procedure. Calling $\sqrt{I}$, x and log M/M$_0$, y, to fit a set of values of x and y to a rectilinear equation of the form y = A + Bx, in which A and B are constants, B is calculated from the formula

$$B = \frac{S(xy) - S(x)S(y)/N}{S(x^2) - S^2(x)/N}$$

S(xy) is the sum of the products of each individual x and its corresponding value of y; that is,

$$S(xy) = (0.687 \times 0) + (0.864 \times 0.0215) + \cdots + (1.447 \times 0.0991)$$

$$= 0.3689$$

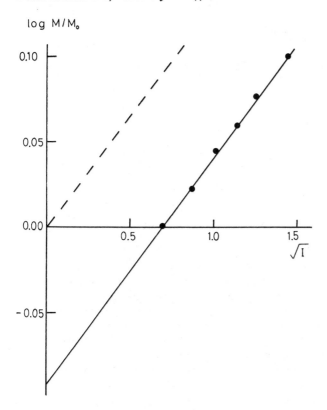

log M/M_o

FIGURE 1.3 Determination of activity coefficients from solubility results; potassium bromate in aqueous sodium chloride solutions.

$S(x)S(y)/N$ is the sum of all the x's [i.e., $(0.687 + 0.864 + \cdots + 1.447) = 6.395$] multiplied by the sum of all the y's [i.e., $0 + 0.0215 + \cdots + 0.0991) = 0.300$] and divided by the number of pairs of x and y (i.e., $N = 6$). Thus

$$\frac{S(x)S(y)}{N} = \frac{6.395 \times 0.300}{6} = 0.3197$$

$S(x^2)$ is the sum of all the squares of each individual x [i.e., $(0.687^2 + 0.864^2 + \cdots + 1.447^2) = 7.187$], $S^2(x)/N$ is the sum of all the x's, squared, and the total divided by the number of pairs of results [i.e., $(0.687 + 0.864 + \cdots + 1.447)^2/6 = 6.816$]. B is now calculated from

$$B = \frac{0.3689 - 0.3197}{7.187 - 6.816} = 0.1325$$

A is calculated by substitution of B and the mean values of x and y ($\bar{x}$ and $\bar{y}$) in the standard equation:

$$\bar{y} = A + B(\bar{x})$$

or

$$A = 0.0500 + 1.066 \times 0.1325 = -0.0911$$

giving the regression equation,

$$\log \frac{M}{M_0} = 0.1325 \sqrt{I} - 0.0911 \qquad \begin{array}{cc} N & r \\ 6 & 0.999 \end{array}$$

N represents the number of pairs of results considered and r is the correlation coefficient. The correlation coefficient varies between zero and 1; the higher the number, the better the correlation. The calculation of the correlation coefficient is usually built into electronic calculator programs for linear regression. The reader is otherwise referred to standard texts on statistics and correlation for the procedure for calculating correlation coefficients.

The activity coefficient at zero ionic strength is unity, so the intercept of the equation should be zero. The equation is therefore rewritten as

$$\log \frac{M}{M_0} = 0.1325 \sqrt{I}$$

which gives a straight line parallel to the previous one, but running through the origin, as indicated by the dashed line in Fig. 1.3. Thus $\log M/M_0$ for NaCl = 0.25 is given by

$$\log \frac{M}{M_0} = 0.1325 \times 0.864 = 0.1145$$

so that

$$\frac{M}{M_0} = \text{antilog } 0.1144 = 1.302 = \frac{f_M^o}{f_M}$$

where f_M^o is the practical activity coefficient at zero concentration and is equal to unity. Hence,

$$f_M = \frac{1}{1.302} = 0.768$$

Activity coefficients for the other solutions are summarized as follows:

$\sqrt{I}$	0.687	0.864	1.011	1.136	1.250	1.447
f_M	0.811	0.768	0.735	0.707	0.683	0.643
$-\ln f_M$	0.209	0.264	0.308	0.347	0.381	0.442

The plot of $\sqrt{I}$ against $-\ln f_M$ is rectilinear over the concentration range covered in the table, giving the equation

$$-\ln f_M = 0.3060 \, \sqrt{I} \; - 0.000972 \qquad \begin{array}{cc} N & r \\ 6 & 1.000 \end{array}$$

from which activity coefficients can be calculated

B. From Distribution Coefficients

The distribution coefficient (K_d) of a nonelectrolyte between water and a water-immiscible solvent, determined experimentally, is the ratio of the concentration in one solvent to that in the other solvent (Chap. 9). This is expressed as

$$K_d = \frac{M_w}{M_0} \qquad (1.31)$$

where M is molar concentration and the subscripts w and o represent water and nonaqueous phase, respectively.

A similar relationship obtains if the aqueous phase contains an electrolyte in addition to the original solute. If the conditions are arranged so that the concentration of the nonelectrolyte in the nonaqueous phase is the same in both systems, the aqueous phases, being in equilibrium with the same nonaqueous phase, are in equilibrium with each other. The chemical potentials (ΔG) are therefore the same in both aqueous solutions; therefore,

$$\Delta G_w = \Delta G'_w = RT \ln a_w = RT \ln a'_w \qquad (1.32)$$

or

$$\ln f'_w = \ln \frac{M_w}{M'_w} + \ln f_w \tag{1.33}$$

The dashed symbols represent the system containing the electrolyte.

It has been stated above that if a solution contains more than one solute, the activity coefficient of one species will be influenced by the presence of the others. The natural log of the resulting activity coefficient follows a power series of the concentrations of the dissolved species. The greatest contribution comes from the first term of the series, so that for the systems under consideration the following equations can be applied.

$$\ln f_w = k_{solute} M_w \tag{1.34}$$

$$\ln f'_w = k_{solute} M'_w + k_{electrolyte} M_{electrolyte} \tag{1.35}$$

k_{solute} and $k_{electrolyte}$ are constants. Subtraction of Eq. (1.34) from Eq. (1.35) gives

$$\ln \frac{f'_w}{f_w} = k_{electrolyte} M_{electrolyte} + k_{solute} (M'_w - M_w) \tag{1.36}$$

which since $(M'_w - M_w)$ is small in comparison with $M_{electrolyte}$, reduces to

$$\ln \frac{f'_w}{f_w} = k_{electrolyte} M_{electrolyte} = \ln \frac{M_w}{M'_w} \tag{1.37}$$

This indicates that a plot of $\ln (M_w/M'_w)$ against $M_{electrolyte}$ will be rectilinear with slope $k_{electrolyte}$ since

$$\ln f'_w = k_{electrolyte} M_{electrolyte} + \ln f_w \tag{1.38}$$

f'_w can therefore be evaluated using a procedure similar to that for solubility, described above.

The experimental procedure involves selecting a range of electrolyte concentrations ($M_{electrolyte}$) and carrying out a series of distribution experiments for each, varying the nonelectrolyte concentration. Simple plots of M'_w, the concentration of nonelectrolyte in the aqueous phase, against M_o', the concentration of nonelectrolyte in the nonaqueous phase, can then be interpolated to give the value of M_w' which corresponds to the same value of M_o' as in the system containing no added electrolyte. It is necessary that the nonelectrolyte concentrations in the aqueous phase be low and that the solvents be completely immiscible. The method could be applied to electrolytes, but the calculations would be more difficult and the end result less reliable.

As will be explained in subsequent chapters, nonelectrolytes sometimes associate with the solvent when taken into solution. The behavior is described as negative deviation, and is characterized by an activity coefficient less than unity. Sykes and Robertson [3] observed this behavior with solutions of the nitrobenzoic acids in isoamyl alcohol (3-methylbutanol). In determining activity coefficients they invoked the following [4]:

$$\frac{(M_o f_o)^n}{M_w f_w} = K_d \tag{1.39}$$

The equation is the same as that used for self-associating solutes (Chap. 9), n in the current case being the ratio of the apparent molecular weights of the solute in the two phases at infinite dilution. Conversion to logs gives

$$\ln M_w = n \ln M_o + (N \ln f_o - \ln f_w) - \ln K_d \tag{1.40}$$

which indicates that a plot of $\ln M_o$ against $\ln M_w$ will be asymptotic with

$$\ln M_w = n \ln M_o - \ln K_d \tag{1.41}$$

Hence if M_o and M_w are measured for a range of concentrations, n can be determined. If the activity coefficient in water (f_w) is unity, as was assumed for the nitrobenzoic acids [3], substitution of n in Eq. (1.40) will give the activity coefficient in the nonaqueous solvent under the ruling experimental conditions. The procedure can then be repeated for determining the activity coefficients of the nonelectrolyte in aqueous electrolyte solutions.

C. From Vapor Pressures

Raoult's law (Chap. 4) states that the partial fugacity of a constituent of a solution is equal to its standard fugacity multiplied by its activity (a). For the conditions normally operating for determining activity coefficients, the vapors can be considered to be ideal, so that vapor pressures can be substituted for fugacities:

$$\bar{p}_1 = p_1^o a_{X,1} \qquad\qquad (1.42)$$

Equation (1.42) indicates that if the saturated vapor pressure of a pure solvent (p_1^o) and its partial pressure in a solution in that solvent ($\bar{p}_1$) are measured, the activity of the solvent can be determined.

In practice the vapor pressure of the solute also has to be taken into consideration, so that the total saturated vapor pressure (p_{tot}) is given by

$$p_{tot} = p_1^o a_{X,1} + p_2^o a_{X,2} \qquad\qquad (1.43)$$

where a_X is the rational activity. If both solute and solvent are volatile, partial pressures cannot be assessed, and it is normal in such situations to use a mean activity coefficient ($f_{X(mean)}$) of the two components, as expressed by

$$p_{tot} = (p_1^o X_1 + p_2^o X_2) f_{X(mean)} \qquad\qquad (1.44)$$

An example of the calculation of the mean activity coefficient of a mixture of two volatile liquids, using Raoult's law, is shown in Chap. 5. If the solute is nonvolatile, as for example with electrolytes and carbohydrates, $p_2^o = 0$, then

$$p_{tot} = p_1^o a_{X,1} \qquad\qquad (1.45)$$

Example

The saturated vapor pressures of a range of solutions of potassium chloride in water are given in the following table. Use this information to prepare an equation for calculating the rational activities of water in aqueous potassium chloride solutions.

[KCl] (M)	0	0.5	1.0	2.0	3.0	4.0
Saturated vapor pressure (Pa)	3166.3	3115.1	3065 5	2964.9	2861.4	2755.3

Solution:

When [KCl] = 0.5 M,

$$\frac{p_{tot}}{p_1^o} = \frac{3115.4}{3166.3}$$

Figures obtained for other concentrations, using the same procedure, are given in the next table. A manual plot of [KCl] against a_1 gives a straight line, with the regression equation

$$\begin{array}{ccc} & N & r \\ a_{M,1} = -0.03238\ M + 1.0003 & 6 & 1.000 \end{array}$$

which provides a means of calculating solvent rational activities for any concentration of potassium chloride. Some of these are given in the table.

p_{tot}/p_1^o $(= a_{M,1})$	1.000	0.984	0.968	0.936	0.904	0.870
$a_{M,1}$(calculated)	1.000	0.984	0.968	0.936	0.903	0.871

Activities of volatile nonelectrolytes can be calculated from the partial pressures of the solute, alone in the solvent, and in a solution of the solute and a nonvolatile solute of the necessary concentration, using

$$\frac{f_{X(2)} X_2}{f_{X(2)}^o X_2^o} = \frac{\bar{p}}{p^o} \tag{1.46}$$

where X_2^o and X_2 are mole fraction concentrations of the solute in pure solvent and solution containing the nonvolatile solute, respectively, and the p's and f_X's are the corresponding partial pressures and activity coefficients. If $X_2 = X_2^o$, the equation simplifies to

$$\frac{f_{X(2)}}{f_{X(2)}^o} = \frac{\bar{p}}{p^o} \tag{1.47}$$

where $\bar{p}$ represents the saturated vapor pressure of a solution containing the same concentration of nonvolatile solute, but no volatile solute. Similarly, $\bar{p}^\circ$ is the saturated vapor pressure of the solution of the volatile solute alone, minus that of the pure solvent.

D. From Depression of Freezing Point

At the melting point (T_m°) of a pure solid, the free energy of the solid $(\Delta \bar{G}_{solid(T_m^\circ)})$ will be equal to the free energy of the liquid "solid" $(\Delta G_{liquid(T_m^\circ)})$. If this is the solvent and a solute is added, the melting point will be depressed (to T_m), and the free-energy change (ΔG) will be represented by

$$\Delta G = \Delta G_{solid(T_m)} - \Delta G_{liquid(T_m)} \qquad (1.48)$$

$$= \Delta G^\circ_{solution(T_m)} + RT_m \ln a_1$$

Application of the Gibbs-Helmholtz equation of classical thermodynamics

$$\frac{d}{dT} \frac{\Delta G}{T} = -\frac{\Delta H}{T^2} \qquad (1.49)$$

gives

$$\frac{d}{dT} \frac{\Delta G^\circ}{T_m} = -\frac{\Delta H^f_{T_m}}{T_m^2} \qquad (1.50)$$

where $\Delta H^f_{T_m}$ represents the enthalpy of fusion of the solvent at

temperature T_m. Substitution from Eq. (1.48) in Eq. (1.50) gives

$$-R \ln a_1 + \frac{\Delta G}{T_m} = -\int_{T_m^\circ}^{T_m} \frac{\Delta H^f_{T_m}}{T_m^2} \cdot dT \qquad (1.51)$$

Integration, and assuming that $T_m T_m^\circ = (T_m^\circ)^2$, gives

$$\ln a_1 = \frac{\Delta H^f_{T_m}}{RT^2} (T_m - T^o_m) \tag{1.52}$$

which since the solution is dilute and $X_1 \cong 1$, provides a means of calculating the activity coefficient of the solvent.

Example

The freezing point of a 0.1 M solution of sodium acetate in water was found to be $-0.36°C$. Given that the enthalpy of fusion of water at $0°C$ is 6090 J mol^{-1}, calculate the activity coefficient of water in this solution. $R = 8.315$ J deg^{-1} mol^{-1}.

Solution:

$$-\ln f_X = \frac{6090 \times 0.36}{8.315 \times 273^2} = 3.538 \times 10^{-3}$$

$$f_X = antilog_e - 3.538 \times 10^{-3} = 0.996$$

The calculation assumes that the enthalpy of fusion at 273 K is equal to that at 272.64 K ($-0.36°C$). Change of ΔH^f with temperature will be discussed later.

E. From Elevation of Boiling Point

Elevation of boiling point data can be used to determine activity coefficients. The procedure is the same as for depression of freezing point, except that enthalpy of vaporization is used in place of enthalpy of fusion.

F. From Osmotic Pressure

The osmotic pressure (Π) of a solution is given by

$$\Pi = iRTM \tag{1.53}$$

where M is the molar concentration and i the van't Hoff factor, which is a correction to allow for deviation from ideality. For strong and nonelectrolytes, in which dissociations are complete and zero, respectively, i is solely a measure of the activity coefficient, but with weak electrolytes it is a composite of activity coefficient and degree

of dissociation. In all cases, as $M \to o$, $i \to n$, where n represents
the number of units per molecule into which the compound dissociates. The ratio i/n is called the osmotic coefficient (ϕ) and is
alternatively defined by

$$\phi = \frac{\text{observed osmotic pressure}}{\text{ideal osmotic pressure}} \qquad (1.54)$$

It is an alternative parameter to activity coefficient and is useful for
expressing the deviation of solvents from ideality. The activity is
often inadequate for this purpose, when it may give a figure close
to unity, in contrast to an activity coefficient markedly different
from unity for the conjugate solute.

The sensitivity of the osmotic coefficient arises from the fact
that it is logarithmically related to concentration. Thus if we consider a solution in equilibrium with its pure solvent, from which it
is separated by a semipermeable membrane, the chemical potential of
the solvent will be the same in both phases and equal to the standard free energy (ΔG°). The corresponding chemical potential for
the solution is determined from the van't Hoff isotherm

$$\Delta G = \Delta G^\circ + RT \ln a_1 \qquad (1.55)$$

plus a free-energy increment arising from the difference between the
osmotic pressures of the two systems. Since the osmotic pressure of
the pure solvent is zero, the difference is equal to the osmotic pressure of the solution. The change in free energy with osmotic pressure can be assessed from the following equation of classical
thermodynamics:

$$\left(\frac{\Delta G}{\Delta \Pi} \right)_T = V_1 \qquad (1.56)$$

so that the total chemical potential is given by

$$\Delta G = \Delta G^\circ + RT \ln a_1 = V_1 , \Pi \qquad (1.57)$$

where V_1 is the molar volume of the solvent. If the right-hand
side of Eq. (1.57) is equated to ΔG°, the standard chemical potential of the solvent is

$$\ln a_1 = \frac{V_1 \Pi_{obs}}{RT} \qquad (1.58)$$

An analogous expression for the corresponding ideal solution is

$$\ln X_1 = \frac{V_1 \Pi_{ideal}}{RT} \tag{1.59}$$

Hence

$$\phi = \frac{\Pi_{obs}}{\Pi_{ideal}} \tag{1.60}$$

Example

A 0.2 m solution of sodium chloride in water was found to have an osmotic pressure of 928 kPa at 25°C. Calculate the osmotic coefficient and the rational activity coefficient of the solvent. $R = 8.315$ J K^{-1} mol^{-1}. Molecular weight of water = 18.02.

Solution:

Since the solution is dilute, it may be considered to be 0.2 M. It is therefore 0.2×10^3 mol m^{-3}.

Ideal osmotic pressure $= 2 \times 0.2 \times 10^3 \times 8.315 \times 298$

$$= 991 \text{ kPa}$$

Therefore,

$$\phi = \frac{928}{991} = 0.936$$

Since the number of molecules of solute in a dilute solution is small compared with the number of molecules of solvent, mole fraction concentration of solute can be expressed in the following simplified form:

$$X_2 = \frac{m_2 W_1}{1000} \tag{1.61}$$

where m_2 represents concentration of solute and W_1 the molecular weight of the solvent. The activity of the solvent is therefore given by

$$\ln a_1 = \phi \ln \left(1 - \frac{n m_2 W_1}{1000}\right) \tag{1.62}$$

Since the solution is dilute, the second term in parentheses will be small compared with 1, so that the standard mathematical form,

$$\ln (1 - x) = -x \tag{1.63}$$

can be applied to give

$$-\ln a_1 = \frac{nm_2 W_1 \phi}{1000} \tag{1.64}$$

Therefore,

$$-\ln a_1 = \frac{2 \times 0.2 \times 18.02}{1000} \times 0.936 = 6.747 \times 10^{-3}$$

$$a_1 = 0.993$$

If the mole fraction concentration of water in the solution is approximated to unity, this corresponds to an activity coefficient of 0.993. Comparison of this figure with the osmotic coefficient illustrates the point made earlier, that the osmotic coefficient is more sensitive to deviation from ideality than the activity coefficient.

The osmotic coefficient can also be calculated through Raoult's law, from which an observed solvent mole fraction concentration $(X_{1(obs)})$ can be calculated using

$$\ln X_{1(obs)} = \ln \frac{p_1}{p_1^o} \tag{1.65}$$

where p_1^o is the saturated vapor pressure of the pure solvent and p_1 that of the solution. The theoretical concentration $(X_{1(calc)})$, using Eq. (1.63), is given by

$$\ln X_{1(calc)} = -\frac{m_2 W_1}{1000} \tag{1.66}$$

but must be multiplied by n to give the mole fraction in terms of the number of ions. The osmotic coefficient can then be obtained as the ratio of these two expressions:

$$\phi = \frac{\ln X_{1(obs)}}{n \ln X_{1(calc)}} = -\frac{\ln (p_1/p_1^o)}{nm_2 W_1} \times 1000 \tag{1.67}$$

$$= \frac{1000}{nm_2 W_1} \ln \frac{p_1^o}{p_1}$$

Example

The vapor pressure of a 0.2 m aqueous solution of sodium chloride was found to be 3.145 kPa at 25°C. Given that the saturated vapor pressure of water at the same temperature is 3.166 kPa, calculate the osmotic coefficient of the solvent in this solution.

Solution:

$$\phi = \frac{1000}{nm_2 W_1} \ln \frac{p_1^\circ}{p_1}$$

$$= \frac{1000}{2 \times 0.2 \times 18.02} \ln \frac{3.166}{3.145} = 0.923$$

Similar calculations can be carried out with elevation of boiling-point and depression of freezing-point data, using the basic equation

$$\phi = \frac{\text{observed colligative property}}{\text{calculated colligative property}} \tag{1.68}$$

The limitation to this variation is the restriction to specific operating temperatures.

G. From Electrical Potential

When a metal is dipped into a solution of its ions, a potential difference is set up between the two phases. Thus, for example, if a copper rod is immersed in an aqueous solution of copper sulfate, metallic copper is capable of passing into solution as cupric ions, leaving the electrons on the metal rod. Similarly, the cupric ions in solution are capable of accepting electrons from the copper rod, depositing metallic copper.

$$Cu^{2+} + 2e \rightleftharpoons Cu \tag{1.69}$$

The process is an equilibrium, and if there is an excess of cupric ions, it moves to the right; if there is a deficiency of cupric ions, it moves to the left. At equilibrium the two processes proceed at the same rate; the rod has a specific electrical potential, and the overall process appears to be stationary. If, however, the copper rod is connected to a conductor that donates electrons, the equilibrium will continue to move to the right until all the cupric ions are exhausted. Similarly, if the conductor accepts electrons, the metallic copper will pass into solution. Thus if a piece of metallic iron is dropped into the equilibrium mixture, it will donate electrons, create ferrous ions, and become coated with metallic copper.

$$Fe + Cu^{2+} = Fe^{2+} + Cu \tag{1.70}$$

The process, stops when the number of ferrous ions reaches a limiting value. It can therefore be seen that the direction in which the electrons flow depends on two factors:

1. The nature of the metal-ion combination, collectively described as an electrode or half cell
2. The concentration, or more correctly, the activity of the ions

The behavior of the electrode is assessed from its standard electrode potential, which is the potential difference between the electrode containing a molar solution of its ions and an electrode consisting of hydrogen gas in conjunction with a hydrogen ion solution of unit activity (hydrogen electrode). The potential of the hydrogen electrode is the baseline of the standard electrode potentials of metals and is placed equal to zero. The system Fe^{2+}, Fe has a standard electrode potential of -0.409 V, and Cu^{2+}, Cu of $+0.340$ V. This means that a standard iron electrode, because its potential is lower, will donate electrons to a standard copper electrode.

The effect of concentration is given by the Nernst equation,

$$E = E° + \frac{RT}{n\Gamma} \ln a \tag{1.71}$$

where n represents the number of electrons involved in the process and Γ is the Faraday, which is equal to 96,487 C mol^{-1}. a is the activity of the ions, which should be divided by the activity of the metal, but this is equal to 1, because elements in their normal state are placed equal to unity, by convention. E is the electrical potential of the half cell, and as the equation suggests, varies with temperature. Most processes are considered at 25°C, for which R, T, and Γ are grouped together as the constant

$$\frac{RT}{\Gamma} = 8.315 \times 298 \div 96,487 = 2.568 \times 10^{-2} \text{ V at } 25°C$$

The potential of a metal, dipping into a dilute solution of an electrolyte having an ion in common with the metal, provides a method for determining ionic activities, and if the solution is saturated, for determing solubilities. It is, however, applicable only to dilute solutions containing low or zero concentrations of other ions.

Example

A potential difference of 321 mV was observed between a lead electrode containing saturated lead sulfate solution and a calomel electrode containing 0.1 M KCl at 25°C. Calculate the activity of the
lead ions in the solution.

Standard electrode potentials (mV):

0.1 M KCl, Hg_2Cl_2, Hg (Calomel) +334

Pb^{2+}, Pb   -126

Solution:

$$E_{Pb^{2+}} = 0.321 - 0.334 = -0.013 \text{ V}$$

$$= E^\circ_{Pb^{2+}} + \frac{RT}{n\Gamma} \ln a_{Pb^{2+}}$$

Therefore,

$$-0.013 = -0.126 - \frac{0.02568}{2} \ln a_{Pb^{2+}}$$

$$\ln a_{Pb^{2+}} = \frac{-0.113 \times 2}{0.02568} = -8.801$$

$$a_{Pb^{2+}} = 1.5 \times 10^{-4} \text{ M}$$

If two Cu^{2+}, Cu electrodes of the type described above, one
containing a weak solution and the other containing a strong solution, are joined together by a salt bridge, as shown in Fig. 1.4a,
the copper rod immersed in the weak solution will have a more negative potential than the other. If the metal rods are connected by a
conductor, electrons will flow along the conductor from the weaker
electrode to the stronger electrode, and coppor ions will pass from
the metal in the weak electrode into solution. In the strong electrode, cupric ions will deposit on the rod, and counterions (SO_4^{2-})
will flow through the salt bridge from the strong solution to the
weak solution.

The salt bridge gives practical problems and can be replaced
by two identical reversible electrodes, as shown in Fig. 1.4b. The
resulting arrangement, called a concentration cell without transport,
provides a convenient means of measuring activity coefficients. The
scope of this procedure has improved with the recent rapid progress in the development of ion-selective electrodes. If the half
cells are labeled A and B, and the mean ionic activities of their
contents are called a_A and a_B, electromotive force (emf) of the
complete cell will be given by

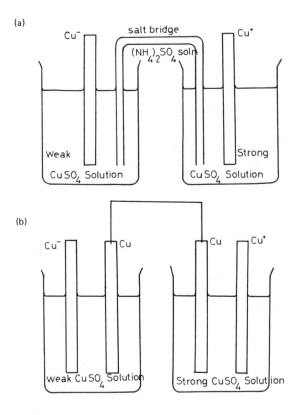

FIGURE 1.4 Potentiometric half cells: (a) with liquid junction;
(b) without liquid junction.

$$E = E_A - E_B = \frac{2RT}{n\Gamma} \ln \frac{a_B}{a_A} \qquad (1.72)$$

The factor 2 is necessary because the current is carried by both
ion and counterion, so that the emf must be doubled. By definition,
the potential of a half cell containing a molar solution is zero. If
in the present situation cell B contains a molar solution, Eq. (1.72)
can be rewritten to give

$$E = E° + \frac{2RT}{n\Gamma} \ln \frac{1}{a_A} \qquad (1.73)$$

or

$$E = E° - \frac{0.0514}{n\Gamma} \ln a_A \tag{1.74}$$

$E°$ can be evaluated by plotting $E + (0.0514/n\Gamma) \ln m$ against a suitable function of m, and extrapolating to m = 0. Substitution in Eq. (1.74) then yields the activity, from which the activity coefficient can be calculated. Extrapolation is sometimes difficult and can be improved by using mf instead of m, estimating the activity coefficient f theoretically.

V. THE GIBBS-DUHEM EQUATION

The free energy (ΔG) of a binary solution is given by

$$\Delta G = \Delta \overline{G}_1 n_1 + \Delta \overline{G}_2 n_2 \tag{1.75}$$

where n_1 and n_2 represent the number of moles of solvent and solute respectively, and $\Delta \overline{G}_1$ and $\Delta \overline{G}_2$ are their partial molar free energies ($\delta \Delta G/\delta n$). If a small quantity of solvent (δn_1) is added such that n_2 can be considered unchanged the change in free energy will be given by

$$\frac{\delta \Delta G}{\delta n_1} = \frac{\delta}{\delta n_1} (\Delta \overline{G}_1 n_1 + \Delta \overline{G}_2 n_2) \tag{1.76}$$

and can be determined by using the mathematical standard form

$$\frac{duv}{dx} = u \frac{dv}{dx} + v \frac{du}{dx} \tag{1.77}$$

giving

$$\frac{d\Delta G}{dn_1} = \Delta \overline{G}_1 + n_1 \frac{d\Delta \overline{G}_1}{dn_1} + n_2 \frac{d\Delta \overline{G}_2}{dn_1} \tag{1.78}$$

Since $\Delta \overline{G}_1 + \delta \Delta G/\delta n_1$

$$n_1 \frac{d\Delta \overline{G}_1}{dn_1} = -n_2 \frac{d\Delta \overline{G}_2}{dn_1} \tag{1.79}$$

Substituting from the van't Hoff isotherm [Eq. (1.16)], and replacing
the number of moles (n) with mole fractions (X), gives

$$-d \ln a_2 = \frac{x_1}{x_2} d \ln a_1 \tag{1.80}$$

which is a form of the Gibbs-Duhem equation.   The equation can be
applied to other thermodynamic functions and expressed in a variety
of forms; for example,

$$\frac{d \ln a_1}{d \ln X_1} = \frac{d \ln a_2}{d \ln X_2} \tag{1.81}$$

and

$$\frac{d \ln f_1}{d \ln X_1} = \frac{d \ln f_2}{d \ln X_2} \tag{1.82}$$

These will be used later.

The following equation applies to solutions containing two or
more components,

$$\Sigma \; X \; \frac{d \Delta G}{dx} = 0 \tag{1.83}$$

The Gibbs-Duhem equation can be used to calculate the activity
coefficient of a solute when the activity coefficients of the solvent
are known over a range of concentrations.

VI.   DETERMINATION OF SOLUBILITY

To the unitiated, solubility would appear to be an easy property to
measure. One has only to prepare a saturated solution, separate it
from excess undissolved solute, and determine the composition of the
resulting solution by a suitable analytical procedure. This assumption is sometimes true, but all too often the procedure is beset with
difficulties and pitfalls. The process will be broken down into three
stages, and these considered in turn.

A. Preparation of Saturated Solutions

1. Analytical Methods. The process of dissolution of a solute
into a solvent was quantified by Noyes and Whitney [5], who derived

$$\frac{dw}{dt} = \frac{AD}{d} \, (c_s - c) \qquad\qquad (1.84)$$

where dw/dt is the increase in weight of solute dissolved with time, A the surface area of the undissolved solute, D the diffusion coefficient of the solute, and d the thickness of the diffusion layer surrounding the undissolved solute. c_s is the solubility of the solute and c is the concentration in solution at time t. The term in parentheses indicates that the change in w with time will be asymptotic, as shown in Fig. 1.5(i). As c increases, $c_s - c$ decreases, the process of dissolution becomes progressively slower, and saturation is theoretically never achieved. One must therefore be content with a situation in which the difference between the actual concentration and saturation is insignificantly small. The problem is not important with solutes that dissolve rapidly, but with slowly soluble materials, the time involved can be excessive.

The solubilities of most nonvolatile solutes increase with temperature. Under these circumstances, a simple means of overcoming the problem of the asymptotic approach to saturation is to carry out the dissolution process initially at an elevated temperature, and then allow the mixture to equilibrate at the temperature of interest. The weight of dissolved solute will increase to a point greater than the solubility at the lower temperature, and on cooling, provided that there is excess undissolved solute, dissolved solute in excess of solubility will crystallize out, leaving a solution that is completely

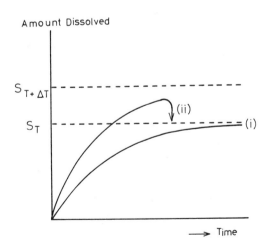

FIGURE 1.5 Asymptotic approach to saturation. S_T, Amount dissolved at temperature of interest; $S_{T + \Delta T}$, amount dissolved at temperature in excess of T.

saturated. The process is shown diagramatically in Fig. 1.5(ii).
Dissolution at elevated temperatures has the added advantage of
increasing the rate of solution through an increased rate of diffusion and a decrease in the thickness of the diffusion layer. One
should, however, be wary of the possibility of decomposition at the
higher temperature.

Equation (1.84) indicates that the rate of solution is proportional
to the area of surface exposed to the solvent, so that it is advan-
tageous to powder solids finely before preparing saturated solutions.
An alternative and obvious way of increasing surface area is to use
more solute, but an unlimited source of solute is a rare luxury.
Large quantities of solute also increase problems involved with trace
impurities. This aspect will be discussed later. Higuchi et al. [6]
suggested that rate of solution could be increased by adding to the
system a small quantity of immiscible liquid in which the solute was
freely soluble. It was anticipated that the solute would rapidly dissolve in the immiscible liquid and that the resultant increase in the
area of contact when the mixture was shaken would bring about an
increase in the rate of solution. They quoted as an example that
if the solvent phase consisted of 100 ml of water and 2 ml of iso-
octane, and 5 mg of norethindrone were added, approximately 40%
of the solute would go into solution in the two solvents. Both solvents would be saturated. The iso-octane layer could then be separated off and the aqueous layer filtered and assayed for norethindrone content. More reproducible results were obtained by this procedure than by traditional methods. This is illustrated by Fig. 1.6,
which compares the method with that involving the preparation of a
saturated solution in water alone. An alternative method is to
evaporate the iso-octane off the aqueous phase. Lewis and Enever
[7] found that for aqueous solubilities under 1 μg g^{-1}, only the

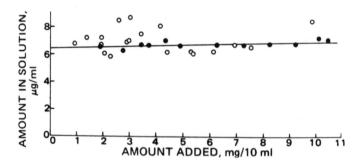

FIGURE 1.6 Phase solubility diagram of norethindrone in water at
25°C. o, 10 ml of water with an equilibrium time of 120 h; •, ml
of water plus 0.5 ml of isooctane, with an equilibrium time of 12 h.
(From Ref. 6.)

slightest contamination with iso-octane could bring about a 10-fold error in solubility.

The crystals comprising a solid, even though they may be of the same morphological form, exist in a spectrum of energy levels, due to differences in surface area and curvature and to cracks and imperfections in individual crystals. The forms with the highest energy will dissolve first, and the observed solubility will correspond to the solubility of the most energetic form still undissolved. True equilibrium in this situation should be checked by approaching saturation through crystallization as well as dissolution.

Solutions of solids in liquids are usually more dense than the solvent alone. Saturated solutions can then be prepared by suspending the solid in a permeable fabric just below the surface of the solvent. As the solute dissolves, the resulting solution falls to the bottom of the container and is replaced by pure solvent or less concentrated solution, which is displaced upward. The process can be assisted by mechanical or occasional manual stirring. This technique is particularly useful for resinous solutes, which sink to the bottom of the vessel to form a sticky, intractable mass.

With gas in liquid and liquid in liquid systems, increased interfacial area can be facilitated by vigorous agitation, which decreases the size of the solute globules. The thickness of the diffusion layer also decreases with increasing agitation. Paddle stirring is probably the most convenient mechanical method of agitation. It is reasonably vigorous and can be used with a container that is suspended in a constant-temperature water bath. If the solute or solvent is volatile, a liquid seal (Fig. 1.7) can be used to prevent vapor loss. Alternatively, a magnetic stirrer can be used and the container sealed, but it should be ensured that the magnetic follower does not react with the solvent. Even with glass-sealed followers, minute cracks in the casing, arising from wear and tear, can permit contact between solvent and the magnetic core. In an alternative process, solvent and solute are sealed in a glass ampule and rotated on a wheel that is immersed in a water bath (Fig. 1.8). Vigorous agitation is not possible with this technique, but it is useful for volatile systems. It is particularly applicable when a large number of samples have to be run, because several ampules can be mounted on the same wheel.

Shaking is another means of agitation, but it has the disadvantage that temperature control is difficult, immersion in a constant-temperature water bath giving rise to troublesome waves and splashes. Baths are available in which the containers are rotated in a horizontal plane, but the agitation is not very efficient and is more appropriate for the microbial incubation procedures for which the apparatus was designed. Alternatively, water at the required temperature can be circulated around a jacketed vessel, containing solute and solvent, and clamped in a mechanical shaker.

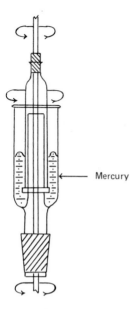

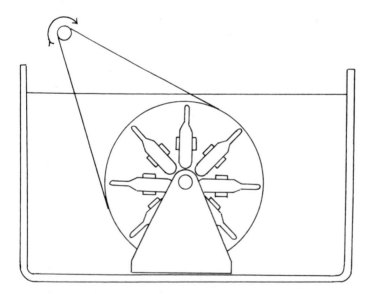

FIGURE 1.7 Liquid seal for paddle stirrer. Mercury is normally used as sealing liquid, but any other suitable liquid may be used in the same way.

FIGURE 1.8 Rotating wheel for preparation of saturated solutions.

Preparation of saturated solutions of liquids in liquids on a macro scale can be achieved using the same techniques as for solids in liquids, provided that the solute is denser than the solution. If the density of the solute is less than that of the saturated solution, dissolution can be carried out in a separatory funnel and samples of saturated solution removed through the tap. In both cases, solute and saturated solution must be made to separate completely and each phase inspected closely for contamination by the other. Unlike solutions of solids in liquids, excess solute cannot be removed from the saturated solution by filtration. On a smaller scale, a glass tube about 0.5 cm in diameter, sealed at the base, is clamped vertically in a constant-temperature bath and solute and solvent introduced. Agitation is provided by a glass rod that is moved vertically up and down the axis of the tube. Racks can be constructed to accommodate banks of tubes, and the attendant glass rods mounted in a similar device so that they can all be operated from one motor. A suitable setup is shown in Fig. 1.9.

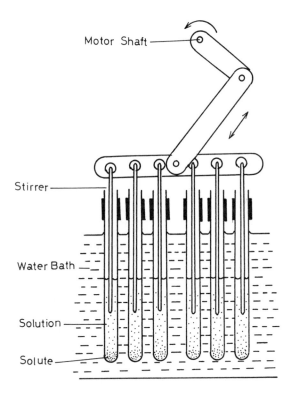

FIGURE 1.9 Open-tube procedure for preparation of saturated solutions.

Most of the methods described so far are suitable for solutes
with low solubilities dissolved in cheap solvents, but with highly
soluble solutes and expensive solvents, prohibitively large quantities of materials are required. Such difficulties can be overcome
by employing percolation. In this process, the solute is powdered
and packed into an open tube and the solvent poured on top. As
the solvent trickles through the powder, each particle is subjected
to a series of dissolution processes. Before the first drops of the
solvent have had time to become saturated, they are replaced by
fresh solvent, the first drops continuing their descent and dissolving more solute from the lower layers of the bed. One of the first
examples of this procedure was described by Fox [8]; the apparatus
is reproduced in Fig. 1.10. The powdered solute was packed on
top of an asbestos plug (D), and the solvent allowed to percolate
through. When all the solvent had passed to B, it was returned

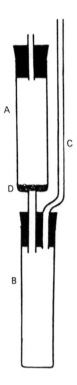

FIGURE 1.10 Percolation apparatus for preparation of saturated
solutions. A, Reservoir for solvent; B, receiving chamber for solution; C, air vent; D, bed of solute resting on porous plate. (From
Ref. 8.)

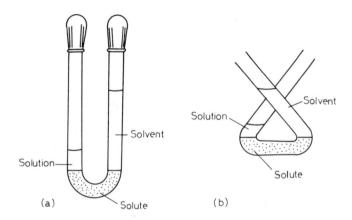

FIGURE 1.11 U-tube methods for preparation of saturated solutions.

to A and percolation continued until the density of the solution remained constant. The apparatus was quite large, and therefore
required large quantities of materials, but can be scaled down by
using glass tubing approximately 0.5 cm in diameter. This is bent
into a U shape, as shown in Fig. 1.11a, and a bed of powdered
solute filled into the base, completely blocking the bend in the tube.
The bed can be kept in position with plugs of glass or cotton wool,
but this is rarely essential. One arm of the tube is then filled with
solvent, which trickles down through the solute until the levels in
the arms of the U tube are equal. Particles displaced from the bed
by the solvent sediment back to their original position, so that most
of the solution in the second arm can be removed with a Pasteur
pipet and returned to the first arm. The procedure is continued
until the concentration of solute in the percolate reaches a constant,
limiting value. The tube is immersed throughout in a constant-
temperature bath with the open ends projecting above the surface.
Problems arise at elevated temperatures and with volatile solvents,
by loss of solvent through the open ends of the tube, and by crystallization of solute in the pipet during transfer from one arm to the
other. This can be overcome by placing Pasteur pipet teats over
the open ends to prevent solvent loss. The solvent can be returned
to the first arm by pressing the appropriate teat. Another refinement uses the tube shown in Fig. 1.11b. By suitable tilting, solvent can be transferred from one arm to the other and back again.

May et al. [9] prepared saturated aqueous solutions of polynuclear aromatic hydrocarbons by pumping water through a column
packed with glass beads that had been coated with the compound
under investigation. The beads had previously been treated with a

solution of the solute in methylene chloride, and the solvent stripped off in a rotary evaporator. However, preparation of crystals by evaporation may lead to a new polymorph, or even an amorphous material on the glass beads.

    2. Synthetic Methods. The general procedure described so far collectively covers what are described as analytical methods, because the saturated solutions are analyzed to determine how much solute has dissolved. Synthetic methods involve the preparation of solute-solvent mixtures of preplanned composition and observing at what concentration the solute fails to dissolve completely. Serial dilution is the simplest version of the general technique. In this, a series of synthetic mixtures of progressively increasing solute concentration are set up and equilibrated at the temperature and pressure of interest. The solubility then lies between the concentrations of the strongest clear solution and the weakest turbid dispersion. This is tedious and imprecise, but it is useful for locating the approximate solubility of a solute, either when an accurate value is not required, or as a preliminary to a more precise determination. The exact solubility can be pinpointed photometrically. When the solubility is exceeded, excess solute appears as a turbidity, which scatters light that passes through it. Therefore, if each tube is placed in turn in an absorptiometer set at a wavelength that is not absorbed by the dissolved solute, those combinations containing less solute than saturation demands will give zero absorbance and those containing more will give finite readings. When the quantities of excess solute are small, absorption of the suspensions will vary uniformly, often rectilinearly, with the quantity of undissolved solute. The plot of extinction against total concentration will therefore exhibit an inflection in the region of the solubility, which may be located precisely by extrapolation back to zero extinction. This technique has been used to measure the solubilities of some aminoalkylphenothiazine tranquilizers and related compounds in water [10].
    In a variation of this technique, solvent is added to solute until a clear solution is obtained, or for liquid-in-liquid solutions, the solute can be placed in a buret and the solvent in the receiving vessel. In this case, the end point will be marked by a transformation from clear to turbid. The method is not easy to use and demands that the solute be rapidly soluble. It is more adaptable to ternary liquid mixtures consisting of a solute, solvent, and "nonsolvent." A typical example involves castor oil, ethanol, and water [11]. Water can be added by buret to a solution of castor oil in ethanol, and the solubility limit observed as the appearance of a turbidity.
    A more refined synthetic method involves subjecting a range of synthetic mixtures to a progressive change in temperature and noting the temperature at which complete solution occurs. If a composition

range is properly chosen, the solubility at the temperature of interest can be located by interpolation. Potter and Clynne [12,13] used this procedure to determine the aqueous solubilities of a range of inorganic salts. For most of these, synthetic mixtures were subjected to increasing temperatures, but salts such as sodium sulfate, whose solubilities decrease with increasing temperature, were cooled. Results were fitted to power series, having the general form

$$\% \, w/w = \sum_{o}^{i} a_i t^i \qquad (1.85)$$

where a_i represents the coefficients for the series and t is temperature in degrees Celsius. As an example, the coefficients for barium chloride dihydrate were $a_0 = 23.304$, $a_1 = 0.16416$, $a_2 = -7.259 \times 10^{-4}$, and $a_3 = 4.595 \times 10^{-6}$, yielding

$$S = 23.304 + 0.16416t - 7.259 \times 10^{-4}t^2 + 4.595 \times 10^{-6}t^3 \qquad (1.86)$$

This equation predicts a solubility of 31.75% w/w at 61.73°C, in comparison with an observed value of 31.65%.

The solvent and solutes for this exercise were cheap and readily available, so that measurements could be carried out on a relatively large scale. Tubes measuring approximately 8×2 cm were used, each with its own stirrer, and since water was the solvent, the tubes could be left unsealed. When Bowen and James [14] determined the solubilities of testosterone propionate in organic solvents at 100°C, smaller quantities had to be used and more stringent precautions taken against evaporation. Glass tubes approximately 12×0.3 cm were used and were sealed at both ends by fusion. The temperature was raised by 1° or less per minute and the tubes agitated manually. Because of the slow rates of solution, results obtained below 60°C were not reproducible, but at temperatures above 70°C the end point was consistent to ±2°C, and above 90°C to ±1°C. Interpolation was implemented through the rectilinear relationship of log solubility with the reciprocal of absolute temperature. A similar procedure was used for the ternary mixture phenanthrene-cyclohexane-methyl iodide by Gordon and Scott [15].

B. Sampling

In the analytical methods it is necessary to withdraw for analysis samples of saturated solution that are not contaminated with undissolved solute. Frequently, this can be achieved by allowing the excess solid to sediment and sampling the supernatant, but such operations should be carried out with caution, with particular attention paid to the possibility of some of the solute floating on the surface of the solution. Excess solute can be removed by filtration, but it must be remembered that if the temperature at which filtration is carried out is markedly different from that at which the saturated solution was prepared, a shift in equilibrium will occur, with a resultant error in the answer obtained. Thus, whereas rapid filtration at room temperature may be adequate for determinations carried out at temperatures near ambient, errors can be anticipated if one is concerned with solubilities at high or low temperatures. A similar criticism can be leveled at procedures in which solute is separated from solution by centrifugation. Authors who use this technique often fail to state that the centrifugation was temperature controlled, and one must therefore assume that it was not.

The guarded pipet is a useful device for withdrawing samples of saturated solution. A small sintered glass disk can be connected to the end of the pipet with flexible tubing and the saturated solution withdrawn through it. The filter and tubing are then removed prior to discharging the liquid. A simpler variation uses a tapered piece of glass tubing containing a small piece of glass or cotton wool. Saturated solutions can also be prepared by equilibrating solute and solvent in a test tube and separating the undissolved solute by pushing a plug of cotton wool down the tube with a glass rod. Samples of saturated solution can then be taken from above the plug.

Cellulose membranes, and therefore presumably cotton wool plugs, can adsorb large quantities of solute from aqueous solutions [16,17]. The quantity adsorbed varies with the filtration medium and the time of contact; for example, Batra [16] found that 96% of progesterone was adsorbed from a 1 μg ml^{-1} aqueous solution by a cellulose acetate membrane, compared with only 23% of estradiol. A glass fiber filter adsorbed only 11% of progesterone. Liu et al. [17] recommend that aqueous suspensions be used to saturate the adsorption sites on the membrane prior to use in solubility determinations. Also, the first few milliliters of filtrate should be discarded.

C. Methods of Analysis

In much of the early solubility work, concentration was determined gravimetrically. A measured aliquot of saturated solution was evaporated to dryness and weighed. The method is accurate but completely unspecific and therefore demands that the solute is pure. It is also of little use with sparingly soluble solutes. Nowadays, saturated solutions are frequently assayed by spectrophotometry, which is almost as unspecific as gravimetric analysis. However, both methods were accepted because it was assumed that if the proportion of impurity was small, the error in the result would be insignificant. Higuchi et al. [6] have pointed out that if the impurity is more soluble than the compound under investigation, it will be preferentially dissolved, and if the method of analysis is unable to distinguish between the substance and its impurity, the apparent solubility will increase with the amount of material used to prepare the saturated solution. It follows that for substances having low solubilities, any advantage gained by increasing the quantity of solute will be counterbalanced by the increased error arising from the impurity. If, for example, 5 mg of a substance having a solubility of 1 mg % and containing 1 % of an impurity having a solubility of 10 mg % is shaken with 10 ml of solvent, the saturated solution will contain 0.1 mg of the substance and 0.05 mg of the impurity. This constitutes a 50% error. Had 50 mg of substance been used, the error would have been 500%.

The problem can be overcome by making a phase solubility correction. A series of apparent solubilities are taken, using the same volume of solvent each time but varying the quantities of solute. A plot of concentration of solute in solution against the total amount added will take the form shown in Fig. 1.12. The initial line represents the dissolution of both solute and impurity, and the second line the dissolution of impurity alone. At the intersection, the solute has reached the limit of its solubility, and extrapolation of the second line back to zero gives the true quantity of solute in solution.

Problems due to impurities are avoided if a specific method of analysis is employed. This is often difficult to achieve, because substances that are difficult to remove in purification processes must, of necessity, have properties similar to those of the substance they

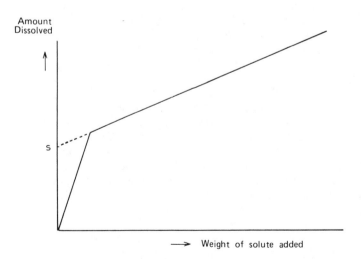

FIGURE 1.12 Phase solubility diagram, showing the influence of the weight of solute, which is not completely pure, on the apparent amount dissolved. S, Solubility of pure material.

are adulterating. A highly discriminating analytical method is therefore necessary. Chromatography often provides the required specificity, and gas-liquid chromatography (GLC) and high-performance
liquid chromatography (HPLC) are popular techniques in this respect, but when the quantity and nature of an impurity is unknown,
one can never be sure that a spot on a plate or a peak on a chart
represents only the isolated, pure solute. One does, however, have
the consolation that if solute and impurity cannot be resolved chroma-
tographically, they should have similar solubilities in the solvent of
interest, so that the error in the observed solubility should be of
the same order as the impurity level. Examples of the use of
chromatography as an analytical tool in solubility determinations
are numerous, for example [9,18].

    With solutes having very low solubilities, the concentration in
the saturated solution may not be sufficient to give an accurate response in the analytical procedure. This occurs most frequently
when aqueous solubilities of large, nonpolar organic molecules are
being investigated. The situation then requires that a more concentrated solution be made from the saturated solution, for example
by liquid-liquid extraction or by evaporating off the solvent and
taking up the residue in a better solvent.

    The process of working up the saturated solution into a more
concentrated form can sometimes be avoided by labeling the solute
with a suitable radioisotope and determining the radioactivity of
the saturated solution. The method is very sensitive and can deal
with dilutions outside the range of most other methods. If an organic compound is to be examined, the experimenter's choice is almost always limited to carbon-14 or tritium. These are both soft β
emitters, so that the most convenient technique is liquid scintillation
counting. This has its attendant problems, in particular poor miscibility of scintillation cocktails with water, and high backgrounds.
The method has been used for cholesterol [19] and other steroids
[16]. There are numerous other examples in the literature.

    The tracer technique has the disadvantage of poor specificity.
Impurities can often be labeled as efficiently as the principal compound during synthesis, and the detector will count the tracer iso-
tope, irrespective of the molecule in which it resides. Also, self-
irradiation renders a labeled compound more susceptible than in-
active materials to contamination. Even soft β emitters are not free
from this problem [20,21]. Particular trouble can be anticipated
with aqueous solubilities, since the radiation can interact with the
water to give aqueous free radicals, which would, in turn, react
with the solute and produce a more water-soluble derivative.

    A further problem associated with tritium is that it can exchange
spontaneously with hydrogen atoms located elsewhere. Even apparently tightly bound tritium can do this, [1,2-^{3}H]methyltestosterone,

for example, will exchange with water [22]. Hawkins [23] recommends freeze drying prior to counting as a means of overcoming this difficulty.

In an investigation of norethindrone derivatives, Lewis and Enever [7,24] found that the aqueous solubilities were below the sensitivity of their analytical methods, and resorted to determining the solubilities in iso-octane, from which they estimated solubilities by using

$$\log \text{ aqueous solubility} = -\log K_d + \log S_{\text{iso-octane}} \tag{1.87}$$

where K_d is the distribution coefficient between iso-octane and water and $S_{\text{iso-octane}}$ is the solubility in iso-octane. Thus the log mass fraction solubility of norethindrone 4-cyclohexyl benzoate was found to be -3.47, and its log distribution coefficient calculated as 6.30, yielding a log aqueous solubility of $-6.30 + (-3.47) = -9.77$. The distribution coefficients were estimated using group contributions calculated from the distribution coefficients of compounds whose aqueous solubilities permitted direct experimental determination. The general approach to this procedure is described in Chapter 9.

D. Determination of Solubilities from Chromatographic Parameters

Schwarz [25] calculated the aqueous solubilities of some slightly soluble organic liquids from the migration of solute-depleted zone in a chromatographic column. The column was packed with Chromosorb P, chosen because the presence of the solute on this material showed up as a pink color. Solute was adsorbed onto the column, eluted off with water, and solubility calculated from

$$x = \frac{S}{\gamma} V + b \tag{1.88}$$

where S is solubility, x the distance traveled by the depleted zone, V the volume of water collected, and b a constant. A plot of x against V will thus be a straight line with slope S/γ, from which the solubility can be calculated. γ is defined by

$$\gamma = \frac{\omega_2 - \omega_1}{L} - \frac{\omega_3 - \omega_2}{L(1 - \rho_{H_2O}/\rho_s)} \tag{1.89}$$

where ω_1 is the weight of the column, ω_2 the weight of the column plus solute, and ω_3 the weight of the column plus solute plus the water occupying the voids. L is the length of the column and ρ_{H_2O} and ρ_s are the densities of water and solute, respectively.

Hafkenscheld and Tomlinson [26] considered that for solutes with poor aqueous solubilities, the use of water alone as eluent is made untenable by excessive retention and low detector sensitivity. They therefore developed a procedure in which mixtures of methanol and water were used as eluent. Their approach was based on

$$\log X_{2sat} = K + \text{a constant} \tag{1.90}$$

and

$$K = K_w + B\phi \tag{1.91}$$

where X_{2sat} is the mole fraction solubility, K the log capacity factor of the eluent, and K_w the corresponding value for water. Capacity factor is defined by

$$K = \frac{t}{t_0} - 1 \tag{1.92}$$

where t is the solute retention time and t_0 the retention time of eluent slightly enriched with water. ϕ is the volume fraction of the organic modifier, in this case, methanol, and B is a constant, characteristic of the experimental conditions. K_w can be obtained for a given solute by repeating the chromatography with a range of combinations of the two eluting solvents, regressing K against ϕ. Data for nine liquid solutes yielded

$$\begin{matrix} & & n & r & \\ -\log X_{2sat} = 1.37 + 1.01K_w & & 9 & 0.993 & \tag{1.93} \end{matrix}$$

but when solids were also considered, an extra parameter (mp − T) had to be included in the equation. mp represents the melting point of the solid and T the temperature at which the measurements were taken, both in degrees Celsius. Following is an example of a correlation covering a sample of 32 liquids and solids:

$$\begin{matrix} & & n & r \\ -\log X_{2sat} = 1.27K_w + 0.0070(mp - 20) + 0.60 & & 32 & 0.956 \; (1.94) \end{matrix}$$

The significance of the expression (mp − T) is discussed in Chapter 4.

Example

The capacity factors for 40 and 70% v/v mixtures of methanol and water, using the chromatographic procedure described by Hafkenscheid and Tomlinson [26] on phenol, were found to be 2.023 and 0.322, respectively, at 20°C. Given that the melting point of phenol is 40.9°C, estimate its solubility in water at 20°C.

Solution:

$\log 2.023 = 0.306 \qquad \log 0.322 = -0.492$

$$0.306 = K_w - 0.4B \qquad\qquad\qquad (a)$$

$$-0.492 = K_w - 0.7B \qquad\qquad\qquad (b)$$

Subtract Eq. (b) from (a) and rearrange:

$$B = \frac{0.306 + 0.492}{0.7 - 0.4} = 2.66$$

Substitute for B in Eq. (a):

$$K_w = 0.306 + 0.4 \times 2.66 = 1.32$$

Substitute for K_w in Eq. (1.94):

$$-\log X_{2sat} = 1.27 \times 1.37 + 0.0070(40.9 - 20) + 0.60$$
$$= 2.49$$

Aqueous solubility at 20°C = antilog $-2.99 = 3.26 \times 10^{-3}$ mole fraction.

E. Determination of Solubilities from Electrical Conductance

Conductance is a useful property for measuring the solubilities of electrolytes in conducting solutions. Basically the procedure is simply one of dipping two parallel platinum plates, a fixed distance apart, into a saturated solution of the electrolyte and measuring its resistance. Conductance is the reciprocal of resistance and is measured in mho or ohm^{-1}. Conductance cells are available commercially and usually take the form of a dip cell with which parallel plates are dipped into the solution, or a cell that acts as a receptacle for the solution.

Temperature must be carefully controlled, and polarization is minimized by coating the plates with platinum black and using an alternating current. Electrolyte impurities, even in trace quantities, will give misleading results. Scrupulous cleanliness is therefore essential, and before use the solvent should be distilled two or three times in all-glass apparatus.

Example

The specific conductance of a saturated aqueous solution of lead sulfate at 18°C is 1.84×10^{-5} mho, and that of the water used, 1.40×10^{-6} mho. The ionic mobilities of $(1/2)Pb^{2+}$ and $(1/2)SO_4^{2-}$ at 18°C are 122 and 136, respectively. Calculate the solubility of lead sulfate. Molecular weight of $PbSO_4$ = 303.

Solution:

Specific conductance of solution = 1.84×10^{-5} mho

Contribution by solvent = $\underline{0.14 \times 10^{-5}}$ mho

Contribution by $PbSO_4$ = 1.70×10^{-5} mho

Molar equivalent conductance = $(122 + 136) \times 2 = 516$ mho

Specific conductance of a molar solution = $\dfrac{516}{1000} = 0.516$

Concentration of saturated solution = $\dfrac{1.70 \times 10^{-5} \times 303}{0.516}$

$$= 9.98 \times 10^{-3} \text{ g dm}^{-3}$$

VII. SIMPLEX SEARCH FOR OPTIMUM SOLVENT BLENDS

When a solution is required as a reagent for a chemical or biological process, the response invariably increases with concentration, and there is a threshold below which the solution does not fulfill its functions effectively. If a specific solvent is required for the solution, it may be that the solute is not soluble enough to meet the threshold and a cosolvent has to be added. If, for example, an aqueous solution of an organic compound is required and water alone is not a good enough solvent to achieve the necessary concentration, it may be possible to raise the solubility by addition of a water-miscible organic liquid. The process of establishing the optimum proportions of the two solvents is often one of trial and error which although simple for mixtures of a solvent and a cosolvent, becomes complicated when there are two or more cosolvents. A simplex search [27] is a useful procedure for dealing with such situations.

A simplex is a geometrical figure, defined by a number of points, which is one more than the number of variables. The simplex for two variables is a triangle, for three variables a four-sided figure, and so on. Suppose that it is required to fix the optimum of three solvents, x, y, and z, for a given solute. Since x + y + z = 100%, once the concentrations of x and y are decided, z becomes fixed and equal to 100 − (x + y). There are therefore only two variables and the number of points in the simplex will be 2 + 1 = 3. Suppose that the three arbitrarily chosen points are given by 1, 2, and 3 in Fig. 1.13 and that their compositions and the solubilities in them are those given in Table 1.2. The solute is least soluble in blend 1, so this point is disregarded and its mirror image plotted across the line

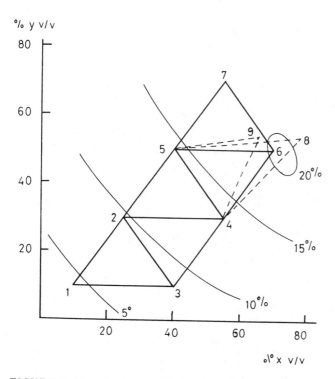

FIGURE 1.13 Simplex path for imaginary ternary solvent system. Coordinates of the points and solubilities are given in Table 1.2. The curves and elipse represent solubility contours.

TABLE 1.2 Coordinates and Solubilities in Ternary Blends of Solvents x, y, and z

Point	1	2	3	4	5	6	7	8	9
Coordinates, (% v/v)									
x	10	25	40	55	40	70	55	76.8	65
y	10	30	10	30	50	50	70	53	47
Solubility (% w/v)	3.5	9.0	7.5	11.0	12.3	22.7	16.4	18.1	17.1

joining 2 and 3 to 4.   This procedure can be carried out geometrical-
ly using a ruler or fitted to mathematical formulas as follows:
The mean coordinates of 2 and 3 are

$$\bar{x}_{2,3} = \frac{x_2 + x_3}{2} = \frac{25 + 40}{2} = 32.5$$

$$\bar{y}_{2,3} = \frac{y_2 + y_3}{2} = \frac{30 + 10}{2} = 20$$

The coordinate of the mirror image (point 4) will therefore be

$$x_4 = \bar{x}_{2,3} + (\bar{x}_{2,3} - x_1) = 32.5 + (32.5 - 10) = 55$$

$$y_4 = \bar{y}_{2,3} + (\bar{y}_{2,3} - y_1) = 20 + (20 - 10) = 30$$

The solubility of the solute in blend 4 must now be determined and
the point in the triangle 2-3-4 with the lowest solubility rejected.
Table 1.2 shows that this is point 3, so a mirror image is drawn
from 3 across the line joining points 2 and 4 to point 5.   The coordinates of this will be $x_5 = 40$ and $y_5 = 50$, as given in Table 1.2.
The curves and elipse in Fig. 1.13 represent the solubility contours of the mixtures and show how the optimization process leads
to the point of maximum solubility.   If the process is continued to
point 7, there is a drop in solubility, compared with point 6, which
indicates that blend 6 is somewhere near the blend of maximum
solubility.
To locate the maximum precisely, point 6 is "accelerated" along
line 2-6 by applying the equation

Coordinates of accelerated point $8 = \bar{x}_{4,5} + \underline{a}(\bar{x}_{4,5} - x_2)$

$\underline{a}$ is an arbitrary expansion factor which must be greater than unity.
Thus if $\underline{a}$ is chosen to be 1.3,

$$x_8 = 47.5 + 1.3(47.5 - 25) = 76.8$$

$$y_8 = 40 + 1.3(40 - 30) = 53$$

If the solubility is lower than in blend 6, as is the case here, point
6 is "contracted" by application of the formula

Coordinates of new point $9 = x_9 = \bar{x}_{4,5} + \underline{b}(\bar{x}_{4,5} - x_2)$

$\underline{b}$ is an arbitrary contraction coefficient which must lie between zero and one. Suppose that 0.7 is chosen:

$$x_9 = 47.5 + 0.7(47.5 - 22.5) = 65$$

$$y_9 = 40 + 0.7(40 - 30) = 47$$

Blend 9 again gives a lower solubility than blend 6, indicating that the maximum is between point 9 and point 8 and that blend 6 is near enough for most practical purposes.

Example

Gould and Goodman [28] used a simplex search to locate the combination of ethanol, propylene glycol, and water that dissolved the most caffeine. Their results [29] are shown in Table 1.3, and the simplex path the authors followed in Fig. 1.14. Their sequence of moves was as follows:

a. Combinations 1, 2, and 3 were arbitrarily chosen for the opening simplex.
b. Point 3 represented the worst solvent mixture, so a mirror image was projected to point 4.
c. The solubilities in 1 and 2 are virtually the same, and therefore lie on approximately the same solubility contour (see Fig. 1.13). Also, caffeine was considerably more soluble

TABLE 1.3 Solubilities of Caffeine in Ethanol, Propylene Glycol, and Water Mixtures

1	—	0	40	24.0
2	—	20	0	26.2
3	—	0	0	17.2
4	Reflection	20	40	44.9
5	Expansion	30	60	17.5
6	Reflection	40	0	52.4
7	Reflection	40	40	36.7
8	Contraction	35	30	52.9
9	Contraction	29	28	53.0

Source: Data from Ref. 29.

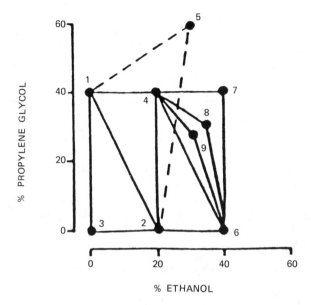

FIGURE 1.14 Simplex path for solubility optimization of caffeine in ethanol-propylene glycol-water mixtures. Coordinates are given in Table 1.3. (From Ref. 28.)

in 4 than in any of the other three. It therefore seemed logical not to choose 1 as the worst solvent mixture of 1, 2, and 4, to project to a mirror image, but to accelerate in the direction of increasing concentration (i.e., from 3 to beyond 4). Point 5 was the result, but it gave a reduced solubility, so it was rejected and the original plan followed. Thus:

d. The mirror image of point 1 across the line joining 2 and 4 led to point 6, which gave an enhanced solubility.

e. Point 2 was the worst solvent in the simplex 2-4-6, and this was imaged across the line joining 4 and 6 to point 7. However, at this point the solubility was lower than in either 4 or 6; therefore,

f. Contraction was carried out along the 2-7 line to points 8 and 9. The solubilities in these two blends were the same and greater than in any of the previous blends. They were therefore considered to bracket the point of maximum solubility.

REFERENCES

1. R. A. Robinson and R. H. Stokes, *Electrolyte Solutions*, Butterworths, London, 1970.
2. C. W. Davies, The extent of dissociation of salts in water: Part VIII. An equation for the mean activity coefficient of an electrolyte in water, and a revision of the dissociation constants of some sulphates, *J. Chem. Soc.*, 2093—2098 (1938).
3. P. H. Sykes and P. W. Robertson, The activity coefficients of the nitrobenzoic acids, *J. Am. Chem. Soc.*, 55, 2621—2625 (1933).
4. B. Cavanagh, Activity measurements by the partition method, I, *Proc. R. Soc. London*, 106A, 243—250 (1924).
5. A. A. Noyes and W. R. Whitney, Die Auflosungsgeschwindigkeit von festen Stoffen in ihren eigenen Losungen (Dissolution rates of solid substances in their solutions), *Z. Phys. Chem.*, 23, 689—692 (1909).
6. T. Higuchi, F. M. L. Shih, T. Kimura, and J. H. Rytting, Solubility determination of barely aqueous-soluble organic solids, *J. Pharm. Sci.*, 68. 1267—1272 (1979).
7. G. A. Lewis and R. P. Enever, Solution thermodynamics of some potentially long-acting norethindrone derivatives: III. Measurement of aqueous solubilities and the use of group free energy contributions in predicting partition coefficients, *Int. J. Pharm.* 3, 319—333 (1979).
8. J. J. Fox, Solubility of lead sulphate in concentrated solutions of sodium and potassium acetate, *J. Chem. Soc.*, 878—889 (1909).
9. W. E. May, S. P. Wasik, and D. H. Freeman, Determination of the aqueous solubility of polynuclear aromatic hydrocarbons by a coupled liquid chromatographic technique, *Anal. Chem.*, 50, 175—179 (1978).
10. A. L. Green, Ionization constants and water solubilities of some aminoalkylphenothiazine tranquillizers and related compounds, *J. Pharm. Pharmacol.*, 19, 10—16 (1967).
11. M. R. Loran and E. P. Guth, A phase study of castor oil, alcohol and water miscibility, *J. Am. Pharm. Assoc. Sci. Ed.*, 40, 465—466 (1951).
12. R. W. Potter and M. A. Clynne, Solubility of highly soluble salts in aqueous media: Part 1. NaCl, KCl, $CaCl_2$, Na_2SO_4 and K_2SO_4. Solubilities to 100°C, *J. Res. U.S. Geol. Surv.*, 6, 701—705 (1978).
13. M. A. Clynne and R. W. Potter, Solubility of some alkali and alkaline earth chlorides in water at moderate temperatures, *J. Chem. Eng. Data*, 338—340 (1979).
14. D. B. Bowen and K. C. James, Solubilities of testosterone propionate in non-polar solvents at 100°, *J. Pharm. Pharmacol.*, 20 (Suppl.), 104S—107S (1968).

15. L. J. Gordon and R. L. Scott, Enhanced solubility in solvent mixtures: I. The system phenanthrene-cyclohexane-methylene iodide, *J. Am. Chem. Soc.*, *74*, 4138—4140 (1952).

16. S. Batra, Aqueous solubility of steroid hormones: an explanation for the discrepancy in the published data, *J. Pharm. Pharmacol.*, *27*, 777—779 (1977).

17. S. T. Liu, C. F. Carney, and A. R. Hurwitz, Adsorption as a possible limitation in solubility determination, *J. Pharm. Pharmacol.*, *29*, 319—321 (1977).

18. C. McAuliffe, Solubility in water of paraffin, cycloparaffin, olefin, acetylene, cycloolefin and aromatic hydrocarbons, *J. Phys. Chem.*, *70*, 1267—1275 (1966).

19. G. L. Flyn, Y. Shah, S Prakongpan, K. H. Kuran, W. I. Higuchi, and A. F. Hofmann, Cholesterol solubility in organic solvents, *J. Pharm. Sci.*, *68*, 1090—1097 (1979).

20. B. Waldeck, [^{3}H]Dopa in [^{3}H]tyrosine with high specific activity: a serious complication in the study of catecholamine metabolism, *J. Pharm. Pharmacol.*, *23*, 64—65 (1971).

21. B. M. Talbert, P. T. Adams, E. L. Bennett, A. M. Highes, M. R. Kirk, R. M. Lemmon, R. M. Noller, R. Oswald, and M. Calvin, Observations on the radiation decomposition of some C^{14}-labeled compounds, *J. Am. Chem. Soc.*, *75*, 1867—1868 (1953).

22. K. C. James, P. J. Nicholls, and L. M. Sanders, Availability of tritium from non-aqueous solutions of [1,2-^{3}H]methyltestosterone, administered orally to rats, *J. Pharm. Pharmacol.*, *32*, 810—814 (1980).

23. D. R. Hawkins, Tracing metabolic fates, *Chem. Br.*, *12*, 379--383 (1976).

24. G. A. Lewis and R. P. Enever, Solution thermodynamics of some potentially long-acting norethindrone derivatives: II. Solutions in 2,2,4-trimethylpentane (iso-octane), *Int. J. Pharm.*, *3*, 275--288 (1979).

25. F. P. Schwaz, Measurement of the solubilities of slightly soluble liquids in water by elution chromatography, *Anal. Chem.*, *52*, 10--15 (1980).

26. T. L. Hafkenscheid and E. Tomlinson, Estimation of aqueous solubilities of organic non-electrolytes using liquid chromatographic retention data, *J. Chromatogr.*, *218*, 409—425 (1981).

27. S. M. Deming and S. L. Morgan, Simplex optimization of variables in analytical chemistry, *Anal. Chem.*, *45A*, 278—283 (1973).

28. P. L. Gould and M. Goodman, Simplex search in the optimization of the solubility of caffeine in parenteral cosolvent systems, *J. Pharm. Pharmacol.*, *35* (Suppl.), 3P (1983).

29. P. L. Gould, Personal communication, 1983.

2

The Liquid State

Although solutions can be solids, liquids, or gases, the liquid is by far the commonest form. It is therefore necessary to consider the liquid state as a preliminary to understanding the properties of liquid solutions and the ways in which they differ from solid solutions and mixtures of gases.

The liquid state is not as amenable to theoretical predictions as
are gases and solids. The molecules in a gas are widely separated,
so that intermolecular forces are very small, and the total molecular
volume is negligible in comparison with the total volume occupied by
the gas. Completely random distribution of the molecules is therefore possible. Intermolecular forces are significant in solids, but
since the molecules in crystalline solids are arranged in a regularly
repeating pattern, the effects of these forces can usually be anticipated. Liquids suffer both disadvantages, intermolecular forces
are significant, and molecules are close together, so that random
distribution is prevented by intermolecular contact. Furthermore,
they do not have the fixed molecular orientation of solids. The approximate behavior of liquids has been evaluated by modeling them
on the two simpler states of matter. Thus liquids have been considered as either quasi-crystalline solids or imperfect, unexpanded
gases. These two models will be considered in turn.

I. THE UNEXPANDED GAS MODEL

Liquids have been treated as imperfect gases on the grounds that
at the critical point liquid and gas are indistinguishable. The ki-
netic theory of gases assumes that gas molecules are random points
having no volume and no forces of attraction or repulsion between
them. The perfect gas laws based on this model fit reasonably well
to expanded real gases (i.e., gases at low pressure and/or high
temperature) because their molecules are widely separated. Thus
at high temperatures and low pressures, gases obey Boyle's law
(PV = a constant) by giving a rectilinear plot of pressure against
volume, as shown in the $T \gg T_c$ isotherm in Fig. 2.1. T_c is critical temperature. If this is expressed in terms of two molecules of
the gas a distance r apart, the energy of interaction between them,
termed the intermolecular pair potential (ΔU), will vary with the
distance of separation in the manner shown in Fig. 2.2. When the
distance of separation is large, the molecules will not exert any influence on each other and ΔU will be zero. This is represented by
line AB in Fig. 2.2, where the plot runs parallel to the distance
axis. Thus, what is happening in region AB of Fig. 2.1 is presented in another way in region AB of Fig. 2.2. The comparison
is not meant to suggest that point B in Fig. 2.1 exactly coincides
with point B in Fig. 2.2, only that these regions in the two figures
represent the same state of matter, and that what can be seen on
the PV diagram (Fig. 2.1) can be explained in terms of intermolecular pair potentials, as depicted in Fig. 2.2.

If pressure is exerted on the gas, the molecules will be forced
closer together, r will decrease, and molecular interactions will

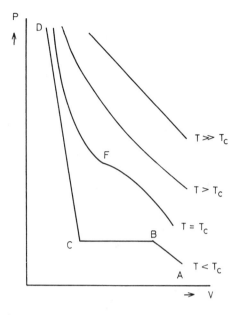

FIGURE 2.1 Isothermals for a simple fluid. T_c, critical temperature.

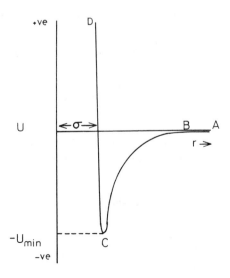

FIGURE 2.2 Intermolecular pair potentials for a simple fluid.

begin to bite, as indicated in Fig. 2.2 by divergence from the distance axis. The molecules will orient so that unlike electrostatic
forces are in apposition, and the net interaction will be one of attraction. The resulting pair potential will therefore be negative
and will decrease progressively with decreasing r to a minimum C.
This energy minimum occurs at the most stable intermolecular distance and is responsible for the process of liquefaction. The attraction involved at this point is expressed as a negative potential
energy and is called the molar cohesive energy ($-U_{min}$). (It is
negative because it is an attractive energy.)

This progression from A to C in Fig. 2.2 can be represented
by the line ABC in Fig. 2.1 ($T < T_c$). AB represents compression
of an expanded gas, but at B the molecules are sufficiently close
for the cohesive energy to reach a value that induces liquefaction.
BC therefore represents a mixture of gas and liquid and follows a
line parallel to the volume axis because the decrease in volume is
due to condensation of gas to liquid, with increasing pressure. CD
in Fig. 2.1 is the PV plot for the liquid; considerable pressure is
required to bring about a small decrease in volume, reflecting the
high resistance of liquids to compression.

The portion CD of the potential energy profile shown in Fig. 2.2
is equivalent to CD in the PV diagram (Fig 2.1) and expresses a
massive increase in potential energy associated with only a small decrease in intermolecular distance. This behavior can be explained
in simple terms as resistance arising from mechanical contact, or
more specifically as repulsion between the electron clouds surrounding the two molecules. At this point, therefore, potential energy is
approximately asymptotic with molecular diameter (σ), and the process
is another way of expressing the influence of the volume of the molecules on the compressibility of a fluid. The intercept of the vertical portion of Fig. 2.2 on the distance axis (σ) is therefore approximately equal to the diameter of the molecules.

If PV isotherms are plotted at progressively increasing temperatures, the horizontal portion represented by BC decreases in length
until at the critical temperature it resolves to a single point F, the
critical point, where liquid and gas are indistinguishable. It is this
identity of liquid and gas at the critical point that is the basis for
modeling the liquid state on an unexpanded gas. At temperatures
above critical, the plot is curved with no inflection ($T > T_c$, Fig.
2.1) and becomes progressively more shallow with increasing temperature until it is rectilinear over a limited region ($T \gg T_c$,
Fig. 2.1).

Van der Waals equation

$$\left(P + \frac{a}{V^2}\right) (V - b) = RT \tag{2.1}$$

is the best known relationship between pressure, temperature, and volume of an unexpanded gas. The constant b is a correction for the volume of the molecules and is subtracted from the total volume V to give the free volume between the molecules. The gas constant can be replaced by Nk, in which N is Avogadro's number and k is the Boltzmann constant, defined as R/N. Attractive forces tend to bring the molecules together, and the observed pressure is therefore less than that expected of a perfect gas. Any correction must therefore be added. The correction is influenced by the total number of molecules in two ways:

1. The greater the number of molecules, the greater the inward pull on any molecule about to collide with the walls of the enclosing vessel.
2. The greater the number of molecules, the greater the number of impacts with the walls.

The correction must therefore be proportional to the square of the number of molecules, or alternatively, to the reciprocal of the square of the molar volume; hence the correction $+ a/V^2$.

Expansion of van der Waals equation gives

$$PV^3 - (Pb + RT)V^2 - aV + ab = 0 \qquad (2.2)$$

which has the form of a cubic equation. It therefore has three roots and at low temperatures takes the form of GHJK in Fig. 2.3, which shows PV plots for carbon dioxide calculated from Eq. (2.1). There are three values of V, corresponding to pressures around those of the horizontal portion BC of the experimental PV plot in Fig. 2.1. Thus in Fig. 2.3, at a pressure of 40 atm, the three volumes are 0.08, 0.12, and 0.39 liters. As the temperature is raised, the three values of V move closer together and coincide at the critical point, giving an inflection in the curve.

The values of a and b for carbon dioxide are 0.364 N m^4 mol^{-2} and 4.27×10^{-5} m^3 mol^{-1}, respectively; ab in Eq. (2.2) is therefore equal to 1.5×10^{-5} m^7 mol^{-3}. The critical temperature of carbon dioxide is 31°C (304 K), so that since the gas constant is 8.32 N m deg^{-1} mol^{-1}, (Pb + RT) is greater than 2700 N m^{-2} at temperatures above critical, even with volumes as low as 1 dm^3 mol^{-1}. The constant ab is therefore considerably less than the V^2 term. Substitution of a and b into the equation gives similar large values for PV^3 compared with ab, so that ab can be ignored in Eq. (2.2), which then reduces to

$$PV^2 - (Pb + RT)V - a = 0 \qquad (2.3)$$

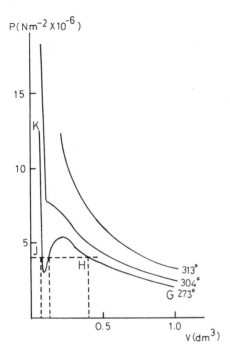

FIGURE 2.3 PV diagram for carbon dioxide.

This is a quadratic equation which predicts a curved PV plot at temperatures exceeding critical, as shown by the 313 K plot in Fig. 2.3.

With expanded gases, V is large, so that a/V^2 is very small and b can be ignored in comparison with V. The second terms in both sets of parentheses in Eq. (2.1) therefore disappear and the equation reduces to PV = RT. The plot of P against V therefore becomes rectilinear. Thus at temperatures around and above critical, the predicted plots have the same form as the experimental results. This can be seen if Fig. 2.1 is compared with Fig. 2.3. Thus the van der Waals equation predicts the behavior of gases adequately except in its failure in the horizontal regions of the PV plots at lower temperatures.

Van der Waals constants have traditionally been expressed using liters and atmospheres as units for volume and pressure, respectively, and older publications quote a and b in this form. Since 1 liter is equal to 10^{-3} m^3, b in m^3 mol^{-1} is equal to b in liters mol^{-1} multiplied by 10^{-3}. One atmosphere is equal to 1.013×10^5 N m^{-2}; therefore, a in N m^4 mol^{-2} is equal to a in 1^2 atm mol^{-2} multiplied by $(10^{-3})^2 \times 1.013 \times 10^5$ or by 1.013×10^{-1}.

Example

Given that $a = 3.59$ liters^2 atm mol^{-2} and $b = 0.0427$ liters mol^{-1} for carbon dioxide, calculate its pressure in SI units at 60°C. $R = 8.32$ N m deg^{-1}.

Solution:

$$a = 3.59 \times 1.013 \times 10^{-1} = 0.364 \text{ N m}^4 \text{ mol}^{-2}$$

$$b = 0.0427 \times 10^{-3} = 4.27 \times 10^{-5} \text{ m}^3 \text{ mol}^{-1}$$

Substitution in the van der Waals equation gives

$$\left[P + \frac{0.364}{(10^{-3})^2} \right] (10^{-3} - 4.27 \times 10^{-5}) = 8.32 \times 333$$

Therefore,

$$P = \frac{8.32 \times 333}{9.57 \times 10^{-4}} - 3.64 \times 10^5 = 2.54 \times 10^6 \text{ N m}^{-2}$$

The van der Waals equation has been discussed in some detail because it is the best known equation of its kind and because it is used to develop equations in regular solution theory. It is, however, only one of many equations of state for unexpanded gases. These have been reviewed by Beattie [1].

Rearrangement of van der Waals equation gives

$$\frac{PV}{RT} = \left(1 - \frac{b}{V} \right)^{-1} - \frac{a}{RTV} \qquad (2.4)$$

Since b is less then V, the second term on the right-hand side can be expanded using the binomial theorem, to give

$$\frac{PV}{RT} = 1 + \frac{b}{V} + \frac{b^2}{V^2} + \frac{b^3}{V^3} + \cdots - \frac{a}{RTV} \qquad (2.5)$$

This is similar to the following virial equation

$$\frac{PV}{RT} = 1 + \frac{B}{V} + \frac{C}{V^2} + \frac{D}{V^3} + \cdots \qquad (2.6)$$

which is used to explain the behavior of gases at high pressures.
B, C, D, and so on, are the second, third, and fourth virial coefficients and form the beginning of a series that can be expanded
indefinitely or until the desired accuracy of prediction of experimental results is achieved. When the volume is not too small and
pressure moderate or low, the coefficients decrease rapidly as the
series is extended. It is therefore normally only the first few coefficients, usually only B/V, which are important. The virial coefficients are temperature dependent and can be evaluated from experimental results. A typical example of their determination has
been given by McGlassan and Potter [2]. The second virial coefficient is negative at low temperatures and increases to a positive
value as temperature is increased. The temperature at which B
equals zero is called the Boyle temperature, because at that point
the gas obeys Boyle's law with reasonable precision.

Comparison of Eq. (2.5) with Eq. (2.6) gives the virial coeffi-
cients in terms of the van der Waals constants, namely, $B = b - a/RT$, $C = b^2$, $D = b^3$, and so on.

Substitution in Eq. (2.4) gives

$$\frac{PV}{NkT} = \frac{V}{V - b} - \frac{a}{VNkT} \tag{2.7}$$

Alter [3] has evaluated these terms for hard spheres, and found
good agreement with experimental results.

At the critical point the PV plot passes through an inflection
corresponding to the critical pressure (P_c) and critical volume (V_c),
at which both dP/dV and d^2P/dV^2 will be equal to zero at constant
(critical) temperature. The solutions to these differentials give three
equations in P_c, V_c, and T_c, from which the critical constants can
be evaluated in terms of a, b, and R, to give the results, $V_c = 3b$,
$T_c = 8a/27Rb$, and $P_c = a/27b^2$. The quotient P_cV_c/RT_c is a dimensionless number, namely 0.375, indicating that P_cV_c/T_c is constant
for all fluids obeying van der Waals equation.

II. THE QUASI-CRYSTALLINE MODEL

The quasi-crystalline approach to liquid structure has a similar claim
to validity as the unexpanded gas theory. Just as the gas and
liquid can be considered identical at the critical point, so is the
structure of a liquid near the melting point not greatly different
from that of the corresponding solid. This conclusion follows from
the very low expansion in passing from solid to liquid, for example,
near the melting point the inter-oxygen spacings are 0.290 nm for
water and 0.286 nm for ice. In general, the increase in volume for
most compounds in passing from solid to liquid is only about 10%.

The crystalline state is an ordered structure. Each molecule occupies a specific position and its only motion is to vibrate about that position. The lattice points are highly specific and can be occupied by only one particular species of molecule or an isomorph of that species. This is in direct contrast to the gaseous state in which all molecules are miscible in all proportions. The high specificity of the crystal lattice is one of the weaknesses of the quasi-crystalline theory of the liquid state, since it does not explain why molecules with widely differing molar volumes are miscible in the liquid state.

If an animal is confined to a large area and has no preference for a particular spot, the probability that it will be found in a given field will depend on the area of that field and not on the position of the field. Similarly, if a molecule that moves in a random manner is confined in a box, the probability that it can be found in a specific space within the box at a given time will be proportional to the volume of the space and independent of where the space is. Thus if the volume of the space is equal to that of the box, the probability of the molecule being found in the space will be 1 in 1; if the volume of the space is half that of the box, the probability will be 0.5, or 1 in 2; and so on. Furthermore, if the box contains more than one molecule, the probability of finding a molecule will increase in proportion to the number of molecules. Put into mathematical terms, if the volume under consideration is δV, the total volume is V, and there are n molecules, the probability of a molecule being found in the volume δV will be $n \, \delta V/V$, or 1 in $V/n \, \delta V$.

The problem could be presented in a different manner. It could be necessary to know how many molecules are likely to be within a distance r or less of a reference molecule situated in V milliliters of an expanded gas containing a total of n molecules. The answer is $(4\pi r^3 n/3V)$, where $(4/3)\pi r^3$ represents the volume of a sphere of radius r, with the reference molecule at its center.

In a similar way, the probability of a molecule having another molecule located a specific distance r away from it can be expressed in terms of the volume of a hollow spherical shell of radius r with the molecule at its center. The total volume will now be represented by the sphere enclosed by the shell, and the probable number of molecules located an exact distance r from the reference molecule will be given by

$$\text{Probability} = \frac{\text{volume of spherical shell}}{\text{volume of sphere enclosed by shell}} \, n \qquad (2.8)$$

$$= n \, \frac{4\pi r^2 \, \delta r}{(4/3)\pi r^3}$$

δr is the thickness of the shell and is assumed to be small in comparison with r. If for any reason the number of particles differs from that predicted by Eq. (2.8), the discrepancy is expressed as the radial distribution function g(r):

$$g(r) = \frac{\text{actual number of molecular centers}}{\text{number occurring in a random distribution}}$$

The plot of radial distribution function against the distance from an arbitrarily chosen molecule is called a radial distribution curve. In an expanded gas, the number of molecules occurring will be the same as that given by Eq. (2.8), so that the radial distribution curve will take the form shown in Fig. 2.4a. g(r) is zero at distances less than the molecular diameter because at this point the molecules would be touching. Distance is assessed as the number of molecular diameters between the center of one molecule and that of another. Molecules are assumed to be spherical.

In closely packed collections of molecules random distribution is restricted by molecular contact. If we assume, for simplicity, a system of equisized spherical molecules, the most compact form they could take would be hexagonal close packing, shown in two dimensions in Fig. 2.5. Each molecule is in contact with 6 molecules in the first surrounding layer, with a second layer of 6 molecules, 6 in the third, and so on. In three dimensions, the first layer would contain 12 molecules. The minimum distance from the center of a reference molecule, at which the center of a neighboring molecule can be found, will be equal to the diameter (σ) of the molecule. At values less than σ, g(r) must be zero. Geometry tells us that g(r) will continue to be zero at values greater than σ, until r = 1.73 σ, when the spherical shell, postulated above, will coincide with 12 molecular centers. The next center occurs at r = 2.00 σ, and so on. The radial distribution curve will therefore take the form of a series of discrete lines, shown in Fig. 2.4b. In the solid state, molecules vibrate about fixed positions. The radial distribution curve of a solid arranged in a hexagonal close-packed lattice would therefore take the form of a series of sharp peaks corresponding to the vertical lines in Fig. 2.4b. Similar models can be developed with body-centered, face-centered, and simple cubic packings. Bernal [4,5] constructed a model consisting of equisized spheres, distributed irregularly, and having the same net density as the corresponding liquid. He noted the existence of fivefold symmetry and pointed out that on geometrical grounds this would not permit a regularly repeating pattern but must give rise to "holes" in the distribution. These holes were mainly tetrahedral and octahedral, occurring in the proportion of 2:1.

(a)

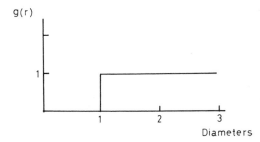

(b)

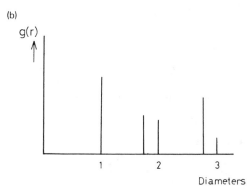

(c)

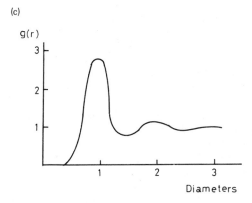

FIGURE 2.4 Radial distribution plots for distributions of unisized spherical molecules: (a) expanded gas; (b) solid with molecules arranged in hexagonal close packing; (c) the liquid state.

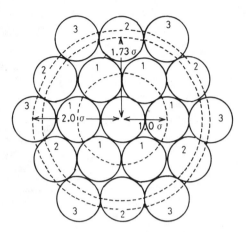

FIGURE 2.5 Hexagonal close packing of identical spherical molecules presented in two-dimensional form. The numbers on the
molecules represent the shells to which they belong.

The precise structure of a crystalline solid can be established
by x-ray diffraction. The orderly arrangement of molecules gives
rise to a series of planes in the crystal, and these can diffract a
beam of x rays directed on to the crystal, giving a diffraction pattern that can be recorded on a photographic plate and observed as
a series of sharp lines. X-ray diffraction patterns for liquids do
not show the same sharp lines as solids, but give rise to two to
three diffuse halos, indicating that each molecule is located in a
slightly ordered arrangement extending to three molecular diameters
and no further. Hence the liquid state is concluded to resemble the
crystalline state in having short-range order but differs from the
crystalline state in the absence of long-range order. The type of
structure that would be anticipated for a distribution of spherical
molecules is shown in two-dimensional form in Fig. 2.6. The first
layer surrounding the reference molecule is slightly disordered but
similar in appearance to that in the hexagonal close-packed form.
There is the suggestion of a second layer, but beyond it there is
little impression of order. The picture represents a structure operating for an infinitely short period of time and changing continuously.
Because of the disorder, molecular centers will not coincide with
specific values of r, so that the radial distribution curve will take
the form of broad bands, as shown in Fig. 2.4c. The peaks diminish with the distance from the chosen molecule and coincide approximately with the vertical lines in Fig. 2.4b.

Radial distribution is depicted in a different way in Fig. 2.4c
from that in Fig. 2.4 a and b. The g(r) axis in Fig. 2.4c represents

all molecules *in contact with* the various hollow spheres, while Fig. 2.4b considers only those molecules *whose centers coincide with* the spherical element. The maxima in the two figures are better illustrated by presenting them in these alternative ways. Figure 2.4a and b would take a similar form to that already shown for Fig. 2.4a, if interpreted in the manner used for Fig. 2.4c.

Example

Calculate the probable number of molecules that are (a) within 1000 nm of and (b) exactly 1000 nm from a reference molecule in an expanded gas containing 0.001 mol dm^{-3}. Avogadro's number = 6.024 × 10^{23}; molecular diameter of gas = 0.34 nm.

Solution:

(a) Volume of sphere of radius 1000 nm $= \dfrac{4}{3} \pi \dfrac{1000^3}{(10^8)^3}$

$$= 4.19 \times 10^{-15} \; dm^3$$

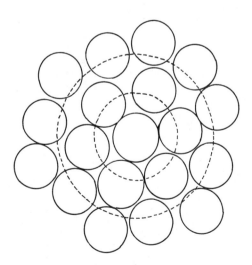

FIGURE 2.6 Two-dimensional representation of identical spherical molecules in the liquid state.

Therefore,

$$\text{Probable number in sphere} = 0.001 \times 4.19 \times 10^{-15} \times 6.024 \times 10^{23}$$

$$= 2.52 \times 10^{6}$$

(b) Any molecules that are *exactly* 1000 nm from a reference molecule will occupy a hollow sphere of radius 1000 nm and thickness 0.35 nm, with the reference molecule at its center. The volume of a hollow sphere of radius r and thickness δr is equal to $4\pi r^2 \delta r$. Therefore, for the conditions operating,

$$\text{Volume of hollow sphere} = 4 \times 3.142 \times 1000^2 \times 0.35 \times (10^{-8})^3$$

$$= 4.40 \times 10^{-18} \text{ dm}^3$$

Since the total volume *enclosed* by the hollow sphere is 4.19×10^{-15} dm^3 and it contains 2.52×10^6 molecules, the probable number occupying the spherical element will be

$$\frac{2.52 \times 10^6 \times 4.40 \times 10^{-18}}{4.19 \times 10^{-15}} = 2.65 \times 10^3$$

The molecular diameter of 0.35 nm has been considered to be negligible in comparison with 1000 nm in these calculations.

Example

Calculate the radial distribution function for the first shell of a hexagonal close-packed structure consisting of one spherical molecule surrounded by 12 identical molecules, all of radius r. (The first shell is that comprising the molecules marked "1" in Fig. 2.5.)

Solution:

$$\begin{array}{l}\text{Volume of sphere enclosed by} \\ \text{and including the first shell}\end{array} = \frac{4}{3}\pi(3r)^3 = 113.1r^3$$

$$\text{Volume of center sphere} = \frac{4}{3}\pi r^3 = 4.2r^3$$

$$\text{Volume of shell} = (113.1 - 4.2)r^3 = 108.9r^2$$

$$g(r) = \frac{12 \times 113.1}{13 \times 108.9} = 0.96$$

Molecular distributions have been treated statistically using the Monte Carlo method [6], which averages the possible configurations of molecules in a random distribution, and the molecular dynamics method [7], which traces the trajectories of the molecules and computes the forces involved. Both are complex mathematical procedures that require the use of high-powered computers.

The quasi-crystalline models described so far do not take the motions of the molecules within their immediate environment into consideration. To allow for this effect, each molecule of a fluid can be considered to be confined in a cavity formed by the surrounding molecules and to vibrate within this space. The difference between the volume of the molecule and its "cage" is the free volume. Free volume can be defined in several ways, for example:

1. The excess of the volume per mole of fluid over the total volume of the individual molecules. This definition is equivalent to $(V - b)$ in the van der Waals equation.
2. The excess of the molar volume of the fluid at the operational temperature over that at 0 K. This is sometimes called the expansion volume.
3. Free volume (V_f) is also defined by

$$\Delta S^V = R \ln \frac{V_g}{V_f} \qquad (2.9)$$

where ΔS^V is the entropy of vaporization and V_g the volume of the gas.

If the cage is considered to be a sphere of radius r and the molecule within it has a radius $\sigma/2$, the free volume will be given by

$$V_f = \frac{4}{3}\pi \left(r - \frac{\sigma}{2} \right)^3 \qquad (2.10)$$

Geometrical considerations tell us that the volume of a hexagonal close-packed structure is $\sqrt{2}$ times the volume of the spheres. The total free volume is therefore $(4/3)\pi\sqrt{2}(r - \sigma/2)^3 = 6(r - \sigma/2)^3$. Constants for other forms of packing are given in Table 2.1.

Quasi-crystalline models are complicated by other factors; for example:

1. Although it is reasonable to anticipate maxima in the radial distribution curves corresponding to those in Fig. 2.5, experimental evidence suggests that actual numbers of molecules involved are less than those anticipated by the models.

TABLE 2.1 Constants for Molecular Packing

	Theoretical nearest neighbors	Factor
Hexagonal close packing	12	$\sqrt{2}$
Face-centered cubic	12	$\sqrt{2}$
Body-centered cubic	8	$\sqrt{3/4}$
Simple cubic	6	$\sqrt{1}$

Differences are usually quoted in terms of coordination number (Z) or number or nearest neighbors.

2. The solute and solvent molecules forming a solution usually have different molar volumes, so that three radial functions $g(r)_{11}$ (solvent to solvent), $g(r)_{22}$ (solute to solute), and $g(r)_{12}$ (solvent to solute) are involved. The magnitude of these functions varies with molecular size and also with relative concentrations of solute and solvent.

3. The quasi-crystalline treatment assumes that the molecules involved are spherical. In practice this is rarely the case.

The process of melting can be considered in the light of the structures just described and occurs when the molecular vibrations are sufficient to break down the highly ordered crystal structure. The molecules in the crystal are so close that displacement of only one molecule causes extensive disorder. Hence the melting point is sharp because it is brought about by a relatively small number of molecules in comparison with the whole mass. After melting, as the temperature rises, the liquid expands and the number of nearest neighbors decreases, resulting in a broadening of the bands in the radial distribution curve. This reaches a climax at the critical point, when the radical distribution curve takes the gaseous form. This gradation in shape of the radial distribution curve, from the discrete vertical lines of the solid to the horizontal line of the gas, explains the success and limitations of the unexpanded gas and quasi-crystalline models of the liquid state. They are effective near the critical point and melting point, respectively, but their predictive properties are limited between these extremes. The radial distribution approach is only slightly less idealistic since molecules rarely bear even a resemblance to spheres, and packing will be highly dependent on shape. Furthermore, in liquid solutions, differences in molecular size and shape between solute and solvent result in less simple molecular arrangements from those described above.

III. INTERMOLECULAR FORCES

Intermolecular forces of attraction can be classified into coulombic
forces, van der Waals forces, hydrogen bonding, charge transfer
forces, coordination bonding, and metallic bonding. The first
three of these will be discussed below. Charge transfer forces and
coordination bonding will be considered later (Chapters 7 and 8)
with respect to their effects on solubility. Metallic bonding is outside the context of this text and will not be considered.

A. Coulombic Forces

Coulombic forces occur between ions in the solid state and in solutions of electrolytes in conducting solvents. Ionically bound compounds are mainly inorganic but also include salts of organic acids
and bases. Since the interaction is between intensely charged
species, the forces are very strong and are of the order of 400
to 800 kJ mol^{-1}.

B. Van der Waals Forces

Van der Waals forces are interactions between covalently bound
molecules. In the dry, gaseous state, hydrogen chloride is a typical nonelectrolyte. By contributing an electron each to the covalent
bond joining them, the hydrogen atom completes its 1s orbit and the
chlorine its 3p sextet, thereby assuming the configurations of helium
and argon, respectively. The electrons in the bond are not evenly
shared; there is an inductive displacement of electrons toward the
chlorine atom, which is more electron attracting than the hydrogen,
giving a partial negative charge to the chlorine and a partial positive charge to the hydrogen. The result of this is that hydrogen
chloride molecules will align themselves in an electric field, with
chlorine directed toward the anode and hydrogen toward the cathode.
They are therefore said to have a dipole moment. When hydrogen
chloride is dissolved in water, the process goes to completion and
the molecules dissociate into ions.

The dipole moment (μ) of a diatomic molecule is the product of
the charge involved multiplied by the distance separating the two
poles. Dipole moments have traditionally been measured in debye
units (D). The SI unit is the coulomb meter. 1 debye = 10^{-18}
electrostatic unit centimeter (esu cm) = 3.336×10^{-30} coulomb
meter (C m).

The dipole moments of molecules which are more complex than
hydrogen chloride are the vector sum of all the bonds and are a
function of the symmetries of the molecules. Thus for the isomeric
dichlorobenzenes the dipole moments are ortho = 8.3, meta = 5.7.

and para = 0, × 10^{-30}Cm. The zero dipole moment of the para
isomer is a result of the individual dipole moments canceling out.
Other examples are carbon tetrachloride and carbon disulfide. Water
has a finite dipole moment because the atoms are not arranged in a
straight line.

Van der Waals forces result from the attraction between the pole
of one dipole and the oppositely charged pole of another. In contrast to ionic interactions, only partial charges are involved, so the
attraction is weaker, varying from 4 to 40 kJ mol^{-1}. They are
classified according to the nature of the dipoles involved.

1. Dipole-Dipole Interaction. Dipole-dipole interaction (Keesom
force) takes place between permanent dipoles. The energy (ΔU) of
two dipoles of moment μ_1 and μ_2, positioned in the most favorable
orientation, depends on the magnitude of the dipole moment. For
strong dipoles at low temperatures, where $\mu_1\mu_2/r^3 >> kT$,

$$\Delta U = - \frac{2\mu_1\mu_2}{r^3} \tag{2.11}$$

k is the Boltzmann constant and r the distance of separation. When
$\mu_1\mu_2/r^3 << kT$,

$$\Delta U = - \frac{2\mu_1^2\mu_2^2}{3r^6} \tag{2.12}$$

2. Dipole-Induced Dipole Interaction. Dipole-induced dipole
interaction (Debye force) occurs between a dipole and an apparently
nonpolar molecule. If a nonpolar molecule, for example Cl_2, is placed
in an electrical field, the electrons in the covalent bond will be attracted toward the anode. The other end of the molecule will be depleted in electrons and develops a partial positive charge, with the
result that a dipole moment is induced on the otherwise nonpolar
molecule. This is called an induced dipole moment, in contrast to
the permanent dipole moment of molecules such as hydrogen chloride.
The effect can also result from the electric field produced by a
neighboring polar molecule. Thus in the chlorination of phenol, a
dipole is induced on the chlorine molecule in aqueous solution by the
electron density of the ortho and para positions of the phenol, giving
the chlorine the necessary electrophilic power to chlorinate the phenol. The ease with which polarization occurs is expressed as the
polarizability (α) and the energy of a pair of polarizable polar molecules A and B given by

$$\Delta U = - \frac{\alpha_A \mu_B^2 + \alpha_B \mu_A^2}{r^6} \qquad (2.13)$$

Therefore, if A has a permanent dipole and B is the induced dipole, the energy of interaction will be given by

$$\Delta U = - \frac{\alpha_B \mu_A^2}{r^6} \qquad (2.14)$$

3.   Intermolecular Attraction Between Nonpolar Molecules (London Forces).   London suggested that the nuclei and electrons in every molecule are in a state of continuous oscillation and attributed the attraction between nonpolar molecules to electrostatic forces between the oscillating dipoles and those induced by them on neighboring molecules.   London derived the following approximate equation for the energy of two such molecules:

$$\Delta U = - \frac{3\alpha_A \alpha_B}{2r^6} \frac{I_A I_B}{I_A + I_B} \qquad (2.15)$$

I is the ionization potential, the energy required to remove the relevant electron from the ground state of the atom to which it belongs. For two identical molecules, Eqs. (2.13) to (2.15) simplify to

$$\Delta U = \frac{-k}{r^6} \qquad (2.16)$$

where k is a constant.   Equation (2.16) is only an approximation and applies to molecules separated by a distance that is considerably greater than the molecule diameter.

When molecules approach very closely, repulsive forces set in rapidly, and the magnitude has been suggested as a high-powered inverse function of the distance of separation (i.e., $\Delta U = j/r^n$). j and n are constants.   This expression can be combined with Eq. (2.16), giving

$$\Delta U = \frac{j}{r^{12}} - \frac{k}{r^6} \qquad (2.17)$$

n has been given the value of 12 for convenience.   Scrutiny of Fig. 2.2 shows that the repulsion increases so steeply that the arbitrary choice of n = 12 would not be expected to give rise to a major error. The Lennard-Jones equation,

$$\Delta U = 4U_{min} \left[\left(\frac{\sigma}{r} \right)^{12} - \left(\frac{\sigma}{r} \right)^{6} \right] \tag{2.18}$$

expresses this in a more precise form. U_{min} is the minimum potential energy and σ the distance of separation when ΔU is zero. These are indicated on Fig. 2.2.

Attraction between polyatomic molecules occurs mainly between adjacent surfaces, so that the outer atoms provide the bulk of the attractive energy. The falloff of London forces with the sixth power of distance indicates that the contribution of the more remote atoms will be very small. It is probable that with polyatomic molecules the attractive energy falls off more steeply than the sixth power of distance.

C. The Hydrogen Bond

The hydrogen bood occurs between certain electronegative atoms and a hydrogen atom whose 1s orbit is already completed by covalent link with another atom. The hydrogen nucleus, because it is small, bears an intense positive charge and is capable of attracting a second electronegative atom toward it while already covalently linked. The ion HF_2^- is a typical example. The stability of the bond is attributed to resonance between the canonical forms.

$$F^- \cdots H\text{-}F \leftrightarrow F^-H^+F^- \leftrightarrow F\text{-}H \cdots F^-$$

Hydrogen bonds occur between hydrogen and oxygen, nitrogen, or fluorine. Other elements are either too electropositive or too large to approach sufficiently closely to the hydrogen atom. Hydrogen bonds have energies ranging from 10 to 30 kJ mol^{-1}.

A hydrogen bond can be intramolecular, as in salicylic acid (Fig. 2.7a); intermolecular between molecules of the same species, as with water (Fig. 2.7b), carboxylic acids (Fig. 2.7c), and alcohols and phenols (Fig. 2.7d); or intermolecular between different molecules, such as chloroform and acetone (Fig. 2.7e). Hydrogen bonding between solute and solvent usually has a greater influence than dipole moment on solubility, and solute molecules that associate by hydrogen bonding are less soluble in nonpolar solvents than their dipole moments suggest. For this reason, groups that are capable of forming hydrogen bonds are frequently classified as polar, even though they may not have a very great influence on the dipole moment of the parent molecule.

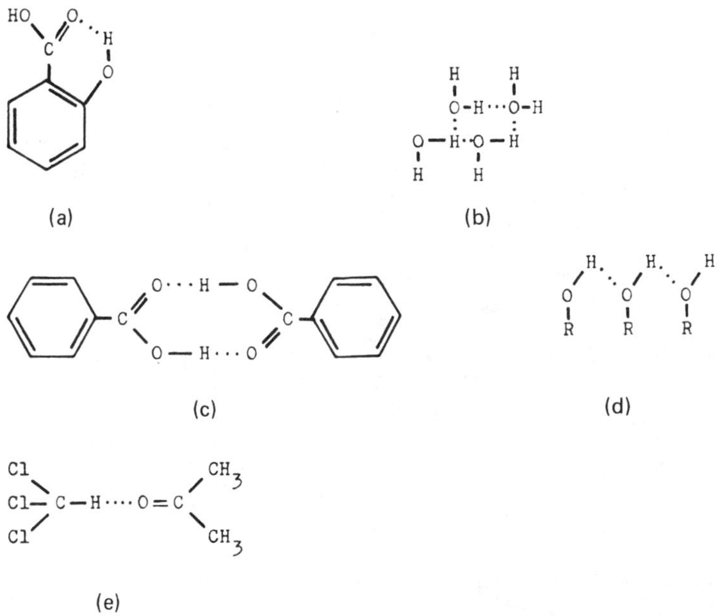

(a)

(b)

(c)

(d)

(e)

FIGURE 2.7 Examples of hydrogen bonds: (a) intramolecular bond
in salicylic acid; (b) intermolecular bonds in water; (c) benzoic acid
dimer; (d) intermolecular bonds between alcohols and phenols; (e)
intermolecular bond between chloroform and acetone.

IV. DIELECTRIC CONSTANT

The dielectric constant is a physical property that is influenced by
interatomic and intermolecular attractions, and is a useful property
with which to classify solvents. The dielectric constant (ε) of a
substance is a measure of its efficiency as an insulator in an electrical condenser. A simple condenser consists of two parallel plates
separated by an insulating medium. The number of coulombs of
electricity (q) the condenser will store is inversely proportional
to the potential difference in volts (v), applied across the plates.
These properties are related by

$$C = qv \qquad (2.19)$$

C is the capacitance of the condenser, which varies with the nature
of the insulator between the plates. Dielectric constant of a fluid x
is the ratio of the capacitance of the condenser when x is the insulator (C_x) to the capacitance when the insulator is a vacuum (C_0), as
given by

$$\varepsilon = \frac{C_x}{C_o} \tag{2.20}$$

The dipole moment of a polar molecule is related to its dielectric constant by the Clausius-Mossotti equation, which is represented by the first two expressions in

$$[P] = \frac{\varepsilon - 1}{\varepsilon + 2}\frac{M}{\rho} = \frac{4}{3}\pi N\alpha + \frac{4}{3}\pi N\frac{\mu^2}{3kT} \tag{2.21}$$

[P] is the molar polarization and is made up of two components, the induced polarization P_i, which is equal to the third term in Eq. (2.21), and the orientation polarization P_o, which is equal to the fourth. A plot of $(\varepsilon - 1)/(\varepsilon + 2)$ against $1/T$ should therefore be rectilinear, so that μ can be evaluated from the slope and α from the intercept. Nonpolar molecules have no permanent dipole moment, so that for these, [P] in Eq. (2.21) is equal to P_i.

Because dielectric constant is a function of permanent and induced dipole moments, together with molecular weight (M) and density (ρ), dielectric constants are not directly related to dipole moment. It can be said, however, that molecules with high dipole moments usually have high dielectric constants, and vice versa. Some examples are shown in Table 3.11.

V. BULK PROPERTIES OF LIQUIDS

Liquids can be classified according to their bulk properties, as: simple fluids (atomic or molecular fluids), inert fluids, and aprotic or protic fluids.

A. Simple Fluids

Simple fluids are the most predictable of the liquid systems, hence the alternative name, *conformal fluids*. The constituent particles are small and symmetrical, and interactions are dependent only on dispersion forces. The particles can be considered as point sources, because they are small, and approximate to spheres, because they are symmetrical. Inert gases in the liquid state are the best examples of simple fluids. Most other examples are gases under normal conditions. The inert gases are *atomic fluids*; the remaining simple fluids are termed *molecular fluids*, so called because they contain at least one covalent bond per molecule. Examples of molecular fluids are methane and sulfur dioxide.

Conformal fluids comply with the empirical relationship

$$\frac{P_c V_c}{T_c} = 0.29R \qquad (2.22)$$

a result that is smaller than the 0.375R predicted by van der Waals equation (2.1). Three peaks can usually be recognized in the radial distribution plot, obtained from refraction measurements, the second and third peaks occurring at around 1.9 and 2.8 times the spacing of the first. The number of nearest neighbors approaches closest packing with decreasing temperature and increasing density. Thus, for example, for xenon, at around 100 K and 0.3 cc g^{-1}, the number is 9 to 10 [8]. Simple fluids conform closely with Trouton's rule. This is an empirically derived generalization which states that the molar enthalpy of vaporization of a fluid, divided by its boiling point, is approximately equal to 21 cal mol^{-1} deg^{-1} (87.9 J mol^{-1} deg^{-1}). This term is equivalent to the entropy of vaporization (ΔS^V), which by inference is a constant, independent of the nature of the fluid.

B. Inert Fluids

Liquids with nonspherical, nonpolar molecules, which interact with other molecules through disperson forces, are classified as inert solvents. The name is given because they are chemically unreactive and consequently are also poor solvents. This group consists almost entirely of hydrocarbons or their halogenated derivatives, and as with conformal fluids, intermolecular attraction comes solely from disperson forces. They differ in having molecules that are too large to act as point sources. Carbon tetrachloride and neopentane (2,2-dimethylpropane) are symmetrical and approximately spherical, but most inert fluid molecules are elongated, for example the liquid *n*-paraffins, or laminar, for example benzene. They give values of $P_c V_c / T_c$ around 0.26R, close to the conformal value, and obey Trouton's rule with reasonable accuracy.

The difference from simple fluids arises from molecular size, so that interactions are between adjacent parts of neighboring molecules rather than between whole molecules. A consequence is that cohesive energies are low. There is little information on intermolecular structure, but benzene and carbon tetrachloride are known to approximate to closest packing [9,10].

C. Aprotic and Protic Fluids

Liquids with significant dipole moments can be subdivided into protic and aprotic fluids. Protic fluids contain at least one proton per

TABLE 2.2 Bulk Properties of Some Gases and Liquids

	Neon, Ne	Nitrogen, N_2	Methane, CH_4	n-Hexane, C_6H_{14}	Benzene, C_6H_6
Melting point, T_m (K)	24.0	63.1	90.7	177.8	278.7
Boiling point, T_b (K)	27.0	77.3	111.7	341.9	353.3
Critical temperature, T_c (K)	44.4	126.1	190.7	507.3	562.1
Critical pressure, P_c(MPa)	2.72	3.39	4.64	3.01	4.90
Critical volume (m^3 mol^{-1} × 10^6)	41.7	90	99	370	259
$P_c V_c / T_c R$	0.31	0.29	0.29	0.26	0.27
Trouton's constant, ΔS^V (JK^{-1} mol^{-1})	64.0	72.3	73.2	84.4	87.0
Dipole moment, μ (C m × 10^{30})	0	0	0	0	0
Dielectric constant (ε)* at 298 K, remainder at 293 K	–	–	–	1.88	2.28
Acceptor number, AN	–	–	–	–	–
Donor number, DN	–	–	–	–	–

Chloroform, $CHCl_3$	Diethyl ether, $C_2H_5OC_2H_5$	Nitro-benzene $C_6H_5NO_2$	Ethanol, C_2H_5OH	Acetic acid, CH_3COOH	Water, H_2O
209.6	156.9	278.9	159.1	289.8	273.2
334.3	307.7	484.0	351.4	391.1	373.2
536.6	466.7	732.0	516.3	594.5	647.4
5.47	3.64	—	6.38	5.78	22.1
239	280	—	167	171	55.2
0.29	0.26	—	0.25	0.20	0.23
104.0	89.3	146.2	144.3	164.4	147.5
3.4	3.8	14.1	5.6	5.8	6.2
4.81	4.34	34.8*	24.6*	6.15*	80.1
23.1	3.9	14.8	37.1	52.9	54.8
—	19.2	4.4	—	—	18.0

molecule, bound to an electronegative atom. Compounds in this group usually enter into hydrogen bonds and will be considered separately. The description *aprotic* embraces the remaining polar molecules. They form a heterogeneous collection and for organic compounds are best described as those liquids not included in the other subgroups. They include esters, tertiary amines, nitro compounds, and partially halogenated hydrocarbons. The effect of polarity on intermolecular forces is not felt as strongly in high molecular weight compounds, where the dipole tends to be deeply embedded within the molecule. Despite their relatively high polarity, these liquids usually follow Trouton's rule reasonably well at the boiling point, although deviations occur when the temperature is reduced.

Aprotic solvents can be assigned donor numbers (DN) and acceptor numbers (AN). The acceptor number is a measure of the readiness to accept electrons and is assessed by NMR shift [11]. Phosphorus pentachloride is the standard acceptor, which is allocated the value of 100; for most aprotic fluids the number is less than 25, for example diethyl ether = 3.9, triethylamine = 1.2, and chloroform = 23.1. The donor number is the energy in $J \, mol^{-1}$ of the bond between the donor molecule and phosphorus pentachloride. Donor numbers are of the same order as acceptor numbers, for example diethyl ether = 19.2, acetone = 17.0, and dimethyl sulfoxide = 29.8. As a consequence of these donor/acceptor activities, aprotic fluids are useful solvents.

Protic fluids have the broadest solubility spectrum of all the fluid groups. They include alcohols, amines, and carboxylic acids, and because they are associated, usually give high Trouton's constants. Dielectric constants are also high. The tendency to hydrogen-bond leads to high donor and acceptor numbers, indicating a readiness to solvate. Hydrogen bonding works against solution of nonpolar solutes, however, due to solvent-solvent association.

Molecular and bulk properties of a selection of liquids are presented in Table 2.2. More comprehensive lists have been published by Marcus [12].

D. Electrostatic Factor

Dack [13] has classified solvents according to their electrostatic factors (EFs), which are the products of dipole moment (in debye units) and dielectric constant. Solvents fall into four groups, as follows:

1. Hydrocarbons: EF = 0 to 2
2. Electron donors: EF = 2 to 20
3. Hydroxylic solvents: EF = 15 to 50
4. Dipolar aprotic solvents: EF = 50+

VI. WATER

Water is considered alone because of its unique standing in our environment. A water molecule contains two hydrogen atoms, each
capable of accepting an electron, and one oxygen atom with a lone
pair of electrons, giving it a capability of forming hydrogen bonds
with two electron acceptor atoms. Water therefore has the capability
of forming a tetrahedral, hydrogen-bonded network, as shown in
Fig. 2.7. Comparison of the physical properties of water with those
of hydrogen sulfide provides evidence for such extensive hydrogen
bonding. The boiling point of hydrogen sulfide is 60°C lower than
that of water, even though their relative positions in the periodic
table suggest that water should be the more volatile compound. Although such structures are well established in ice, it would be il-
logical to assume a similar rigid network in a liquid. Present-day
thought considers that liquid water takes the form of flickering
clusters [14]. An irregularly structured network exists in the form
of "icebergs" suspended in a "sea" of individual water molecules,
and there is a continuous interchange of molecules between the icebergs and the sea. Diffraction measurements give radial distribution
peaks at 1.0 and 1.6 times the O-O spacing of ice at 277 K, with
4.4 nearest neighbors. The dielectric constant is high (80.4), but
it is accompanied by a rather low dipole moment (6.2×10^{-30} C m).
The acceptor number of water is among the highest encountered,
but its donor number is only 18. This low figure is probably misleading since because of its small molar volume, more than one water
molecule can be associated with a solute cation, thereby increasing
the electron density properties of the solvent.

VII. ASSESSMENT OF POLARITY FROM MOLECULAR
     STRUCTURE

Kier [15] has attempted to classify 36 liquids ranging in polarity
from cyclohexane to water, by comparing a series of physical properties related to polarity with first-order molecular connectivity, a
parameter that is assessed from the molecular structure of the molecule (Chap. 9). A good correlation between polarity and connectivity was claimed, and the procedure recommended because connectivity is easily calculated and does not require the availability of the
actual liquid.

VIII. SUPERCRITICAL FLUIDS

At the critical point, liquid and gas are in equilibrium, one form
merging into the other as the critical point is crossed. In the

region of the critical point, the gas completely fills the vessel it occupies, but because it is subjected to a high pressure, has a density similar to that of a liquid. In this form the gas is called a supercritical fluid and is capable of dissolving materials, usually in substantially greater quantities than in the normal liquid state. It is therefore possible to extract large quantities of a solute with a supercritical fluid and then induce the fluid to precipitate the solute by reducing the pressure or increasing the temperature. By manipulation of these two thermodynamic parameters, one is able to achieve separations by a process analogous to fractional distillation.

Extraction with supercritical fluids is useful for volatile and thermolabile solutes. The solvent is usually a substance that is gaseous at ambient temperatures. Particular success has been achieved with carbon dioxide, which has the added bonuses of being odorless, noncorrosive, nonflammable, and nontoxic. For further information the reader is referred to the following references [16—19].

REFERENCES

1. J. A. Beattie, The computation of the thermodynamic properties of real gases and mixtures of real gases, *Chem. Rev.*, *44*, 141—192 (1949).
2. M. L. McGlassan and D. J. B. Potter, An apparatus for the measurement of the second virial coefficients of vapours; the second virial coefficients of some *n*-alkanes and some mixtures of *n*-alkanes, *Proc. R. Soc. London*, *267A*, 478—500 (1962).
3. B. J. Alder and T. E. Wainright, Phase transition of a hard sphere system, *J. Chem. Phys.*, *27*, 1208—1209 (1957).
4. J. D. Bernal, A geometrical approach to the structure of liquids, *Nature*, *183*, 141—147 (1959).
5. J. D. Bernal, The structure of liquids, *Proc. R. Soc. London*, *280A*, 299—322 (1964).
6. N. Metropolis, A. W. Rosenbluth, M. N. Rosenbluth, A. H. Teller, and E. Teller, Equation of state calculations by fast computing machines, *J. Chem. Phys.*, *21*, 1087—1092 (1953).
7. B. J. Alder and T. E. Wainright, Studies in molecular dynamics: 1. General method, *J. Chem. Phys.*, *39*, 459—466 (1959).
8. J. A. Campbell and J. H. Hildebrand, The structure of liquid xenon, *J. Chem. Phys.*, *11*, 334—337 (1943).
9. A. H. Narten, M. D. Danford, and H. A. Levy, Structure and intermolecular potential of liquid carbon tetrachloride derived from X-ray diffraction data, *J. Chem. Phys.*, *46*, 4875—4880 (1967).
10. A. H. Narten, Diffraction pattern and structure of liquid benzene, *J. Chem. Phys.*, *48*, 1630—1634 (1968).

11. V. Guttmann, *Coordination Chemistry in Non-aqueous Solutions*, Springer-Verlag, Vienna, 1968, p. 19.

12. Y. Marcus, *Introduction to Liquid State Chemistry*, Wiley, New York, 1977.

13. M. R. J. Dack, The influence of solvent on chemical reactivity, in *Solutions and Solubilities*, Part II (M. R. J. Dack, ed.), *Techniques of Chemistry*, Vol. 8, Wiley, New York, 1976.

14. G. Nemethy and H. A. Scheraga, Structure of water and hydrophobic bonding in proteins: 1. A model for the thermodynamic properties of liquid water, *J. Chem. Phys.*, *36*, 3382–3400 (1962).

15. L. B. Kier, Quantitation of solvent polarity based on molecular structure, *J. Pharm. Sci.*, *70*, 930–933 (1981).

16. P. A. Peaden and M. L. Lee, Supercritical fluid chromatography: methods and principles, *J. Liq. Chromatogr.* 5 (Suppl. 2), 179–221 (1972).

17. W. Worthy, Supercritical fluids offer improved separations, *Chem. Eng. News*, *59*(31), 16–17 (1981).

18. M. Gitterman and I. Procaccia, Quantitative theory of solubility in supercritical fluids, *J. Chem. Phys. 78*, 2648–2654 (1983).

19. I. Procaccia and M. Gitterman, Supercritical extraction at atmospheric pressures, *J. Chem. Phys. 78*, 5275–5276 (1983).

3

A Qualitative Treatment
of Solubility

I. THE LIKE-DISSOLVES-LIKE CLASSIFICATION OF SOLUBILITIES

It is rarely possible to predict the extent to which a given solute will dissolve in a particular solvent, but one can anticipate from experience the type of solvent which will be most suitable for that solute. Further, we can frequently designate the approximate degree

of solubility, using vague terms such as "very soluble" or "sparingly soluble". The *British Pharmocopoeia* and *United States Pharmacopoeia* have attempted to rationalize the procedure by assigning
approximate solubilities to some such expressions, as follows:

Descriptive phrase	Approximate quantities of solvent by vol- for 1 part of solute by weight
Very soluble	Less than 1 part
Freely soluble	From 1 to 10 parts
Soluble	From 10 to 30 parts
Sparingly soluble	From 30 to 100 parts
Slightly soluble	From 100 to 1000 parts
Very slightly soluble	From 1000 to 10,000 parts
Practically insoluble	More than 10,000 parts

The instinctive selection of a solvent is usually based on the
principle "like dissolves like"; that is, a solute will dissolve in a
solvent having similar properties. The concept is frequently expressed in the form of two rules:

1. Polar solutes dissolve in polar solvents.
2. Nonpolar solutes dissolve in nonpolar solvents.

The term *polar* is used in an empirical manner which considers water
the most "polar" of the common solvents, and diethyl ether, carbon
tetrachloride, and fixed oils examples of "nonpolar" solvents.

The rules become confusing when one tries to define the terms
polar and *nonpolar* in a rigorous manner. The term *polar* has electrostatic origins. A polar molecule is one having a dipole moment,
which results from the properties, position, and number of its substituent groups. Electron-withdrawing groups such as nitro or chloro,
and electron-donating groups such as hydroxy- or methoxy, have a
marked influence on the dipole moments of the molecules to which they
are attached and are therefore polar groups. An electron-donating
group balanced against an electron-withdrawing group will create a
dipole moment in the parent molecule. Two groups which are both
electron withdrawing or both electron attracting will bring about a
similar, but smaller effect, provided that the degree of electronic
influence is different. Even identical groups can induce a dipole
moment, provided that they do not exert their influence in exactly

opposite directions; for example, *o*- and *m*-dichlorobenzenes have finite dipole moments, but the para isomer does not. Similarly, carbon disulfide and carbon tetrachloride have zero dipole moments. Hydrocarbons also have zero or low dipole moments, due to a combination of symmetry and the low influence of the C-H bond on dipole moment.

Polarity, so defined, is loosely related to solubility, since nonpolar solutes do dissolve in nonpolar solvents, and solutes with ionizable groups, and therefore with infinite dipole moments, dissolve in conducting solvents. Similarly, solutes tend to dissolve in solvents with similar dipole moments. However, when hydrogen-bonding groups are considered, the concept is stretched outside the limits defined by electrostatic considerations.

The terms *polar* and *nonpolar*, as used in the like-dissolves-like rules quoted above, are dependent on the number, properties, and position of substituent groups in the molecules, but the polarities of these groups have been judged not on their contributions to dipole moments, but on their influence on the solubilities of the molecules to which they may be attached. In other words, if the presence of a given group was known to promote solubility in water, it was considered to be a polar group, irrespective of the fact that it may contribute little to dipole moment. Confusion arose because hydrogen bonding, which is usually of greater importance to solubility than polarity, was not considered, and because hydrogen-bonding groups were designated polar on the basis of their contribution to aqueous solubility. Ambiguities invariably result, for example in terms of solubility, amino was said to be more "polar" than nitro, because aniline is three times more soluble in water than nitrobenzene. In contrast, the electrostatic "polarities" are reversed, aniline has a dipole moment of 5.1×10^{-30} C m and that of nitrobenzene is 14.1×10^{-30}.

An infinite dipole moment results when the bond joining the two polar groups breaks heterogeneously, giving two oppositely charged ions. This of course constitutes an electrolyte. Electrolytes dissolve in conducting solvents because there is a strong electrostatic interaction between the solute ions and the ions and dipoles of the solvent.

The term *polar* is best avoided when speaking of substituent groups in the context of their influence on solubility. A better procedure follows the terminology of surface chemistry and classifies groups as hydrophilic and hydrophobic, according to the way in which they affect solubility. Some common groups are arranged in this manner in Table 3.1. The vertical columns fall naturally into the four groups of a more comprehensive "like dissolves like" classification as follows:

TABLE 3.1 Classification of Substituent Groups[a]

Conducting (a)	Hydrophilic (b)	Weakly hydrophobic (c)	Strongly hydrophobic (d)
–O'	–OH	–NO$_2$	Various alkyl groups
–COO'	–COOH	–Cl	
–SO$_3'$	–NH$_2$	–Br	
–NH$_3{}^+$	–F	–(CH$_2$)$_3$O–	
Other charged amine groups	C=O		
	–CH$_2$CH$_2$O–		

[a]Like-dissolves-like classification.

1. Electrolytes dissolve in conducting solvents.
2. Solutes containing hydrogen capable of forming hydrogen bonds dissolve in solvents capable of accepting hydrogen bonds, and vice versa.
3. Solutes with significant dipole moments dissolve in solvents having significant dipole moments.
4. Solutes with low or zero dipole moments dissolve in solvents with low or zero dipole moments.

Overlap occurs between groups, for example water, which ionizes and therefore belongs to group 1, is capable of forming hydrogen bonds, and so also belongs to group 2. Similarly, chloroform, which belongs to group 3 because it has a significant dipole moment, also belongs to group 2 because its hydrogen atom is capable of hydrogen bonding with electron donors.

Fundamentally the "like dissolves like" generalization depends on the relative values of the intermoleuclar pair potential energies (U) of solute and solvent. These can be expressed in an elementary way in terms of the "attraction" between the different types of molecule in the solution, if the solvent is A and the solute B, and the three possible types of attraction are represented by A-A, B-B, and A-B, one of three conditions will arise.

1. If A-A >> A-B, that is, the affinity of a molecule of solvent for its own kind is markedly greater than its affinity for a solute molecule. The solvent molecules will be attracted to each other and form a loose aggregation from which the solute is excluded.

2. If B-B >> A-B, the solvent will not be able to break the bonds between the solute molecules in order to disperse them.
3. If A-B > A-A and B-B or is of the same order, the solute will be dispersed to form a solution.

Classification into groups of solute-solvent combinations goes only part way toward providing a comprehensive scheme for qualitatively assessing solubilities. The procedure is adaptable to simple molecules, but increasing molecular weight is accompanied by increasing complexity, involving combinations of groups with differing hydrophobic and hydrophilic influences. Furthermore, specific solutes and solvents have their own exceptions to general rules. Solubility will therefore be considered in a complementary manner, by considering chemical groups of solutes and solvents, fitting them into the like-dissolves-like classification, and examining their individual peculiarities. When the terms *soluble* and *insoluble* are used without reservation, they are employed in a completely subjective manner, the criterion being whether or not a solution of usable concentration is possible at ambient temperature.

A. Conducting Solvents

Since other conducting solvents are of limited use, water will be the only solvent considered in this section. Carboxy acids, which are also conducting solvents, will be mentioned briefly later. Water ionizes according to

$$nH_2O \rightleftharpoons (H_2O)_{n-1}H^+ + OH^-$$ (3.1)

For convenience, n is usually placed equal to 2.

Electrolytes dissolve in water because there are strong interactions between the charges on the solute molecules and the ions and dipoles of water. Water is therefore the solvent of choice for inorganic salts, most of which are more soluble in water than in any other solvent. Similarly, salts of organic acids and bases are usually very soluble in water, because they are completely ionized in aqueous solution. The aqueous solubility of organic molecules is increased more by the possession of an ionizing group than by any other single group. The affinity of solute ions for the solvent is so great that even ions containing relatively large hydrophobic contributions are freely soluble. Phenobarbital (I), for example, is such a weak acid that it is almost completely nonionized and is therefore virtually insoluble in water (1 in 1000 at 20°C). At pH values above about 8.3, however, it becomes very soluble (1 in 3 at 20°C), because it is converted to its fully ionized anion, in accordance with

$$\begin{array}{c} \text{NH--CO} \quad C_2H_5 \\ / \qquad \backslash / \\ O=C \qquad \quad C \qquad + \text{ OH}^- \rightleftharpoons \\ \backslash \qquad / \backslash \\ \text{NH--CO} \quad C_6H_5 \end{array} \qquad \begin{array}{c} \text{NH--CO} \quad C_2H_5 \\ / \qquad \backslash / \\ O=C \qquad \quad C \qquad + \text{ H}_2O \qquad (3.2) \\ \backslash \qquad / \backslash \\ N=CO^- \quad C_6H_5 \end{array}$$

(I)

A hydrogen-bonding solvent, donor or acceptor, is necessary to dissolve the undissociated acid. Ethanol, diethyl ether, and chloroform are examples. In a similar way, atropine is soluble in 400 parts of water at 20°C, while its sulfate is soluble in 1 part of water at 20°C. Once again ethanol diethyl ether, or chloroform would be suitable solvents for the nonionized base.

Highly hydrophobic compounds can sometimes be made soluble in water by making a derivative with a dibasic acid, leaving one of the carboxyl groups free for ionization. Hydrocortisone, for example, is almost completely insoluble in water. Esterification of its 21-hydroxyl group with succinic acid produces the hemisuccinate (II),

Hydrocortisone Hemisuccinate

(II)

which is soluble in aqueous alkali and forms a sodium salt that is soluble in 3 parts of water at 20°C. This derivative provides a means of administering a corticosteroid by aqueous injection. Carbenoxolene (III), the disodium salt of the hemisuccinate of glycyrrhetic acid, is another example. The glycerrhetate anion is too large and hydrophobic to be rendered water soluble by only one carboxylate group, but the second ionizing group makes up the deficit, with the result that carbenoxolone is soluble in about 3 parts of water at ambient temperature.

Carbenoxolone

(III)

B. Water

1. Water as a Hydrogen-Bonding Solvent. Water is capable of extensive hydrogen bonding. Each molecule contains two hydrogen atoms which can accept electrons and form hydrogen bonds, and one oxygen atom capable of contributing electrons to two hydrogen bonds. There is therefore an exact balance between electron donors and electron acceptors, and as a result water is able to form a three-dimensional hydrogen-bonded lattice, as shown in Fig. 2.7. The precise conformation of the lattice changes continuously with time. This structure resists entry of potential solute molecules, as described in condition 1 above (A-A) >> (A-B). A water-soluble solute must therefore have a high affinity for water molecules and be able to fit into the three-dimensional network.

2. Water as a Solute. There is considerable evidence [1] which indicates that when water is dispersed in such nonpolar solvents as aliphatic and aromatic hydrocarbons, it exists almost exclusively as monomers. The result is that water is more soluble in these solvents than the solvents are in water. In more polar solvents, such as the partially halogenated hydrocarbons, water exists mainly as dimers and trimers, and the difference between the mutual solubilities narrows. This behavior is illustrated by the results in Table 3.2 [2].

C. Alcohols

1. Alcohols as Solutes. The hydroxyl group is strongly hydrophilic because it is similar to the water molecule, and its atoms are

TABLE 3.2 Mutual Solubilities of Water and Some Organic Solvents

| Solvent | Mole fraction solubility (X_2) | | |
	In water	Water in	Ratio
Cyclohexane	1.18×10^{-5}	4.67×10^{-4}	39
n-Hexane	1.98×10^{-6}	5.32×10^{-4}	269
Benzene	4.12×10^{-4}	2.73×10^{-3}	6.6
Toluene	1.01×10^{-4}	1.71×10^{-3}	17
Carbon tetrachloride	9.01×10^{-5}	8.56×10^{-4}	9.5
Chloroform	1.24×10^{-3}	4.76×10^{-3}	4.0
1,2-Dichloroethane	1.48×10^{-3}	8.16×10^{-3}	5.5
Diethyl ether	1.54×10^{-2}	5.79×10^{-2}	3.8

accepted into hydrogen bonds by water molecules as readily as aqueous hydrogen and oxygen. It is the group attached to hydroxyl that limits aqueous solubility. If a monohydric alcohol has a low molecular weight, it will dissolve in water, its hydroxyl group forming part of the three-dimensional network of water molecules, and its alkyl group, because it is small, fitting into the gaps. Thus methanol, ethanol, and propanol are all completely miscible with water. At butanol, the bulkiness of the alkyl group sets up a strain on the network, so that the aqueous solubility is diminished. Both 1- and 2-butanol are soluble in water at ambient temperature to the extent of only about 1 M.

As the homologous series of normal fatty alcohols is ascended further, the influence of the lipophilic nature of the alkyl group increases and the aqueous solubilities fall with increasing carbon number. The relationship between carbon number and solubility is approximately exponential, as shown in Table 3.3 Even when the aqueous solubility is negligible, the hydroxyl group continues to exert its influence. Molecules in excess of solubility then form an insoluble, unimolecular film, the hydroxyl groups forming part of the aqueous surface layer.

The hydrophobic influence of a large alkyl group can be compensated by additional hydroxyl groups. As an example, the solubility of glucose (IV) in water is about seven times that of cyclohexanol (V). Both are six-membered ring compounds and contain six carbon atoms, but glucose contains more hydroxyl groups. These interact with the water molecules, and the entire glucose

Glucose (IV)

Cyclohexanol (V)

molecule can be considered to slot into the hydrogen-bonded network like a piece into a jigsaw puzzle. The difference between the solubilities would be greater if glucose happened to be a liquid. This is a factor that has not been mentioned so far. Energy is needed to liquify a solid solute before it dissolves, with the consequence that solids tend to be less soluble than liquids. This generalization embraces all liquid solutions.

The influence of hydroxy groups on aqueous solubility is sometimes exploited when choosing an acid anion for the salt of a base. Quinidine (VIa), for example, is a large, basic, hydrophobic molecule, having a solubility of 1 in 2000 parts of water at 20°C.

TABLE 3.3 Solubilities of *n*-Fatty Alcohols in Water at Ambient Temperature

$$(C_nH_{2n+1}OH)$$

n	t (°C)	% w/w	mol liter^{-1}
4	25	7.35	0.99
5	25	2.21	0.25
6	25	0.57	0.056
7	25	0.181	0.016
8	25	0.0586	0.0045

(VIa) n = 1; X = zero   Quinidine

(VIb) n = 2; X = $H_2SO_4 \cdot 2H_2O$ Quinidine Sulfate

(VIc) n = 1;

Quinidine Gluconate

Conversion to a salt increases its aqueous solubility, because the positive charges on the quinidine cation have a strong affinity for water (electrolytes dissolve in conducting solvents). Thus the sulfate (VIb) is more soluble (1 in 80), a big improvement on the base, but still not very encouraging. A further increase is achieved by using gluconic acid to neutralize the base (VIc). The hydroxyl groups in the anion give an added affinity for water, and the salt is very soluble. Similarly, chlorhexidine acetate and hydrochloride have aqueous solubilities of 1 in 55 and 1700 at 20°C, respectively, while the gluconate has a solubility of more than 1 in 4.

An interesting variation of this principle concerns the solubilities of the *n*-alkyl sulfate detergents. Sodium lauryl sulfate (VIIa) has

$$C_{12}H_{23} \cdot OSO_3^- \; X^+$$

(VIIa) X = Na   Sodium Laurylsulfate

(VIIb) X - $H_3N \cdot CH_2CH_2OH$ Monoethanolamine Laurylsulfate

(VIIc) X = $H_2N(CH_2CH_2OH)_2$ Diethanolamine Laurylsulfate

(VIId) X = $HN(CH_2CH_2OH)_3$ Triethanolamine Laurylsulfate

only a moderate solubility in water, so that solutions of strength
suitable for shampoo formulations crystalize out at low temperatures.
In contrast, the ethanolamine salts (VIIb to VIId) enjoy higher solubility in water, and strong solutions do not separate on cooling.
This difference must be due to the presence of the hydroxyl groups
on the cation.

In some cases the presence of hydroxyl groups can work against
solution in water. Cellulose is a linear polymer of D-glucose residues, each bearing three hydroxyl groups. The polymer chains are
long, and the positions of the hydroxyl groups are such that there
is strong OH···OH hydrogen bonding between adjacent chains, with
the result that cellulose is a highly insoluble material, and as such,
forms the main skeletal tissue of most vegetable matter.

However, the hydroxyl groups are chemically reactive and can
be nitrated, for example, to give a derivative that is soluble in organic solvents. The enhanced solubility is attributed to a reduction
in the number of hydrogen bonds between the polymer chains. The
degree of substitution of the derivatives is indicated by the ds value,
the number of substituted hydroxyls per glucose residue. Thus
cellulose has a ds of zero, and a fully substituted derivative would
have a ds of 3. Solubility depends on the ds value; cellulose ace-
tates of ds 2 to 2.5, for example, are insoluble in water, but those
with ds values of 0.5 to 1.0 are soluble. Methylcellulose, sodium
carboxymethyl cellulose, and cellulose acetate are commonly used
water-soluble polymers of this type.

2. Alcohols as Solvents. The most popular solvents in this
group are methanol, ethanol, and isopropanol. Ethanol will be used
as an example and is typical of the other two. There are two principal ways, with respect to the process of solution, in which ethanol
differs from water. They influence the solvent properties of ethanol
in opposite ways; thus:

1. Ethanol does not ionize, and its dielectric constant is significantly lower than that of water. It is therefore less
   able to break up aggregations of solute molecules in order
   to disperse them.
2. Ethanol molecules contain only two atoms capable of hydrogen
   bonding. Ethanol therefore associates in the form of chains
   rather than a network, and is more readily infiltrated by
   other molecules.

The result of this combination of properties is that ethanol is a
good solvent for organic liquids and solids capable of donating electrons to or accepting electrons from hydrogen bonds, provided that
the solute-solute intermolecular forces of attraction are not too strong.

It is capable of dissolving molecules whose moderate lipophilic contents give them low solubilities in water; for example, benzyl alcohol, chloramphenicol, and camphor are not soluble in water to any great extent but are readily soluble in ethanol. It is a poor solvent for more lipophilic molecules, such as aromatic and higher aliphatic hydrocarbons, although good solubility in alcohols usually results when molecular weights are similar; for example, n-octane and n-octanol are miscible in all proportions. Similarly, fats and fixed oils have negligible solubility in ethanol, although castor oil, whose principal components are esters of ricininolic acid, which contains a hydroxyl group, is soluble in ethanol but not in solvents, such as chloroform and carbon tetrachloride, normally used for glycerides. Volatile oils are normally readily soluble in ethanol.

Undissociated weak electrolytes are soluble in ethanol provided that the lipophilic influence in the solute molecule is not too great. Phenols, aromatic acids and amines, and most alkaloids, for example, enjoy good solubility in ethanol.

Since hydrogen bonding is the principal factor involved in the solution of carbohydrates in water, it seems surprising that alcohols are poor solvents for these compounds. The reason is given in condition 2 above, namely that B-B >> A-B. The abundance of hydroxyl groups, and their ability to hydrogen bond, build up strong forces of attraction between carbohydrate molecules, resulting in relatively hard crystaline solids, more in keeping with an electrolyte than with an electrically neutral molecule. These forces are too great to be broken by organic solvents; water, however, has a sufficiently high dipole moment to do so. Inorganic salts are insoluble in ethanol for the same reason.

Polyols, in particular glycerol and propylene glycol, are useful solvents for hydrogen-bonding solutes. They find use as cosolvents for bringing hydrophilic solutes into lipid solutions [3] or for bringing water-insoluble solutes into aqueous solution [4]. In this respect, solid polyalcohols, such as sorbitol, are useful cosolvents in aqueous systems [4].

D. Carboxy Acids

1. Carboxy Acids as Solutes. Like the hydroxyl group, the carboxy group is capable of forming more than one hydrogen bond with water. The fatty acids therefore behave in a manner similar to the fatty alcohols. The first four members of the homologous series, formic (C_1) to n-butyric (C_4), are miscible with water in all proportions, valeric acid (C_5) has a finite aqueous solubility, and subsequent homologs show declining aqueous solubilities with increasing molecular weight. The higher fatty acids form insoluble films on water.

The carboxy acids differ from the alcohols in that their solubilities are pH dependent. Carboxy acids are weak electrolytes. At
neutral and low pH values they are largely undissociated, and their
aqueous solubilities are dependent on the hydrophilic properties of
the undissociated carboxy group. At high pH values, the carboxy
group ionizes and the mechanism of solution moves from a hydrogen-
bonding solute dissolving in a hydrogen-bonding solvent to an electrolyte dissolving in a conducting solvent. The enhanced effect on
aqueous solubility can be illustrated by reference to stearic acid
and its sodium salt. Stearic acid has negligible solubility in water,
but sodium stearate is universally known to be highly soluble. The
picture is not as simple as it seems, however; the *true* solubility of
sodium stearate in water is small, although not as small as that of
stearic acid. The "supersaturated" solutions are actually colloidal
dispersions of micelles, aggregates with the alkyl chains in the interior, protected from the water, and the carboxylate groups facing
outward. This behavior further illustrates the enhancement of hydrophilic properties by ionization. The surface activity of undissociated stearic acid is limited to formation of an insoluble film on water.

2. Carboxy Acids as Solvents. The lower fatty acids are useful
solvents. They are miscible with a wide range of liquids and can be
blended with aprotic solvents (see Section V.C in Chapter 2) to introduce a greater hydrogen-bonding component to the mixture. Formic and acetic acids are widely used in chromatography in this capacity. The lower fatty acids conduct electricity; acetic acid, for
example, ionizes as follows:

$$2CH_3COOH \rightleftharpoons CH_3COOH_2^+ + CH_3COO' \qquad (3.3)$$

and is used as a protogenic (proton-donating) solvent in nonaqueous
titrations. Bases tend to become indistinguishable in strength in
protogenic solvents, so that weak bases, such as pyridine and
adrenaline, can be titrated against perchloric acid, giving sharp
end points with acid-base indicators.

E. Phenols

Phenols share the properties of alcohols and carboxy acids. In organic solvents and neutral and low-pH aqueous solutions, they behave
in a similar manner to alcohols. Unlike the lower fatty alcohols, none
of the phenols is freely soluble in water, because all phenols are
attached to bulky, hydrophobic aromatic groups, and also because
phenols are solids at ambient temperatures. Phenolic hydroxyl is
mildly hydrophilic, of the same order as alcoholic hydroxyl. Phenols

ionize at high pH values, and the affinity of the phenoxy ion for water is such that phenols of moderately high molecular weight are soluble in strongly alkaline aqueous solutions.

The aqueous solubilities of polyols are seen to increase roughly with the number of hydroxyl groups. The situation is not as simple with polyphenols. The aqueous solubilities of a selection of phenols are shown in Table 3.4 and indicate that the positions of substitution are a critical factor. No simple relationships can be detected, and the overall pattern must be dependent on a combination of factors, such as melting point, mesomerism, and intramolecular hydrogen bonding.

F. Ethers

1. Ethers as Solutes. Ethers contain an oxygen atom bearing two pairs of unshared electrons. They are therefore capable of hydrogen bonding with solvents containing hydrogen atoms which are able to accept electrons, in particular, with the hydrogen atoms of water. This affinity of the oxygen atom for water is opposed by the hydrophobic forces operating in alkyl groups attached to the oxygen. The influence of the ether group on aqueous solubility is not quite counterbalanced by two methylene groups, so that the oxyethylene group (CH_2CH_2O) has a small residual affinity for water. Polyethylene glycols, having the general formula $CH_2(OH)[CH_2CH_2O]_n$ CH_2OH, are made by condensation of ethylene oxide and water under controlled conditions. Viscous liquids, unctious semisolids, and waxy

TABLE 3.4 Aqueous Solubilities of Some Phenols

Compound	Solubility (% w/w at 20°)	Melting point (°C)
Phenol	8.2	42
1,2-Benzenediol (catechol)	31.1	104
1,3-Benzenediol (resorcinol)	63.7	118
1,4-Benzenediol (quinol)	6.7	169
1,2,3-Benzenetriol (pyrogallol)	38.5	133
1,3,5-Benzenetriol (phloroglucinol)	1.1	218

solids are obtained depending on the value of n, producing materials with rheological properties characteristic of lipids, but highly soluble in water. They therefore provide useful topical bases when hydrophilic properties are required.

Wool fat or lanolin is a lipid material obtained from the wool of the sheep and consists mainly of fatty acid esters of cholesterol and other high molecular weight alcohols. The free alcohols are obtained by saponification of wool fat and are collectively known as wool alcohols. Monographs describing wool alcohols appear in most pharmacopoeias; their chemistry has been reviewed by Motiuk [5]. Although the wool alcohols are highly lipophilic and have negligible solubility in water, they can be made soluble by condensation of polyethylene oxide chains to the hydroxyl groups. Numberous products that depend on this principle are available commercially. McCarthy and Schlossman [6] have described the effects of ethyloxylation on the physical properties of wool alcohols.

A third methylene group attached to ether oxygen is sufficient to change the balance from one that favors water to one that is opposed to water. Consequently, the aqueous solubilities of polypropylene polymers decrease with increasing molecular weight. The poloxalkols are copolymers of ethylene oxide and propylene oxide, having the general formula

$$HO(CH_2CH_2O)_a(CH_2CH_2CH_2O)_b(CH_2CH_2O)_cH$$

have solubilities dependent on the balance between the hydrophilic nature of ethoxy and the hydrophobic nature of propoxy (i.e., the values of a and b) and range from very soluble to almost completely insoluble in water.

The solubilities of ethers are influenced by the configuration of the bonds attached to the oxygen atom. Diethyl ether is soluble in about 10 parts of water at 20°C, but tetrahydrofuran (VIII), which contains the same number of carbon and oxygen atoms, is miscible

$$\begin{array}{ccc} CH_2 & \!\!\!\!—\!\!\!\! & CH_2 \\ | & & | \\ CH_2 & & CH_2 \\ & \diagdown \; \diagup & \\ & O & \end{array}$$

Tetrahydrofuran (VIII)

in all proportions with water. The reason is probably steric, associated with the exposure of the unshared electrons on the oxygen atom, resulting from the fixed position of the two covalent bonds attached to the oxygen. Dioxane (IX) is a similar molecule and is

```
              O
            /   \
    CH 2       CH 2
      |          |
    CH 2       CH 2
        \      /
           O
```

Dioxane (IX)

also completely miscible with water. However, furan (X) is only soluble in 100 parts of water, probably because the molecule is aromatic, and the unshared electrons form part of the resonating system.

```
    CH —— CH
    ‖        ‖
    CH      CH
      \    /
        O
```

Furan (X)

2.   Ethers as Solvents.   Ethers particularly diethyl ether, are useful solvents and have a solubility spectrum similar to that of the alcohols but biased toward more lipophilic solutes.   Ethers are capable only of donating electrons to hydrogen bonds, so their usefulness is limited with solutes that are exclusively electron donors, for example, carbonyl compounds.   Diethyl ether enjoys the two advantages that it is only slightly miscible with water and that it is volatile.   It is therefore a useful solvent for extracting solutes from aqueous solutions.

G.   Sulfur-Containing Compounds

Sulfur occurs farther down the periodic table from oxygen.   Sulfur is therefore a more electropositive element and its unshared electrons less attracted to water than oxygen.   This factor becomes evident when the solubilities of sulfur and oxygen compounds are compared; thus ethyl mercaptan (C_2H_5SH) is almost insoluble in water, while ethanol is completely miscible with water.   Similarly, thiourea

(NH_2CS NH_2) is soluble in 11 parts of water, whereas urea
(NH_2CO NH_2) requires only 1 part of water in which to dissolve.
A second consequence of the position of sulfur in the periodic
table is that the sulfhydryl group (SH) is more acidic than hydroxyl. Mercaptans are therefore soluble in aqueous alkali.

It has already been mentioned that a bulky hydrophobic molecule containing a hydroxyl group can be converted into a water-
soluble derivative by condensation with a polybasic acid and neu-
tralization of the remaining acid hydrogens to give an alkali metal
salt. There are numerous examples of drugs that have been treated
in this way, but sulfuric acid does not seem to have been a popular choice of polybasic acid in this respect. However, it is used
extensively as a hydrophilic group in surfactant molecules. The
sodium alkyl sulfates are the best known examples. The ionized
sulfate group is capable of bringing long alkyl chains into solution.

As a charged species, the sulfonate ion has a powerful poten-
tiating effect on aqueous solubility. The hydrophilic properties
of the sulfonate group have been exploited in the development of
dyestuffs. Apparent aqueous solubilities of a selection of azo dyes
are given in Table 3.5 [7,8]. If we assume that the unsubstituted
compounds are completely insoluble in water and that the hydroxyl
group has a negligible effect on their aqueous solubilities in comparison with the sulfonate group, the data indicate that each sodium sulfonate is capable of bringing the equivalent of three benzene rings into solution in cold water. This generalization is followed by many azo dyes.

The examples quoted for sulfates and sulfonates all represent
a powerful hydrophilic group balanced against a large hydrophobic
unit. In such cases the molecules are invariably surface active, and

TABLE 3.5 Aqueous Solubilities of Some Azo Dyes

Dye	Substituents		Apparent aqueous solubility
Orange II	(XI)	$4'\text{-}SO_3Na$	Soluble in cold water
Fast Red A (roccelline)	(XII)	$4'\text{-}SO_3Na$	Soluble in hot water
Fast Red B (Bordeax B)	(XII)	$3,6\text{-}(SO_3Na)_2$	Soluble in cold water
Amaranth	(XII)	$3,4',6\text{-}(SO_3Na)_3$	1 in 15 of cold water
Sunset yellow	(XI)	$4',6\text{-}(SO_3Na)_2$	1 in 5 of cold water

(XI)

(XII)

the so-called solutions are actually colloidal dispersions of micelles. For this reason, the figures quoted in Table 3.5 are described as *apparent* aqueous solubilities.

Because sulfonic acids are strong acids, the undissociated SO_3H group also exerts a significant hydrophilic influence, although not as strong as that of the sodium salt. Thus benzenesulfonic acid is very soluble in water, whereas benzoic acid has a solubility of only 1 in 350 parts of water. Sulfonates are also much less sensitive to pH changes than are the salts of carboxylic acids. Sodium sulfonates usually require mineral acid to precipitate the free acid.

H. Nitrogen-Containing Compounds

Amine groups are capable of accepting electrons to form hydrogen bonds and are therefore hydrophilic in nature. The lower aliphatic amines, like the corresponding alcohols and carboxy acids, are completely miscible with water, but as the homologous series is ascended solubility falls, because of the increasing influence of the hydrophobic alkyl group. Thus the aliphatic amines up to pentylamine are miscible with water. Secondary and tertiary amines behave similarly; diethylamine and triethylamine are completely miscible with water, but higher homologs are not. The uncharged nitrogen atom therefore appears to be capable of taking five to six methylene groups into aqueous solution. Cyclic amines containing five or six ring atoms, except pyrrole, are also miscible with water. Like phenolic OH, the primary amine group confers only limited aqueous solubility on aromatic amines; aniline, for example, is soluble in 29 parts of cold water.

An amine is capable of accepting a proton to become a positively charged ion. The charged nitrogen atom is highly hydrophilic and

TABLE 3.6 Solubilities of Some Amines, Sulfacetamide, and Their
Salts in Water

Salt	Empirical formula of ion	Aqueous solubility[a] (%)	
		Salt	Nonionized form
Cocaine hydrochloride	$C_{17}H_{22}O_4N^+$	71 (25)	0.17 (25)
Procaine hydrochloride	$C_{13}H_{21}NO_2N^+$	50 (20)	0.33 (20)
Strychnine hydrochloride	$C_{21}H_{23}NO_2N^+$	29 (15)	0.01 (20)
Sulfacetamide sodium	$C_8H_9NO_3SN^-$	67 (20)	0.67 (20)

[a]Numbers in parentheses represent the temperatures (°C) at which
solubilities were determined.

capable of taking large hydrophobic groups into aqueous solution.
Some examples are given in Table 3.6. Secondary and tertiary
amines behave in the same way, but all three are weak bases, so
that the free base is precipitated from an aqueous amine salt solution if the pH is allowed to rise too far. The critical value varies
with the nature of the base; it is usually between pH 7 and 9 but
can be less than 7. Most amine drugs, in particular alkaloids,
antihistamines, and local anesthetics, are administered as salts because of the enhanced aqueous solubility brought about by protona-
tion of the nitrogen atom.

Quaternary amines are strong bases and their ionization is sensitive only to highly alkaline media. The quaternary amine group
is strongly hydrophilic and is responsible for the aqueous solubility
of most cationic surfactants.

The amide group has a lesser hydrophilic influence and is roughly equivalent to that of the nonionized carboxy acid group. Benzoic acid and benzamide, for example, have similar aqueous solubilities.
These and other examples are shown in Table 3.7.

The nitrogen of the amide group bears a residual negative charge,
but the charge is usually too small to form salts. In the sulfonamides,
however, it is sufficiently large to form an electrovalent linkage with
a cation. Sulfonamides are therefore soluble in aqueous alkaline
solutions. They are weak acids, however, and are precipitated at
low pH values.

TABLE 3.7 Solubilities of Amides and Related Compounds in Water at 20°C

Compound	Solubility	Compound	Solubility
 Benzamide (CONH$_2$)	1 in 170*	 Benzoic Acid (COOH)	1 in 290
 Paracetamol (OCONH$_2$, NH$_2$)	1 in 70	 p-Aminobenzoic Acid (COOH, NH$_2$)	1 in 170
 Salicylamide (CONH$_2$, OH)	1 in 500	 Salicylic Acid (COOH, OH)	1 in 550
 Sulfanilamide (SO$_2$NH$_2$, NH$_2$)	1 in 170	 Sulfanilic Acid (SO$_2$OH, NH$_2$)	1 in 170

*At 12°C.

I. Amino Acids and Proteins

Most naturally occurring amino acids have good aqueous solubilities; some of these are shown in Table 3.8. Aqueous solubility decreases as the proportion of lipophilic groups in the molecule increases. Needham et al. [9] have demonstrated a relationship between aqueous

TABLE 3.8   Aqueous Solubilities of Amino Acids

$$
\begin{array}{c}
H \\
| \\
R-C-COOH \\
| \\
NH_2
\end{array}
$$

Name	R	Molecular weight	Molar solubility
1. Glycine	H--	75	3.3
2. Alanine	CH_3-	89	1.9
3. Serine	$HO \cdot CH_2-$	105	0.48
4. Valine	$(CH_3)_2CH-$	117	0.76
5. Threonine	CH_3 ⟍ CH- ⁄ HO	119	1.7
6. Leucine	$(CH_3)_2CH \cdot CH_2-$	131	0.19
7. Isoleucine	CH_3CH_2CH- $| CH_3$	131	0.31
8. Aspartic acid	$-CH_2COOH$	133	0.38
9. Glutamic acid	$--(CH_2)_2COOH$	147	0.059
10. Phenylalanine	$C_6H_5CH_2-$	165	0.18
11. Tyrosine	$HO-\langle\text{ring}\rangle-CH_2-$	181	0.0025
12. Methionine	CH_2CH_2- $| S \cdot CH_3$	149	0.23
13. Cystine	$-S \cdot S \cdot CH_2CH \cdot COOH$ $| NH_2$	240	0.0004
14. Tryptophan	(indole ring) $C \cdot CH_2$ ‖ CH NH	204	0.056

solubility and carbon number in five amino acids, but their correlation necessitated allocation of a carbon number of 3 for the benzene group in phenylalanine. A plot of ln molar solubilities, taken from Table 3.8, against carbon number is shown in Fig. 3.1. The amino acids are considered as α-substituted glycines, and the numbers on the abcissa represent the number of carbon atoms in the substituent group. The aliphatic groups, containing carbon and hydrogen only, give a reasonable rectilinear plot, and the positions of the remaining points relative to the line give an indication of the effects of other substituents. Thus if the point for phenylalanine is moved two to three carbon number units to the left, it coincides with the line, confirming the suggestion of Needham et al. [9] that the benzene ring of phenylalanine is equivalent to only three carbons. The presence of sulfur and carboxyl reduces aqueous solubility, as also does, surprisingly, hydroxyl. The effect is particularly marked with tyrosine and could well be a consequence of solute-solute complexation

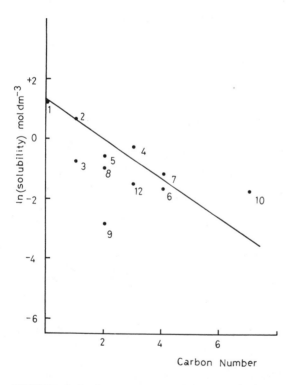

FIGURE 3.1 Aqueous solubilities of amino acids. The key to the numbers is given in Table 3.8. The straight line is the regression line through amino acids 1, 2, 4, 6, and 7.

(Chapter 7). Aqueous solubilities of amino acids are facilitated by the charged amino and carboxyl groups and are therefore highest at extremes of pH. Glycine, for example, has a solubility in water of 32.9% at pH 2.7, and of 29.6% at pH 9.3, both at 25°C, but the solubility is only 21.8% at pH 6.2. The effects of hydroxy as in serine and threonine, and a second carboxyl as in aspartic and glutamic acids, on the aqueous solubility of an amino acid have been considered to be a secondary consequence of its effect on the pK_a value. This should make little contribution, however, since the groups are separated from the amino and carboxyl groups by at least two carbon atoms, with the result that the pK_a values vary very little. Alanine, for example, has pK_a values of 2.34 and 9.69 and an isoelectric point of 6.01, compared with 2.21, 9.15, and 5.68 for serine. This conclusion is supported by the fact that plots of solubility against pH for amino acids tend to be truncated, the minimum solubility spreading over a range of several pH units.

Solubilities of amino acids in organic solvents are generally poor; glycine, for example, is soluble in about 10,000 parts of methanol and isopropanol and about 25,000 parts of ethanol at 25°C. Solubilities in nonpolar solvents increase with the proportion of lipophilic groups in the molecule; thus proline, with a large lipophilic component, has a solubility of 67% in ethanol. Fauchere et al. [10] have increased the lipid solubilities of glycine and alanine by attaching large lipophilic groups, such as adamantyl (XIII) and neopentyl (XIV).

Adamantyl (XIII)   Neopentyl (XIV)

Globular protein molecules are considered to fold under the influence of hydrophobic interactions (Section IV in Chapter 7) in an aqueous environment, so that the nonpolar fragments are buried within the mass of the protein and are surrounded by a layer rich in polar residues. Nozaki and Tanford [11] have classified the hydrophobicities of amino acids in terms of the free energy of transfer from water to ethanol, as expressed by

$$\text{Hydrophobicity} = \Delta G = -RT \ln \frac{\text{solubility in water}}{\text{solubility in ethanol}} \qquad (3.4)$$

and Meirovitch et al. [12] according to the orientation of the amino acid within the protein molecule. If the side chain were directed toward the center of the molecule, the parent acid was hydrophobic, and if it pointed toward the periphery, it was hydrophilic. The magnitude of the effect was scaled according to the size of the angle of orientation. Amino acids classified as hydrophilic according to these criteria were found to be more numerous in the outer reaches of the protein molecule, while the lipophilic amino acids were predominent on the inside.

The situation is reversed in water-insoluble proteins. Keratin is an example, taking the form of a helix, with the hydrophobic parts of the constituent amino acids pointing outward and the hydrophilic groups located within the spirals. The loops of the helix are held together by hydrogen bonds between the polar groups, so that access to the hydrophilic regions of the molecule is prevented, resulting in an insolubility, much appreciated by the owners of skin and hair, in water. The lipophilic exterior of the helix gives rise to an affinity for oils, which wet the skin, and a resistance to water, which rolls off in the form of droplets. The dielectric properties of oils are too small to break down the structure of keratin and thereby take it into solution.

Globular proteins sometimes require the presence of electrolyte to take them into aqueous solution. This process of "salting in" prevents association of the protein molecules by accumulating on the surface, thereby increasing the degree of hydration. An excess of electrolyte will salt out the protein, the electrolyte competing with the protein for the solvent.

J. Steroids

The hydrocarbon skeletons of the steroids exert a powerful hydrophobic influence on their solubilities. Substitution with strongly hydrophilic substituents, such as the ionized carboxyl groups of the bile salts, and hydrocortisone hemisuccinate (II), or the polyoxyethylene chains of some lanolin derivatives, is necessary to achieve reasonable aqueous solubilities. The common hydrophilic groups associated with steroids, carbonyl and hydroxyl, are not sufficiently powerful to bring about such an effect, even when the molecule contains several such substituents. Hydroxyl would be expected to increase aqueous solubility to some extent, but its effect is variable; thus, for example, esterification of the hydroxyl group of testosterone results in an anticipated decrease in aqueous solubility, whereas 17α hydroxylation of progesterone decreases solubility.

Hydrocarbons are not usually good solvents for steroids, despite the preponderence of carbon-carbon and carbon-hydrogen from the cyclopentanophenanthrene nucleus, particularly when the steroid

molecule contains one or more hydroxyl groups. The best solvents
are those which are capable of hydrogen bonding with the solute.
Chloroform, which is able to accept electrons from carbonyl and
hydroxyl oxygen, is usually one of the best solvents, and alcohols
are effective for the same reason. Electron-donating solvents, such
as ethers, are good solvents for steroids containing hydroxyl groups,
but are less effective with steroids, which have no electron-accepting
groups. Aromatic solvents appear to function as electron donors
with hydroxyl groups [13] and as electron acceptors with carbonyl
groups [14].

Steroid solubilities are indirectly influenced by melting point
through its effect on ideal solubility [15], and in consequence,
solubility can vary according to the polymeric form in which the
solute occurs. Solubility can also be influenced by solvate formation [16] or by steric orientation between solute and solvent [17].

II. BALANCE BETWEEN HYDROPHILIC AND
HYDROPHOBIC GROUPS

In discussing the influence of hydrophilic groups on aqueous solubility, it was shown that as a homologous series is ascended, the
influence of the alkyl group increases, so that the homologs become
progressively less soluble in water and develop greater preference
for solvents with low or zero dipole moments. The fall-off in aqueous solubility with carbon number varies with the nature of the
hydrophilic group; thus n-alkanols are completely miscible with
water up to propanol (C_3), whereas the normal fatty acids are completely miscible up to butyric acid (C_4). Similarly, benzenesulfonic
acid is very soluble in water, whereas benzoic acid is not. It
therefore appears that the sulfonic acid group is more hydrophilic
than carboxyl, which in turn is more hydrophilic than hydroxyl.

The aqueous solubility of a compound containing several hydrophilic groups should be greater than an equivalent molecule containing only one such group. The solubilities of cyclohexanol (V)
(0.6 M at 20°C) and d-glucose (IV) (1.3 M at 20°C) provide an
example. The generalization has reservations; polysubstitution with
hydrophilic groups is invariably accompanied by an increase in melting point, and if one is comparing a monosubstituted liquid with a
polysubstituted solid, it should be borne in mind that the additional
hydrophilic influence is counterbalanced by the energy required to
liquefy the solid. Thus n-butyric acid (C_3H_7COOH), which is a
liquid, is miscible in all proportions with water at 20°C, while succinic acid ($C_2H_4(COOH)_2$), which is a solid, has an aqueous solubility of only 0.5 M at 20°C, even though it contains two carboxyl
groups, compared with butyric acid's one. Similarly, the difference

between cyclohexanol and d-glucose cited above would be more significant if d-glucose, like cyclohexanol, were a liquid at 20°C.

Substitution of a solute molecule with hydrophilic groups reduces its solubility in low-polarity solvents. Castor oil is a classical example. Fixed oils, which are long-chain fatty acid esters of
glycerol, have a solubility profile characteristic of their chemical
structure. They are freely soluble in light petroleum, but almost
completely insoluble in ethanol. However, castor oil is miscible with
ethanol and has only a limited solubility in light petroleum. The
difference is due to the presence of a hydroxyl group on the alkyl
chain of ricinoleic acid (XV), the fatty acid of castor oil. Lipophilic

$$CH_3(CH_2)_5 \underset{\underset{OH}{|}}{CH} \cdot CH_2 CH=CH(CH_2)_7 COOH$$

Ricinoleic Acid   (XV)

groups have the opposite effect, reducing aqueous solubility and
increasing solubility in solvents with low dipole moments. Electronic
interactions and intramolecular hydrogen bonding between groups in
solute molecules can also influence solubilities, making them markedly
different from what one would expect from the relative hydrophilic
and hydrophobic influences of substituent groups. This applies particularly to aromatic compounds.

The solubility of a compound can thus be considered to be controlled by the balance between the hydrophilic and hydrophobic
groups making up the molecule. This concept is not new and has
long been recognized with surface-active agents. The best known
parameter of this type is the hydrophilic-lipophilic balance (HLB)
value, devised by Griffin [18]. Griffin assigned arbitrary numerical
values for nonionic surfactants, by dividing the percentage by weight
of hydrophilic groups in the molecule by 5. The general procedure
is given by

$$HLB = \frac{E + P}{5} \tag{3.5}$$

where E is the percentage by weight of ethylene oxide chain and P is
the percentage by weight of alcoholic hydroxyl. Thus for polyethylene glycol 300 (XVI), m is 5 to 6; if we suppose that m is 6, the

$$HOCH_2(CH_2 O \cdot CH_2)_m CH_2 OH$$

Polyethylene Glycol 300   (m = 5 or 6)   (XVI)

molecular weight will be $[(CH_2CH_2O)_6 = 264] + [(OH)_2 = 34] + [(CH_2)_2 = 28]$, giving

$$HLB = \frac{100(264 + 34)}{5(264 + 34 + 28)} = 18.3$$

The 5 is in the denominator to reduce the range of the values. A 100% lipophilic molecule would have the hypothetical HLB of 20, so a 0 to 20 HLB scale was devised on the basis of this formula. A surfactant with a low HLB value therefore has an affinity for lipids, and those with values approaching 20 form clear, colloidal dispersions in water. The magnitude of an HLB value designates the most favorable application of the surfactant; an antifoaming agent, for example, must spread on an air-aqueous solution interface. It must therefore be almost completely lipophilic, but there must be some hydrophilic activity; otherwise, it will not spread on the surface. E + P must therefore be low, but not zero. Griffin assigned an HLB value of 1 to 3 for antifoaming agents.

HLB values can be calculated from group numbers, some of which are reproduced in Table 3.9. These were derived by Davies by analyzing the structures of a large number of surfactants of known HLB. Each group number indicates the contribution of the substituent it represents to HLB value, which is calculated from

$$HLB \text{ value} = 7 + \text{sum of group numbers} \tag{3.6}$$

These parameters provide an approximately quantitative indication of the influence of substituent groups on solubility. Ionized groups, such as SO_4' and COO', have high positive values and therefore make a powerful contribution to aqueous solubility. The influence

TABLE 3.9 Group Contributions to HLB Values

Group	Number	Group	Number
SO_4' Na^+	38.7	$-CH-$	
COO' K^+	21.1	$-CH_2-$	-0.475
COO' Na^+	19.1	$-CH_3$	
Ester	2.4	$-(CH_2CH_2O)-$	0.33
COOH	2.1	$-(CH_2CH_2CH_2O)-$	-0.15
OH	1.9	$-N$	9.4
$-O-$	1.3		

of SO_4' is greater than that of COO'. Alkyl groups oppose aqueous solubility to the extent of 0.475 unit per carbon atom, so that five methylene groups are necessary to counter the aqueous affinity of nonionized carboxyl, and four methylenes are required for hydroxyl. These conclusions correspond to the observed aqueous solubilities of the respective homologous series, as discussed above. Similarly, the ether group is equivalent to between two and three methylene groups, in line with the known solubilities of the polyethylene glycols and the poloxalkols, and with the group numbers given for ethoxy and propoxy. The ester group does not appear to fit this comparison. The contributions of the ionized groups are higher than anticipated from known aqueous solubilities, an observation that is not unexpected, since HLB values calculated from Davis numbers for surfactants containing these groups are invariably in excess of the theoretical maximum of 20.

A similar scheme can be derived from the solubilities of the lower, liquid members of homologous series. If a single carbon atom attached to hydrogen(s) is given the arbitrary value of -1, and a compound that is completely miscible with water at ambient temperature, considered to have a positive value, approximate contributions for hydrophilic groups can be evaluated. A positive contribution would indicate that the group is hydrophilic, and the magnitude of the number indicates the extent of the hydrophilic influence. Thus since n-butyric acid is completely miscible with water and valeric is only partially miscible, a value of 3 can be assigned to the carboxyl group. Consideration of the lower n-fatty alcohols gives the same value to hydroxyl. Methyl formate is the only ester that is completely miscible with water, and therefore the ester group is assigned a value of 1. Ethers are difficult to assess, since the lower homologs are gases, but the contribution of ether oxygen is less than 4, because diethyl ether is only partially miscible with water. General experience indicates that the hydrophilic influence is less than that of carboxyl or hydroxyl but more than ester, suggesting a contribution of 2. Griffin assigned a contribution of 9.4 to the tertiary amine group, making it equivalent to nearly 20 methylenes. This figure is probably excessive where aqueous solubilities are concerned, since it suggests that dimethylaniline and diethylaniline should be freely soluble in water, which they are not. However, its contribution is in excess of 6, because triethylamine is completely miscible with water. These and similar considerations lead to the results summarized in Table 3.10, in which the parameters are termed *hydrophilic contributions*, to avoid confusion with Davis's group contributions.

The information from which these figures have been obtained is very scanty, but the contributions are sufficient to give a guide to the balance between hydrophilic and hydrophobic forces within

TABLE 3.10 Hydrophilic Contributions of Substituent Groups

Group	Contribution	Group	Contribution
OH	3	CH	
COOH	3	CH_2	-1
Ester	1	CH_3	
—O--	2	(CH_2CH_2O)	1
N—	6	$(CH_2CH_2CH_2O)$	-0.5
·NH	5		
--NH_2	5		
C=O	3		

a molecule. The scheme is not meant to be quantitative, nor does
it take heats of fusion into account. Ionizing groups have not been
considered for this reason, since molecules containing charged
groups are usually solids with high melting points, but it can be
assumed that they make high contributions to aqueous solubility.
Thus comparison of the solubilities of heptadecane and sodium stearate indicates that the carboxylate group is equivalent on the hydrophilic contribution scale to something in the region of 17 methylene
groups. Such high contributions introduce the added complication
that in attempting to balance the hydrophilic tendency against an
equivalent hydrophobic influence, one is moving out of the sphere
of solutions into that of colloidal electrolyte dispersions. Some examples of the balance concept will now be quoted.

Assignment of hydrophilic contributions to polyvinylpyrrolidone
(PVP) (XVII) indicates that each monomer makes a positive contribution to aqueous solubility. PVP is, in fact, readily soluble in water.

$$
\left[
\begin{array}{c}
CH_2 \!-\!\!-\! CH_2 \\
| \qquad | \\
CH_2 \quad C\!=\!O \\
\diagdown \; \diagup \\
N \\
| \\
-CH\!\cdot\!CH_2-
\end{array}
\right]_n
$$

Polyvinylpyrrolidone   (XVII)

When it was introduced in 1953, it created interest in the cosmetic industry because not only was it the first completely synthetic com- pound to be used in hair lacquers and setting lotions, but it also had most of the properties desirable for such preparations [19]. An aqueous or alcoholic solution is applied to the hair, to leave an envelope of polymer on each fiber after the solvent evaporates, thereby retaining the style that was intended. The principal dis- advantage of PVP is that it is susceptible to humid conditions and becomes tacky in wet weather.

Vinyl acetate forms a polymer (XVIII) which is virtually insoluble in water. This again is predicted by summing the hydrophilic con- tributions of the groups in the monomer, which results in a net negative value. Copolymers of vinylpyrrolidone and vinyl acetate are random combinations of the two monomers and have a range of aqueous solubilities ranging progressively from the high solubility of polyvinylpyrrolidone to the negligible solubility of polyvinyl ace- tate. Increasing quanties of ethanol or isopropanol are therefore

$$
\left[
\begin{array}{l}
CH_3 \\
| \\
C{=}O \\
| \\
O \\
| \\
-CH \cdot CH_2-
\end{array}
\right]_n
$$

Polyvinyl Acetate   (XVIII)

required as cosolvent as the proportion of vinyl acetate increases. At the same time, susceptibility to atmospheric conditions decreases, but other adverse properties, such as brittleness of the film and loss of substantivity to hair, come into play.

Other copolymers behave in a similar manner, for example, maleic anhydride-ethylvinyl ether copolymer (XIX). Treatment with

$$
\left[
\begin{array}{c}
CH_3 \\
| \\
O \\
| \\
-CH_2-C-C = C- \\
|\ \ |\ \ \ \ | \\
H\ \ C\ \ \ \ C \\
\diagup\!\diagdown \diagup\!\diagdown \\
O\ \ \ O\ \ \ O
\end{array}
\right]_n
$$

Maleic Anhydride-Methylvinyl Ether Copolymer (XIX)

an aqueous solution of a base hydrolyzes the anhydride group and neutralizes the resulting carboxy groups. The number of groups neutralized depends on the concentration of the base, so that a spectrum of aqueous solubilities can be obtained, depending on the proportions of copolymer and base. The solubility change is reflected in the susceptibility to moisture uptake [20].

III. DIELECTRIC CONSTANT

Dielectric constant (ε) is a physical property dependent on electronic distribution and is therefore influenced by interatomic and intermolecular attractions. Because of this dependence, it is a useful property with which to classify solutes and solvents with respect to potential mutual solubilities. A selection of dielectric constants is given in Table 3.11; they are grouped according to the like-dissolves-like classification. Water, which is a conducting solvent, has a high dielectric constant, and the very hydrophobic solvents have low values. Between these extremes, the dielectric constants decrease progressively from group a to group d, although the trend is not uniform. There are also exceptions; for example, acetic acid, which is a conducting solvent, has a value of only 6.15 at 20°C, and nitrobenzene has a higher value than ethanol, contrary to their behavior as solvents.

TABLE 3.11 Dipole Moments and Dielectric Constants

Like-dissolves-like group	Solvent	Dielectric constant	Dipole moment, C_m
a. Conducting	Water	80.4	6.2
	Acetic acid	6.15	5.8
b. Hydrogen bonding	Ethylene glycol	43.0	7.6
	Ethanol	25.7	5.6
	Acetone	21.4	9.6
	Isopropanol	18.3	5.5
c. Significant dipole moment	Nitrobenzene	34.8	14.1
d. Low or zero dipole moment	Benzene	2.3	0
	Carbon tetrachloride	2.2	0
	Cyclohexane	2.0	0

Dielectric constant is a function of both permanent and induced dipole moment, together with molecular weight and density, and therefore although substances with high dielectric constants usually have high dipole moments, the two properties do not necessarily have the same relative values. This can be seen from Table 3.11, in which dielectric constants are compared with dipole moments.

Dielectric constants therefore serve as a useful aid to the choice of solvent for a given solute. They also provide a means for quantitating the selection of solvent blends. Moore [21] calculated approximate dielectric constants from

$$\text{Dielectric constant} = \frac{(\% \text{ solvent A}_A) + (\% \text{ solvent B}_B) + \cdots}{100} \qquad (3.7)$$

Volume-to-volume proportions were employed because these were more convenient, although the author believed that calculation on a weight basis would have been more precise. It was, in fact, found that calculated and experimental dielectric constants could disagree. Moore found that phenobarbitone and pentabarbitone were most soluble in blends having a dielectric constant around 57. Equation (3.7) applies when the solvent blend is an ideal solution, and therefore gives only approximate dielectric constants with real systems. Measured dielectric constants for water-ethanol-glycerol and water-ethanol-propylene glycol blends were found to be linearly related to volume composition, but agreement with values calculated from Eq. (3.7) was poor, except at dielectric constants of 40 to 50 [22]. Predictions were better than those calculated on a weight basis.

Lordi et al. [23] introduced the parameter dielectric requirement defined as the dielectric constant at which the solubility of the solute was maximal. It was considered to be independent of the solvents used and was dependent only on the nature of the solute. However the solubility of a solute would not be the same in all solvents having the necessary dielectric requirement. Subsequent investigations have revealed a degree of solvent dependence; for example, caffeine gave a dielectric requirement around 40 for aqueous ethanol and around 50 for aqueous methanol [27]. Some dielectric requirements are given in Table 3.12. The concept of dielectric requirement has thus not lived up to its original promise. Rogers and Nairn [30] examined the solubilities of chloramphenicol palmitate in water-propylene glycol mixtures and found that the solubility did not increase significantly until the propylene glycol concentration reached 60% of the solvent mixture, corresponding to a fall in dielectric constant to around 50. They suggested that this threshold was a more meaningful parameter than dielectric requirement.

TABLE 3.12 Dielectric Requirements

Solute	Dielectric requirement	Solvent system	Reference
Phenobarbitone	27–30	Propylene glycol-ethanol	
		Glycerol-ethanol	23
		Water-ethanol	
Salicyclic acid	15 and 25		24
Benzoic acid	20		25
Caffeine	40–43	Ethanol-water	26
	50–55	Methanol-water	26
	30–34	Dioxane-water	26
	40	Ethyl Cellusolve-water	27
Theophylline	30–34	Dioxane-water	26
	40–43	Ethanol-water	26
	50–55	Methanol-water	26
	30	Ethyl Cellusolve-water	27
Theobromine	30–34	Dioxane-water	26
	50–55	Ethanol-water	26
	50–60	Methanol-water	26
Methyl to propyl parabenz	10	Dioxane-water	28
Methyl to butyl parabenz	14	Methanol to butanol-water	29

Paruta [31] used sucrose to reduce the dielectric constant of water and was able to achieve increases in the solubilities of substances that are sparingly soluble in water alone.

REFERENCES

1. S. D. Christian, A. A. Taha, and B. W. Gash, Molecular complexes of water in organic solvents and in the vapor phase, *Chem. Soc. Q. Rev., 24,* 30–36 (1970).
2. J. A. Riddick and W. B. Bunger, Organic solvents, physical properties and methods of purification, in *Techniques of Chemistry*, Vol. 2, 3rd ed., Wiley-Interscience, New York, 1970.
3. J. Ostrenga, C. Steinmetz, and B. Poulsen, Significance of vehicle composition: I. Relationship between topical vehicle composition, skin penetrability and clinical efficacy, *J. Pharm. Sci., 60,* 1175–1179 (1971).
4. J. J. Sciarra and D. Elliott, A solubility study of the boric acid glycerol complex, I, *J. Am. Pharm. Assoc. Sci. Ed., 49,* 115–117 (1960).
5. K. Motiuk, Wool wax alcohols: a review, *J. Am. Oil Chem. Soc., 56,* 651–658 (1979).
6. J. P. McCarthy and M. L. Schlossman, Ethoxylated lanolin derivatives—some properties of and their effect on cosmetic applications, *J. Soc. Cosmet. Chem., 26,* 523–530 (1975).
7. D. M. Marmion, *Handbook of U. S. Colorants for Foods, Drugs, and Cosmetics*, Wiley, New York, 1979.
8. J. F. Thorpe and R. P. Linstead, *The Synthetic Dyestuffs*, 7th ed., Charles Griffin, London, 1933.
9. T. E. Needham, A. N. Paruta, and R. J. Gerraughty, Solubility of amino acids in pure solvent systems, *J. Pharm. Sci., 60,* 565–567 (1971).
10. J. L. Fauchere, K. Q. Do, P. Y. C. Jow, and C. Hansch, Unusually strong lipophilicity of "fat" and "super" amino acids, including a new reference value of glycine, *Experientia, 36,* 1203–1204 (1980).
11. Y. Nosaki and C. Tanford, The solubility of amino acids and two glycine peptides in aqueous ethanol and dioxane solutions. Establishment of hydrophobicity scale, *J. Biol. Chem., 246,* 2211–2217 (1971).
12. H. Meirovitch and H. A. Scheraga, Empirical studies of hydrophobicity: 2. Distribution of the hydrophobic, hydrophilic neutral and ambivalent amino acids in the interior and exterior layers of native proteins, *Macromolecules, 13,* 1406–1414 (1980).
13. K. C. James and M. Ramgoolam, Complexation of some 3-keto-17-hydroxy-steroids in polar solvents, *Spectrochim. Acta, 31A,* 1599–1604 (1975).

14. K. C. James and P. R. Noyce, An infrared study of solute-solvent interactions of testosterone propionate, *J. Pharm. Pharmacol.*, *22 (Suppl.)*, 109S–113S (1970).
15. K. C. James and M. Roberts, The solubilities of the lower testosterone esters, *J. Pharm. Pharmacol.*, *20*, 709–714 (1968).
16. M. Gharavi and K. C. James, The properties of testosterone and related androgens crystallized from normal alkanols, *Int. J. Pharm.*, *14*, 325–331 (1983).
17. M. Gharavi, K. C. James, and L. M. Sanders, Solubilities of mestanolone, methandienone, methyltestosterone, nandrolone and testosterone in homologous series of alkanes and alkanols, *Int. J. Pharm.*, *14*, 333–341 (1983).
18. W. C. Griffin, Classification of surface active agents by "HLB," *J. Soc. Cosmet. Chem.*, *1*, 311–326 (1949).
19. H. A. Shelanski, M. V. Shelanski, and A. Cantor, Polyvinyl-pyrrolidone (PVP)—A useful adjunct in cosmetics, *J. Soc. Cosmet. Chem.*, *5*, 129–139 (1954).
20. R. S. McGee and N. M. Morse, Polymer evolution—from natural to synthetic, *J. Soc. Cosmet. Chem.*, *22*, 27–41 (1971).
21. W. E. Moore, The use of an approximate dielectric constant to blend solvent systems, *J. Am. Pharm. Assoc. Sci. Ed.*, *47*, 855–857 (1958).
22. D. L. Sorby, R. G. Bitter, and J. G. Webb, Dielectric constants of complex pharmaceutical solvent systems: I. Water-ethanol-glycerol and water-ethanol-propylene glycol, *J. Pharm. Sci.*, *52*, 1149–1153 (1963).
23. N. G. Lordi, B. J. Sciarrone, T. J. Ambrosio, and A. N. Paruta, Dielectric constants and solubility, *J. Pharm. Sci.*, *53*, 463–464 (1964).
24. A. N. Paruta, B. J. Sciarrone, and N. G. Lordi, Solubility of salicylic acid as a function of dielectric constant, *J. Pharm. Sci.*, *53*, 1349–1353 (1964).
25. A. N. Paruta, B. J. Sciarrone, and N. G. Lordi, Correlation between solubility parameters and dielectric constants, *J. Pharm. Sci.*, *51*, 704–705 (1962).
26. A. N. Paruta and S. A. Irani, Solubility profiles for the xanthines in aqueous alcoholic mixtures: I. Ethanol and methanol, *J. Pharm. Sci.*, *55*, 1055–1059 (1966).
27. A. N. Paruta and S. A. Itani, Solubility profiles for the xanthines in aqueous solutions of a glycol ether: II. Ethyl cellusolve, *J. Pharm Sci.*, *55*, 1060–1064 (1966).
28. A. N. Paruta, Solubility of the parabens in dioxane-water mixtures, *J. Pharm. Sci.*, *58*, 204–206 (1969).
29. A. N. Paruta, Solubility of parabens in alcohols, *J. Pharm. Sci.*, *58*, 216–219 (1969).

30. J. A. Rogers and J. G. Nairn, Solubility and dielectric constant. Correlations of the systems chloramphenicol palmitate-propylene glycol-water, *Can. J. Pharm. Sci.*, *8*, 75—77 (1973).

31. A. N. Paruta, Solubility of several solutes as a function of the dielectric constant of sugar solutions, *J. Pharm. Sci.*, *53*, 1252--1254 (1964).

4

Ideal Solutions

Fundamentally, the like-dissolves-like generalization depends on the relative values of the intermolecular cohesive energies (c). Calling the cohesive energies between solvent and solvent, solute and solute and solvent and solute c_{11}, c_{22}, and c_{12}, respectively, three situations can be described, according to the relative values of these terms. When c_{11} or c_{22} is greater than c_{12}, the solute tends not to dissolve, but when c_{12} is greater than either c_{11} or c_{22}, solution occurs. The concept has been explained in more detail in Chapter 3. The simplest model for a liquid solution is one in which intermolecular forces of attraction can be ignored. This occurs in ideal solutions, which are dispersions of molecules in which unlike molecules have the same affinity for each other as they do for their own kind. Thus, in terms of cohesive energies, ideal solutions result when $c_{11} = c_{22} = c_{12}$. Ideal solutions are analogous to perfect gases, but whereas in perfect gases there is no intermolecular attraction, intermolecular attraction is significant in ideal solutions, but is uniform throughout.

Strictly speaking, the ideal solution is a theoretical concept, but mixtures consisting of nonpolar and/or low-polarity molecules often have properties that agree closely to ideal conditions. Intermolecular attraction between nonpolar molecules occurs because the electrons of the molecules are in a continuous state of oscillation, and result from the electrostatic forces between the oscillating dipoles and those induced by them on neighboring molecules. These are termed London or dispersion forces; they are weak, and approximately constant from one type of nonpolar molecule to another. It is for this reason that such mixtures often behave ideally.

I. IDEAL SOLUTIONS OF LIQUIDS IN LIQUIDS

Liquids that mix to form ideal solutions do so without energy change and are miscible in all proportions. There is no volume change on mixing, and the components obey Raoult's law. Concentration and activity are equal in ideal solutions. If it is assumed that fugacities are equal to vapor pressures, then

$$a_1 = \frac{\bar{p}_1^i}{p_1^o} = X_1^i \tag{4.1}$$

where a is activity and X concentration, both expressed in mole fraction terms. $\bar{p}_1^i$ is the partial pressure of the solvent in the solution and p^o the saturated vapor pressure of the pure solvent. The symbol i denotes ideal. Rearrangement of Eq. (4.1) gives

$$\bar{p}_1^i = p_1^o X_1^i \tag{4.2}$$

which is Raoult's law. The same relationship applies to the solute. Variation of the total vapor pressure of an ideal binary liquid mixture with composition is shown in Fig. 4.1. At all concentrations the vapor pressure of the system is equal to the sum of the partial pressures calculated by Raoult's law. The plot represents mixtures of benzene and diethyl ether, which deviate only marginally from ideal behavior.

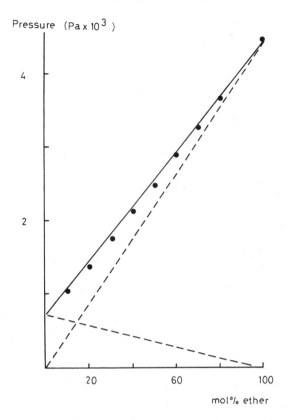

FIGURE 4.1 Saturated vapor pressures of benzene-diethyl ether
mixtures. ———, Total pressure; ----, partial pressures; ●, observed
results.

Example

It is required to change the package of an established aerosol preparation containing 60% w/w dichlorodifluoromethane and 40% trichlorofluoromethane, from metal to glass. The propellant mixture obeys
Raoult's law and is completely immiscible with the other constituents,
which have negligible concentrations and vapor pressures. Determine if the glass container, which is capable of withstanding a maximum pressure of 4.8×10^5 Pa (70 lb/in.[2]), can be used with safety.*

---

*Pressures are usually quoted in pounds per square inch in aerosol
technology. These values are given in parentheses.

Saturated vapor pressures: dichlorodifluoromethane = 8.07 × 10^5 Pa (117 lb/in.^{2}), trichlorofluoromethane = 6.21 × 10^4 Pa (9 lb/in.^{2}).

Solution:

Molecular weights:

Dichlorodifluoromethane = 12 + (19 × 2) + (35.5 × 2) = 121

Trichlorofluoromethane = 12 + 19 + (35.5 × 3) = 137.5

Mole fractions:

Dichlorodifluoromethane = $\dfrac{0.6/121}{(0.6/121) + (0.4/137.5)}$ = 0.63

Trichlorofluoromethane = 1 − 0.63 = 0.37

therefore,

Total vapor pressure = (0.63 × 8.07 × 10^5) + (0.37 × 6.21 × 10^4)

= 5.31 × 10^5 Pa

Conclusion: The glass container cannot be used.

II. IDEAL SOLUTIONS OF SOLIDS IN LIQUIDS

When ideal solutions of solids in liquids are formed, energy is necessary to liquefy the solute. The process of liquefaction can be considered as an equilibrium between liquid and solid. The enthalpy of fusion ΔH^f is the energy of the transition, and the ideal solubility (X_2^i) is equivalent to the equilibrium constant. Application of the van't Hoff isochore gives

$$\frac{d \ln X_2^i}{dT} = \frac{\Delta H^f}{RT^2} \tag{4.3}$$

and if ΔH^f is assumed to be independent of temperature, integration leads to

$$\ln X_2^i = \frac{-\Delta H^f}{RT} + \text{constant} \tag{4.4}$$

At the melting point (T_m), the solid solute becomes a liquid, so that $X_2^i = 1$, and $\ln X_2^i = 0$. Substitution in Eq. (4.4) then gives

$$\text{Constant} = \frac{\Delta H^f}{RT_m} \tag{4.5}$$

which leads to

$$\ln X_2^i = \frac{-\Delta H^f}{R} \frac{T_m - T}{T_m T} \tag{4.6}$$

Equation (4.6) has been used to determine ideal solubilities of benzoic acid and related compounds [1] and sulfonamides [2].

ΔH^f normally varies with temperature, however, due to the difference (ΔC_p) between the heat capacities of solid and supercooled liquid. The change is governed by the Kirchoff equation of classical thermodynamics,

$$\frac{d \Delta H^f}{dT} = \Delta C_p \tag{4.7}$$

which on integration between T_m and T yields

$$\Delta H_T^f = \Delta H_m^f - \Delta C_p (T_m - T) \tag{4.8}$$

ΔH_m^f and ΔH_T^f represent heats of fusion at the melting point and at the temperature of interest, respectively. Substitution of ΔH_T^f from Eq. (4.8) for ΔH^f in Eq. (4.3), and integration between T_m and T gives

$$\ln X_2^i = \frac{-\Delta H_m^f}{R} \frac{T_m - T}{T_m T} + \frac{\Delta C_p}{R} \frac{T_m - T}{T} - \Delta C_p \ln \frac{T_m}{T} \tag{4.9}$$

Ideal solubilities of iodine [3] and benzoic acid [4] have been calculated using this equation. Bowen and James [5] have pointed out that as T approaches T_m, the correction term becomes very small, and Eq. (4.9) reduces to Eq. (4.6), in which ΔH_m^f is substituted for ΔH^f.

Heat of fusion can be measured with a differential scanning calorimeter [6,7]. The instrument is designed to apply heat to a sample so that its temperature rises precisely, at a predetermined rate. The energy required to maintain the sample at the required temperatures is recorded on a chart, which is geared to the temperature rise. The output is therefore a plot of heat absorbed by the

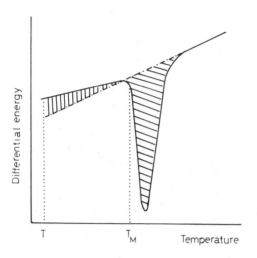

FIGURE 4.2   Typical differential scanning calorimetry thermogram
for a solid.   T, Temperature of interest; T_M, melting point.

sample against temperature.   A typical example for a solid in the
region of its melting point is shown diagramatically in Fig. 4.2.
Heat of fusion can be calculated from the area under the maximum,
shown by the diagonal hatching in the figure.   Before melting, the
energy input increases only gradually, satisfying the heat capacity
of the solid.   Similarly, the post-peak plot represents the heat capacity of the liquid.   If the plot for the liquid is extrapolated backward,
an approximately triangular area, indicated by the vertical hatchings
in Fig. 4.2, is formed between the solid and the supercooled liquid, representing ΔC_p and its variation with temperature.   Thermograms in
which the heat capacity of the supercooled liquid is greater than that of
the solid also occur, and occasionally the vertically hatched area is so
small that it may be ignored.   James and Roberts [8] obtained thermograms of the first type when measuring the heats of fusion of some testosterone esters, indicating that ΔC_p is not constant, as Eq. (4.7) suggests. ΔC_p can be measured on the thermogram for any required
temperature.

   Figure 4.2 indicates that ΔC_p is a rectilinear function of temperature, and therefore follows a relationship typified by

$$\Delta C_p = a + b(T_m - T) \qquad\qquad (4.10)$$

where a and b are constants, and can be evaluated from data abstracted
from the thermogram.   Substitution of ΔC_p from Eq. (4.10) into Eq.
(4.7) gives

$$\Delta H_T^f = \Delta H_m^f - a(T_m - T) - \frac{b}{2}(T_m - T)^2 \tag{4.11}$$

which on substitution in Eq. (4.3) and integration leads to

$$\ln X_2^i = \frac{1}{R}\left[\frac{(-\Delta H_m^f + aT_m + 0.5bT_m^2)(T_m - T)}{T_m T} \right.$$
$$\left. - (a + bT_m)\ln\frac{T_m}{T} + 0.5(T_m - T) \right] \tag{4.12}$$

James and Roberts [8] used this equation to calculate the ideal solubilities of some testosterone esters, and obtained figures which correlated with the observed solubilities in organic solvents, and other physical properties.

A similar relationship can be derived when the heat capacity of the supercooled liquid exceeds that of the solid. Richardson [9] has described a procedure for the analysis by computer of the output from a differential scanning calorimeter, thus affording a less tedious method of abstracting data for the calculation of a and b.

Example

Calculate the ideal mole fraction solubility of benzoic acid at 25°C

Enthalpy of fusion $(\Delta H_{298}^f) = 17.3$ kJ mol^{-1}, melting point = 122°C,

R = 8.315 J mol^{-1} deg^{-1}.

Solution:

$$-\log X_2^i = \frac{\Delta H^f}{2.303R}\frac{T_m - T}{T_m T}$$

$$= \frac{17.3 \times 10^3 \times (395 - 298)}{2.303 \times 8.315 \times 298 \times 395}$$

$$= 0.7445$$

Therefore,

$$X_2^i = \text{antilog } -0.7445 = 0.18$$

Example

The enthalpy of fusion of testosterone propionate at its melting point $(T_m = 120°C)$ is 21.74 kJ mol^{-1}. What is the enthalpy of fusion at 25°C? ΔC_p is given by the empirical equation

$$\Delta C_p = C_{p(\text{liquid})} - C_{p(\text{solid})} = 2.88(T_m - T) - 52.76 \text{ J deg}^{-1}$$

Solution:

$$\frac{d \Delta H^f}{dT} = \Delta C_p = C_{p(\text{products})} - C_{p(\text{reactants})}$$

Therefore,

$$\frac{d \Delta H^f}{dT} = 2.88 \times 393 - 2.88T - 52.76 = -2.88T + 1079$$

Cross-multiply and integrate between T_m and T:

$$\int_T^{T_m} d \Delta H^f = \int_T^{T_m} \Delta C_p \ dT = \int_T^{T_m} -2.88T + 1079$$

$$\left[\Delta H^f \right]_{298}^{393} = \left[\frac{-2.88}{2} T^2 + 1079T \right]_{298}^{393}$$

$$\Delta H^f_{393} - \Delta H^f_{298} = (-2.2241 + 4.2405 + 1.2788 - 3.2154) \times 10^5$$

$$= 7980 \text{ J mol}^{-1}$$

$$\Delta H^f_{298} = (21.74 - 7.98) \times 10^3 \text{ J mol}^{-1}$$

$$= 13.76 \text{ kJ mol}^{-1}$$

Heats of fusion can be obtained by differential thermal analysis. In this technique, a gradually increasing temperature is applied to sample and reference, but no attempt is made to maintain them at a programmed temperature, as with differential scanning calorimetry. The result is that in an endothermic transition such as melting, the sample temperature drops in comparison with the reference and is recorded on a chart as a plot of differential temperature (ΔT) against system temperature (that of the reference) or time. A typical thermogram is shown in Fig. 4.3. The enthalpy of the transition is proportional to the area under the peak. The method is described in more detail elsewhere [10].

Walden [11] suggested that molar heat of fusion divided by melting point was roughly constant for nonassociated substances and equal to 13.5 cal deg^{-1} mol^{-1} (56.5 J deg^{-1} mol^{-1}). The failure of associated substances to follow the rule was used to estimate degree of association, by dividing the experimentally obtained ratio by 13.5.

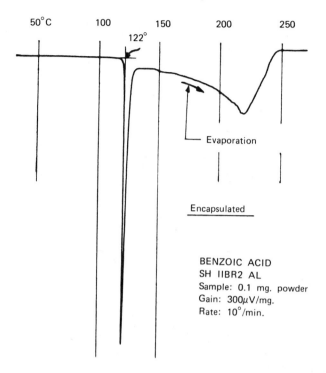

FIGURE 4.3 Differential thermal analysis thermogram for benzoic acid.

Walden's rule has been used to estimate heats of fusion for use in solubility calculations [1]. The practice is not highly accurate, because constants frequently deviate from the anticipated value and cannot even be relied to stay constant within groups of related compounds, as shown in Table 4.1. However, the principle is useful for estimating rough solubilities. This is done by substitution of the Walden constant for $\Delta H^f/T_m$ in Eq. (4.6), to give

$$-\ln X_2^i = \frac{56.5}{R} \frac{T_m - T}{T} \tag{4.13}$$

The example given below illustrates this point.

Example

The enthalpy of fusion of phenobarbitone is 2.78×10^4 J mol^{-1} [12]. Its melting point is given by the *British Pharmacopoeia* as 174 to

TABLE 4.1 Thermal Data and Ideal Solubilities

Compound	Melting point (K)	Heat of fusion (kJ mol^{-1})	Walden's constant (J deg^{-1})	Ideal mole fraction solubility (298 K)		
				Eq. (4.6)	Eq. (4.13)	Eq. (4.15)
Testosterone						
Acetate	413	22.5	54.5	0.08	0.07	0.10
Propionate	393	22.1	56.2	0.12	0.11	0.15
Butyrate	382	25.3	66.2	0.11	0.15	0.19
Anthracene	490	28.8	58.8	0.01	0.01	0.02
Phenanthrene	369	18.6	50.4	0.24	0.20	0.24
Benzene	279	9.87	35.4	–	–	–
Naphthalene	353	18.8	53.3	0.31	0.29	0.33
Phenobarbitone	449	28.6	63.7	0.02	0.03	0.05
Amylobarbitone	430	26.5	61.6	0.04	0.05	0.07
Barbitone	463	25.2	54.4	0.03	0.02	0.04

Source: Steroid results taken from Ref. 8; barbiturate results taken from Ref. 2.

177°C. Estimate its ideal solubility at 25°C (a) using the enthalpy of fusion, and (b) using Walden's constant (56.5 J deg^{-1} mol^{-1}). Gas constant = 8.315 J deg^{-1} mol^{-1}.

Solution:

(a) Using the upper limit of the melting-point range yields

$$T_m = 177 + 273 = 450 \text{ K}$$

$$\ln X_2^i = \frac{-2.78 \times 10^4}{8.315} \left(\frac{450 - 298}{450 \times 298} \right) = -3.79$$

$$X_2^i = 2.3 \times 10^{-2}$$

Similarly, for the lower limit of the melting-point range,

$$X_2^i = 2.4 \times 10^{-2}$$

The 3°C range of temperature therefore results in a 4% range in estimated solubility.

(b) Using the upper limit of the melting-point range gives us

$$\ln X_2^i = \frac{-56.5}{8.315} \left(\frac{450 - 298}{298} \right) = -3.47$$

$$X_2^i = 3.1 \times 10^{-2}$$

Similarly, for the lower limit of the melting-point range,

$$X_2^i = 3.3 \times 10^{-2}$$

giving a similar percentage range in predicted solubility to that observed with the melting points. In contrast, there is a 35% gap between the predictions of the two methods. It can therefore be concluded that although the Walden constant will not give a precise ideal solubility, it is a useful means of providing an estimate. Some other examples are given in Table 4.1.

Walden's concept of a constant entropy of fusion has been criticized from time to time, usually on the grounds that in practice it is not constant. However, a study of 84 disubstituted benzenes [13] found the entropy of fusion to be independent of molecular shape, size, or dipole moment, and also of intra- or intermolecular hydrogen bonding. In contrast, enthalpy of fusion and melting point showed a definite dependence on molecular properties. In an analysis of various molecular properties that could contribute to entropy of fusion, Yalkowsky [14] accepted a constant figure of 56.5 J deg^{-1} mol^{-1} for rigid molecules, but proposed

$$\Delta S^f = 56.5 + 10.5(n - 5) \text{ J deg}^{-1} \text{ mol}^{-1} \tag{4.14}$$

for flexible molecules. n represents the number of atoms, except hydrogen, forming the flexible chain. Thus for heptyl-p-amino-benzoate (XX), n = 9 giving

$$\Delta S^f = 56.5 + 10.5 \times 4 = 98.5 \text{ J deg}^{-1} \text{ mol}^{-1}$$

COO(CH$_2$)$_6$CH$_3$

(XX)

NH$_2$

Yalkowsky [15] has rewritten Eq. (4.6) in the form

$$-\ln X_2^i = \frac{\Delta H^f}{R} \frac{mp - 25}{(273 + mp) \times 298} \qquad \text{at } 25°C \tag{4.15}$$

where mp represents the melting point in degrees Celsius. He further suggested that, since ΔH^f is usually of the order of 12.5 kJ mol^{-1}, and varies only slightly in comparison with melting point, it can be considered constant, and since mp is of much less importance in the denominator than in the numerator, Eq. (4.15) can be written as

$$\ln X_2^i \cong 0.02(25 - mp) \tag{4.16}$$

or

$$\log X_2^i \cong 0.01(25 - mp)$$

Ideal solubilities calculated from Eq. (4.15) are given in Table 4.1 and show good agreement with the answers obtained with the other equations.

The mathematical standard form,

$$\frac{d \ln T}{dT} = \frac{1}{T}$$

expressed here in terms of temperature (T), may be used to rewrite the van't Hoff isochore, as follows:

$$\frac{d \ln X_2^i}{dT} = \frac{\Delta H^f}{RT} \frac{1}{T} = \frac{\Delta H^f}{RT} \frac{d \ln T}{dT} \qquad (4.17)$$

which yields the following equation for ideal saturated solutions:

$$R \frac{d \ln X_2^i}{d \ln T} = \frac{\Delta H^f}{T} \qquad (4.18)$$

Enthalpy of fusion increases with temperature, because the heat capacity of the supercooled liquid is greater than that of the solid. The increase is roughly equivalent to the increase in temperature, so that $\Delta H^f/T$ is reasonably constant; for example, $\Delta H^f/T$ for iodine changes only 2.8% in moving from 25°C to 50°C. Ln X_2^i should therefore be rectilinearly related to ln T. Straight lines are in fact frequently obtained experimentally when ln X_2 is plotted against ln T, even with real saturated solutions. The second derivative of Eq. (4.18) is given by

$$\frac{d^2 \ln X_2^i}{(d \ln T)^2} = T \frac{d}{dT} \frac{d \ln X_2^i}{d \ln T} = T \frac{d}{dT} \frac{\Delta H^f}{RT} \qquad (4.19)$$

obtained by substituting for d ln T from Eq. (4.16), and for d ln X_2^i/d ln T from Eq. (4.18). Further substitution, this time for ΔH^f from Eq. (4.8), gives

$$\frac{d^2 \ln X_2^i}{(d \ln T)^2} = T \frac{d}{dT} \frac{\Delta H_m^f - \Delta C_p T_m + \Delta C_p T}{RT} \qquad (4.20)$$

which on integration leads to

$$\frac{d^2 \ln X_2^i}{(d \ln T)^2} = \frac{\Delta C_p}{R} - \frac{\Delta H_m^f}{RT} \qquad (4.21)$$

Since Eq. (4.18) represents a straight-line relationship, the second derivative is equal to zero, leading to

$$T_m \, \Delta C_p = \Delta H_m^f \tag{4.22}$$

The free energy of fusion (ΔG_m^f) is zero at the melting point, because liquid and solid are in equilibrium; therefore,

$$\Delta G_m^f = \Delta H_m^f - T \, \Delta S_m^f = 0 \tag{4.23}$$

so that

$$\Delta H_m^f = T_m \, \Delta S_m^f = T_m \, \Delta C_p \tag{4.24}$$

Substitution of ΔS_m^i from Eq. (4.24) into Eq. (4.18) gives

$$R \, \frac{d \ln X_2^i}{d \ln T} = \Delta S_m^i \tag{4.25}$$

and integration of Eqs. (4.18) and (4.25) between T_m and T gives

$$\ln X_2^i = \frac{\Delta H^f}{R T_m} \ln \frac{T}{T_m} \tag{4.26}$$

and

$$\ln X_2^i = \frac{\Delta S^f}{R} \ln \frac{T}{T_m} \tag{4.27}$$

providing alternative equations for expressing ideal solubilities.

It can be argued that the involvement of ΔC_p in the derivation of Eqs. (4.26) and (4.27) will partially correct for the failure to consider ΔC_p in Eq. (4.6), although which of these equations gives the best prediction of ideal solubility has yet to be established.

III. MELTING POINT

All the foregoing equations for the calculation of ideal solubilities contain the melting point of the solute. Melting point therefore has an influence on solubility. Unexpected solubilities within a group of otherwise related solutes, or even differences between results obtained with what are assumed to be identical materials, can frequently

be traced to peculiarities in the transformation of solid solute to
liquid solute. Some common examples are described below.

A. Polymorphism

Polymorphism occurs when a compound is capable of existing in two
or more solid states. The various states are called polymorphs; they
are different crystalline forms of the compound, which are distin-
guishable in the solid state, but are identical in the liquid state and
the gaseous state. Physical properties vary from one polymorph to
another, and the most important physical properties in the present
context are melting point and enthalpy of fusion. As a result, solubilities frequently vary from one polymorph to another, but the situation is not always as complicated as it seems, because often only
one polymorph is stable in the presence of the particular solvent.
Under these circumstances the equilibrium between solid and solvent
will be independent of the polymorph employed, although it may take
considerable time for the unstable polymorph to transform completely
into the other. The polymorphs of cortisone acetate for example,
all revert to form IV when suspended in water, but the process takes
up to 2 weeks to reach completion [16].
    When a solid that occurs in two crystalline forms with a transi-
tion point T_t is mixed at a temperature below T_t, with a solvent in
which it is soluble, excess solid in equilibrium with the saturated
solution will adopt the form that is stable at temperatures below T_t.
Suppose that this is polymorph A, and the other is polymorph B.
If the temperature is raised, at T_t, A will be transformed to B,
which then becomes adopted by the solid in equilibrium with the solution. If ΔC_p is ignored, the energy required to produce an ideal
saturated solution will be that required to transform polymorph A
to polymorph B, plus the energy required to liquefy polymorph B.
The variation of solubility with temperature can be expressed by

$$\frac{d \ln X_2^i}{d \ln T} = \frac{\Delta S_A^f}{R} = \frac{\Delta S_{AB}^t + \Delta S_B^f}{R} \tag{4.28}$$

where ΔS_{AB}^t represents the entropy of the transition from A to B,
and ΔS_B^f is the entropy of fusion of polymorph B. The variation
of solubility with temperature at temperatures above T_t is given by

$$\frac{d \ln X_2^i}{d \ln T} = \frac{\Delta S_B^f}{R} \tag{4.29}$$

Since $\Delta S_{AB}^t + \Delta S_B^f$ is greater than ΔS_B^f, a plot of ln X_2^i against ln T will take the form of two straight lines, intersecting at T_t, the pre-T_t line having the steeper slope. Extrapolation of the pre-T_t plot to $X_2^i = 1$ gives the metastable melting point of polymorph A.

B. Solvates

Solutes can crystallize in a form in which molecules of solvent are incorporated in the crystal lattice. The phenomenon is called pseudo-polymorphism, and the solid that separates from the solution is described as a solvate. Like polymorphs, solvates have different physical properties from each other and from polymorphs of the pure solute, with a resulting difference in solubility. A good example of this behavior is seen in the aqueous solubility plot of sodium carbonate, shown in Fig. 4.4. At lower temperatures the solubilities represent the equilibria between water and sodium carbonate decahydrate. The solubilities increase with temperature, and if the saturated solution is cooled, the decahydrate will crystallize out. At 32°C there is an inflection, above which solubilities decrease with increasing temperature, and this portion of the plot represents equilibria between water and the anhydrous salt.

Flynn et al. [17] observed odd-even alternations in the solubilities of cholesterol in the *n*-alkanols from methanol to heptanol. The

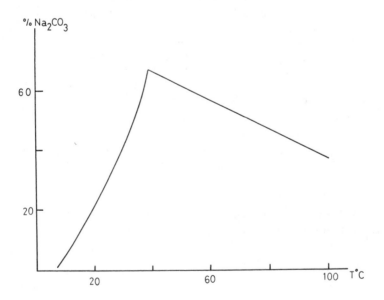

FIGURE 4.4 Aqueous solubilities of sodium carbonate.

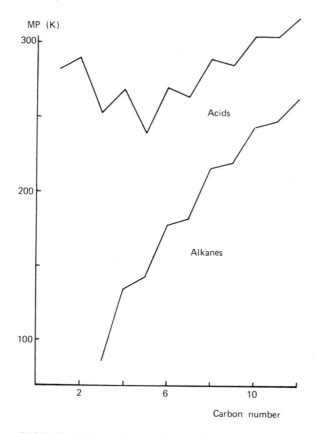

FIGURE 4.5 Melting points of *n*-alkanes and *n*-fatty acids.

fusion behavior of the crystals obtained by crystallizing cholesterol
from these solvents varied markedly from one alkanol to another, indicating that solvates, characteristic of each solvent, were formed.
It was suggested that the crystalline properties of the solvates exhibited odd-even alternations in their fusion energetics, analogous
to those observed with solid hydrocarbons (see below).

C. Odd-Even Alternation in Compounds with Long
Alkyl Chains

The physical properties of homologs frequently change irregularly
with increasing carbon number, but progress uniformly if the odd
and even carbon number homologs are considered separately. Typical examples are given in Fig. 4.5, which shows the melting points

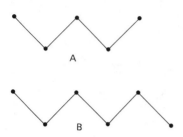

FIGURE 4.6 Configuration of *n*-alkanes: (A) *n*-pentane; (B) *n*-hexane.

of the lower *n*-alkanes and *n*-fatty acids. This odd-even effect must be remembered when using the solubilities of one or more homologoues to speculate on the solubilities of others. Odd-even behavior is attributed to differences between the packing of the two types. Each carbon atom has tetrahedral bonds, with the result that alkyl chains have a "zigzag" structure. The difference between the stackings of the odd and even homologs arises from the difference between the relative orientations of the terminal bonds. The terminal bonds of even-numbered chains will lie parallel, while in the odd-numbered chains the bonds will be at an angle to each other. This is illustrated in Fig. 4.6.

D. Stacking Between Steroid Nuclei

When an alkyl chain is attached to a bulky group, such as a steroid nucleus, the bulkiness of the chain may influence the crystallography of the molecule. The lower *n*-fatty acid esters of testosterone are an example of this. Lattice spacings of the acetate to valerate esters, shown in Table 4.2, suggest that the esters can be arranged into two groups, acetate and propionate, and butyrate and valerate, according to their b and c spacings. The difference between the two pairs has been associated with the orientation of the ester chains [8], the butyrate and valerate groups being too bulky to assume the same configuration as the lower two esters. The melting points can be classified into the same two groups. The difference between the melting points of acetate and propionate is attributed to α-to-α face attraction. The α face presents a large, comparatively flat surface, and the area of α face-to-α face contact is considered to be the largest factor influencing the melting point. This theory was supported by the fact that the ratio of the melting point to the area per molecule of an α face adjacent to the α face of a neighboring molecule was the same for acetate and propionate. A similar relationship obtained for butyrate to valerate.

TABLE 4.2 Crystallographic Data for Testosterone Esters

Ester	m.p. (K)	Spacings (nm)			Area of α face adjacent to those of neighboring molecules (nm^2)	Area $\dfrac{\text{m.p.} \times 10^{-3}}{}$
		a	b	c		
Acetate	413	1.26	1.81	0.78	0.77	1.86
Propionate	393	1.26	2.03	0.76	0.63	1.60
Butyrate	382	1.23	1.63	1.03	0.88	2.30
Valerate	380	1.23	1.67	1.03	0.89	2.34

Source: Ref. 8.

IV. "REALLY" AND "NEARLY" IDEAL SOLUTIONS

Ben-Naim [18] considered that there are three different types of ideal solutions in practice: ideal gas mixtures, symmetrid ideal solutions, and dilute ideal solutions. Mixtures of ideal gases form ideal solutions because their radial distribution functions are equal to 1.

Symmetric ideal solutions occur when the components have zero or near-zero dipole moments and are similar to each other. Such systems are sometimes termed *nearly ideal solutions*. Thus Ellis and Chao [19] reported only 2.4% deviation from ideal behavior for an equimolar mixture of *n*-hexane and 1-hexene, and observed similar adherence to the ideal state for other alkane mixtures. Even when the components are not isomers, mixtures of liquids sometimes follow Raoult's law reasonably well, as is shown in Fig. 4.1. Close adherence to ideal behavior by symmetric mixtures is rare, occurring only with mixtures of optically active isomers.

It therefore appears that the ideal solution is a very rare phenomenon in real situations. It is, in fact, almost entirely a theoretical concept, but it is a necessary concept because it provides the baseline upon which corrections can be applied in order to explain nonideal behavior.

REFERENCES

1. F. A. Restaino and A. N. Martin, Solubility of benzoic acid and related compounds in a series of *n*-alkanols, *J. Pharm. Sci.*, *53*, 636–639 (1964).
2. C. Sunwoo and H. Eisen, Solubility parameter of selected sulfonamides, *J. Pharm. Sci.*, *60*, 238–244 (1971).
3. J. H. Hildebrand and C. A. Jenks, Solubility: IV. Solubility relations of naphthalene and iodine in the various solvents, including a method for estimating solubility data, *J. Am. Chem. Soc.*, *42*, 2180–2189 (1920).
4. M. J. Chertkoff and A. N. Martin, The solubility of benzoic acid in mixed solvents, *J. Pharm. Sci.*, *49*, 444–447 (1960).
5. D. B. Bowen and K. C. James, Solubilities of testosterone propionate in non-polar solvents at 100°, *J. Pharm. Pharmacol.*, *20* (*Suppl.*), 104S–107S (1968).
6. J. L. McNaughton and C. T. Mortimer, Differential scanning calorimetry, in *IRS, Physical Chemistry Series 2*, Vol. 10, Butterworths, London, 1975.
7. S. Watson, M. J. O'Neill, J. Justin, and N. Brenner, A differential scanning calorimeter for differential thermal analysis, *Anal. Chem.*, *34*, 1233–1238 (1964).

8. K. C. James and M. Roberts, The solubilities of the lower testosterone esters, *J. Pharm. Pharmacol.*, *20*, 709–714 (1968).

9. M. C. Richardson, Precision differential calorimetry and the heat of fusion of polyethylene, *J. Polym. Sci.*, *Part C*, *38*, 251–259 (1972).

10. P. Pacor, Applicability of the Du Pont 900 DTA apparatus in quantitative differential thermal analysis, *Anal. Chim. Acta*, *37*, 200–208 (1967).

11. P. Walden, Uber die Schmelzwarme, spezifische Kohasion und Molekulargrosse bei der Schmelztemperatur (Regarding the heat of fusion, specific cohesion and molecular weight at the melting point, *Z. Elektrochem.*, *14*, 713–724 (1908).

12. C. Treiner, C. Vaution, and G. N. Cavé, Correlations between solubilities, heats of fusion and partition coefficients for barbituric acids in octanol + water and in aqueous micellar solutions, *J. Pharm. Pharmacol.*, *34*, 539–540 (1982).

13. E. Martin, S. H. Yalkowsky, and J. E. Wells, Fusion of disubstituted benzenes, *J. Pharm. Sci.*, *68*, 565–568 (1979).

14. S. H. Yalkowsky, Estimation of entropies of fusion of organic compounds, *Ind. Eng. Chem.*, *Fundam.*, *18*, 108–111 (1979).

15. S. H. Yalkowsky and S. C. Valvani, Solubility and partitioning: I. Solubility of non-electrolytes in water, *J. Pharm. Sci.*, *69*, 912–922 (1980).

16. J. E. Carless, M. A. Moustafa, and H. D. C. Rapson, Cortisone acetate crystal forms, *J. Pharm. Pharmacol.*, *18 (Suppl.)*, 190S–197S (1966).

17. G. L. Flynn, Y. Shah, S. Prakongpan, K. H. Kwan, W. I. Higuchi, and A. F. Hofmann, Cholesterol solubility in organic solvents, *J. Pharm. Sci.*, *68*, 1090–1097 (1979).

18. A. Ben-Naim, Molecular origin of ideal solutions and small deviations from ideality, in *Solutions and Solubilities*, Part I (M. R. Dack, ed.), *Techniques of Chemistry*, Vol. 8, Wiley, New York, 1976, pp. 20–103.

19. J. A. Ellis and K. C. Chao, Vapor pressures and interaction constants of some nearly ideal solutions, *J. Chem. Eng. Data*, *18*, 264–266 (1973).

5

Regular Solutions

I. SOLUTIONS OF LIQUIDS IN LIQUIDS

The effective partial vapor pressures of the liquid components of nonideal binary liquid systems are different from those predicted by Raoult's law. The higher the effective partial vapor pressure of a component, the more easily it will volatilize into the atmosphere above the mixture. *Escaping tendency* is an alternative term for this readiness to volatilize. Deviations can be either positive or negative.

A. Negative Deviation

Figure 5.1 represents the vapor pressure-composition curve of chloroform-diethylether mixtures and shows negative deviation. The total vapor pressure passes through a minimum and is always less than that predicted by Raoult's law. The escaping tendency is therefore negative. The hydrogen of chloroform bears a partial positive charge, due to the inductive effect of the chlorine atoms, while the oxygen of diethylether is negative. There is no strong negative site in chloroform nor strong positive site in diethyl ether, so that intermolecular attractive forces in the pure liquids are not unusually great. However, when the two are mixed, a strong hydrogen bond is formed between the two oppositely charged centers. The consequent affinity of chloroform for diethylether reduces the escaping tendency, or alternatively, can be said to exert an "inward pull," which reduces the partial vapor pressure.

The activity (a) of a component in a nonideal solution is expressed by

$$a = fX \tag{5.1}$$

where X is mole fraction concentration and f is the activity coefficient, characteristic of the component and of its concentration. Substitution for a from Eq. (5.1) into Raoult's law (page 128) yields

$$\frac{\text{observed vapor pressure}}{\text{saturated vapor pressure}} = fX \tag{5.2}$$

Vapor Pressure (MPa)

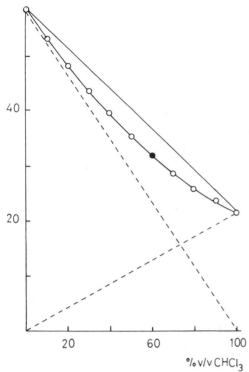

FIGURE 5.1 Vapor pressures of chloroform-diethyl ether mixtures (showing negative escaping tendency). ----, Partial vapor pressures predicted by Raoult's law; —o—, observed vapor pressures; ——, total vapor pressure predicted by Raoult's law.

and provides a method of calculating activity coefficients. Taking the black circle in Fig. 5.1 as an example, this represents:

Component 1 (diethyl ether): $X_1 = 0.4$; $p_1^o = 58.9$ MPa

Component 2 (chloroform): $X_2 = 0.6$; $p_2^o = 21.7$ MPa

giving

$p_{(observed)} = 31.9$ MPa

$p_{(calculated)} = (X_1 p_1^o + X_2 p_2^o)f = 36.6f$

yielding a mean activity coefficient of

$$f = \frac{31.9}{36.6} = 0.87$$

It should be noted that the value is less than unity, which is characteristic of negative deviation. Activity coefficients greater than 1 indicate positive deviation.

One would anticipate that the partial pressures of the components in Fig. 5.1 would follow bow-shaped curves, similar to that obtained with the observed total pressures, each component contributing equally to the negative deviation. The following are used for calculating activity coefficients in binary liquid systems:

$$\ln f_2 = \beta_2 X_1^2 \tag{5.3}$$

$$\ln f_1 = \beta_1 X_2^2 \tag{5.4}$$

where β is a parameter, dependent on temperature, and derived from the constants a and b in the van der Waals equation. Equations (5.3) and (5.4) permit an easier understanding of the term β, since as X_1 approaches unity β_2 becomes equal to $\ln f_2$. We may therefore say that β_1 is the value of $\ln f_1$ as X_1 approaches zero and β_2 is the equivalent value for the other component. If β_2 is given arbitrary values, corresponding values of f_1 can be calculated, and substitution in Eq. (5.2) yields equivalent values of p_1/p_1^o. These are plotted against mole fraction concentration in Fig. 5.2. Butler et al [1] used experimental vapor pressures to calculate partial pressures of methanol, ethanol, n-propanol, and n-butanol in alcohol-water mixtures and obtained similar profiles. The curves are unsymmetrical, becoming more so as β deviates positively or negatively from unity, and indicate that the components do not contribute equally to the reduction in vapor pressure, the relative contributions varying with concentration.

A significant feature of Fig. 5.2 is that as the mole fraction concentration of a component approaches unity, the true partial vapor pressure approaches that predicted by Raoult's law. Raoult's law can therefore be applied to the solvent in real solutions of liquids in liquids, provided that the solution in dilute. It is for this reason that the standard for activity coefficients in nonelectrolyte solutions is normally the pure liquid (i.e., when $f_1 = 1$).

The change of a property of a component of a binary liquid mixture with concentration is related to that of the other component by the Gibbs-Duhem equation (see Section V in Chapter 1), of which the following is a form.

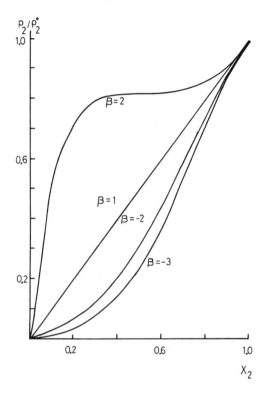

FIGURE 5.2 Partial vapor pressures in binary liquid mixtures.

$$\frac{d \ln \theta_1}{d \ln X_1} = \frac{d \ln \theta_2}{d \ln X_2} \tag{5.5}$$

θ can be activity, entropy, free energy, and so on. Application to dilute solutions, since the solvent behaves ideally, gives

$$\frac{d \ln a_1}{d \ln X_1} = \frac{d \ln a_2}{d \ln X_2} = 1 \tag{5.6}$$

which leads to

$$d \ln a_2 = d \ln X_2 \tag{5.7}$$

Integration of Eq. (5.7) gives

$$a_2 = K X_2 \tag{5.8}$$

where K is a constant. Substitution of a_2 from Raoult's law leads to

$$p_2 = Kp_2^{o}x_2 \qquad\qquad (5.9)$$

which is Henry's law. Thus in dilute solutions, the solvent obeys Raoult's law and the solute obeys Henry's law. It therefore follows that in dilute real solutions the partial pressures of both solute and solvent are proportional to their concentrations, but it is only with the solvent that the proportionality constant is the saturated vapor pressure of the pure liquid.

The same conclusion follows from scrutiny of the geometry of Fig. 5.2. As the mole fraction concentration approaches zero, the true partial vapor pressure profile approximates a straight line and

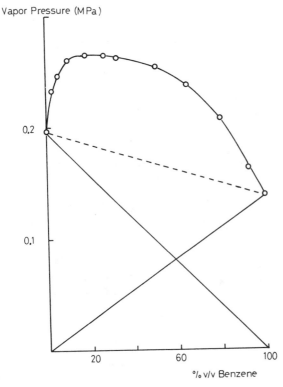

FIGURE 5.3 Vapor pressures of benzene-ethanol mixtures (showing positive escaping tendency). ——, partial vapor pressures predicted by Raoult's law; –o–, observed vapor pressures; - - -, total vapor pressures predicted by Raoult's law.

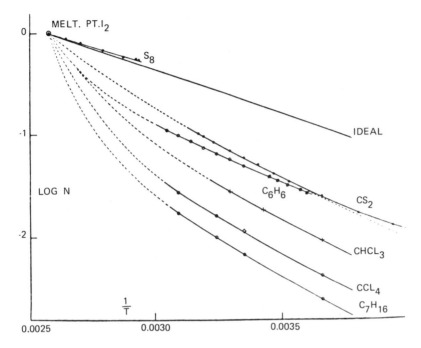

FIGURE 5.4 Regular solubilities of iodine. (From Ref. 2.)

meets the ideal plot at an angle, indicating that ideal pressure is proportional to real pressure at a given dilute concentration. This is another way of expressing Henry's law.

B. Positive Deviation

Positive deviation occurs when the pair potential energy between un-like molecules (u_{12}) is greater than the energies between similar molecules (u_1 and u_2). The net effect, in comparison with that in the pure liquids, is one of repulsion and an increase in the escaping tendency. In simple terms, each component is giving the other an "extra push." Since the observed pressure is greater than calcu-lated, activity coefficients will be greater than 1, characteristic of all mixtures showing positive deviation. Benzene-ethanol mixtures behave in this way; a vapor pressure-composition plot is shown in Fig. 5.3. Total vapor pressures are in excess of that of either pure component, so that an azeotropic mixture would separate on fraction-al distillation. The mutual solubility of mixtures that exhibit very high positive deviation is limited to specific concentration ranges, outside which separation into conjugate solutions occurs.

Hildebrand suggested that when deviation from Raoult's law, either positive or negative, is not too great, thermal movement in the mixture will be sufficient to keep the molecules randomly dispersed. He designated these regular solutions. Hildebrand first noted the existence of solutions of this type when investigating the solubilities of iodine in a series of solvents [2]. When log solubility was plotted against the reciprocal of temperature, those solvents forming violet solutions gave lines running parallel to the ideal solubility curve, whereas those giving brown (solvated) solutions did not. His results are reproduced in Fig. 5.4. The former were therefore named *regular*, because they formed a regular family of curves, and the name has persisted. The activity of a regular solution depends on the energy of mixing, but the energy involved is small and is provided by thermal motion arising from the heat of the surroundings. Because the molecules are randomly dispersed, the entropy of mixing is ideal.

II. ENERGY OF MIXING OF REGULAR SOLUTIONS

When the intermolecular forces between solvent and solute are unequal, work must be done to overcome uneven mixing and maintain random distribution. Equations for the energy of mixing have been evaluated using the unexpanded gas, quasi-crystalline, and distribution function models. All give similar results.

A. The Unexpanded Gas Model

The term a/V^2 in van der Waals equation accounts for the fall in internal pressure arising from the intermolecular attraction between molecules. Pressure multiplied by volume has the dimensions of energy, so that a/V represents the internal energy due to intermolecular attraction. In pure liquid solvent, the energy involved between one molecule and all the other molecules in the population will be $(n_1 - 1)a_1/V_1$, which since n_1, the total number of molecules, is large, approximates $n_1 a_1/V_1$. If this is summed for all the molecules, the total energy will be $n_1^2 a_1/V_1$. The corresponding energy for pure solute will be $n_2^2 a_2/V_2$. If 1 and 2 are mixed, a new factor is introduced due to interaction between solute and solvent molecules. If this is represented by a_{12}, the total energy of the solution (ΔU_{total}) will be given by

$$\Delta U_{total} = \frac{n_1^2 a_1 + n_2^2 a_2 + 2n_1 n_2 a_{12}}{\text{total volume of mixture}} \qquad (5.10)$$

In the van der Waals equation, b is the volume occupied by the molecules. In unexpanded systems this is approximately equal to the sum of the partial molar volumes

$$b = n_1 V_1 + n_2 V_2 \tag{5.11}$$

so that Eq. (5.10) can be expressed in the form

$$\Delta U_{total} = \frac{n_1^2 a_1 + n_2^2 a_2 + 2n_1 n_2 a_{12}}{n_1 V_1 + n_2 V_2} \tag{5.12}$$

The energy of mixing will be equal to the total energy less the energies of the individual solute and solvent and is given by

$$\Delta U^m = \frac{\Delta U_{total}}{V_{total}} - \frac{n_1 a_1}{V_1} - \frac{n_2 a_2}{V_2} \tag{5.13}$$

Substitution for ΔU_{total} and V_{total} from Eqs. (5.11) and (5.12) leads to

$$\Delta U^m = \frac{n_1^2 a_1 + n_2^2 a_2 + 2n_1 n_2 a_{12}}{n_1 V_1 + n_2 V_2} - \frac{n_1 a_1}{V_1} - \frac{n_2 a_2}{V_2} \tag{5.14}$$

Multiplication of the top and bottom of the second and third terms on the right-hand side by $(n_1 V_1 + n_2 V_2)$ gives

$$\Delta U^m = \frac{-n_1 n_2}{n_1 V_1 + n_2 V_2} \left(a_1 \frac{V_2}{V_1} + a_2 \frac{V_1}{V_2} - 2a_{12} \right) \tag{5.15}$$

Further simplification is possible by multiplying the expression outside the parentheses by $V_1 V_2$ and the expression inside by $1/V_1 V_2$, giving

$$\Delta U^m = \frac{-n_1 n_2 V_1 V_2}{n_1 V_1 + n_2 V_2} \left(\frac{a_1}{V_1^2} + \frac{a_2}{V_2^2} - \frac{2a_{12}}{V_1 V_2} \right) \tag{5.16}$$

which, since volume fraction concentration (ϕ) is defined in general terms as $n_i V_i / (n_i V_i + n_j V_j)$, reduces to

$$\Delta U^m = -\phi_1 \phi_2 \left(\frac{a_1}{V_1^2} - \frac{2a_{12}}{V_1 V_2} + \frac{a_2}{V_2^2} \right) \tag{5.17}$$

The partial energy of mixing of the solute $(\Delta \overline{U}_2^m)$ is the energy change when a small amount of solute is dissolved in a large volume of solvent (i.e., Δn_2 is significant compared with n_2, but n_1 is constant). It can therefore be calculated by differentiating the energy of mixing with respect to n_2, keeping n_1 constant, as in

$$\Delta \overline{U}_2^m = \left(\frac{d \, \Delta U^m}{dn_2} \right)_{n_1} \tag{5.18}$$

Thus differentiation of Eq. (5.16) with respect to n_2 gives*

$$\Delta \overline{U}_2^m = \frac{-n_1^2 V_1^2 V_2}{(n_1 V_1 + n_2 V_2)^2} \left(\frac{a_1}{V_1^2} + \frac{a_2}{V_2^2} - \frac{2a_{12}}{V_1 V_2} \right) \tag{5.19}$$

or

$$\Delta \overline{U}_2^m = -\phi_1^2 V_2 \left(\frac{a_1}{V_1^2} + \frac{a_2}{V_2^2} - \frac{2a_{12}}{V_1 V_2} \right) \tag{5.20}$$

---

*Differentiation is based on the theorem

$$\frac{d}{dx} \frac{u}{v} = \frac{v(du/dx) - u(dv/dx)}{v^2}$$

$$\frac{d}{dn_2} \frac{-n_1 n_2}{n_1 V_1 + n_2 V_2} = \frac{-(n_1 V_1 + n_2 V_2)n_1 + n_1 n_2 V_2}{(n_1 V_1 + n_2 V_2)^2}$$

$$= (-n_1^2 V_1 - n_1 n_2 V_2 + n_1 n_2 V_2)/(n_1 V_1 + n_2 V_2)^2$$

$$= -n_1^2 V_1/(n_1 V_1 + n_2 V_2)^2$$

B. The Quasi-Crystalline Model

Suppose that a pair of solvent molecules and a pair of solute molecules, each joined by attractive forces, are separated into their individual molecules and then combine to form two unequal pairs of solute + solvent molecules. This is shown diagrammatically in Fig. 5.5. The energy required to make the change will be $w_{11} + w_{22} - 2w_{12}$, where w_{11} and w_{22} are the work required to separate the respective pairs of like molecules, and $-w_{12}$ is the energy that is restored when a molecule of 1 is joined to a molecule of 2. Hildebrand and Salstrom [3] used this approach to derive an expression for the energy of mixing of silver chloride and alkali metal halides in the molten state. A system of $n_1 + n_2$ ions was considered, and each ion was assumed to be surrounded by q immediate neighbors, q' in the second layer, q" in the third layer, and so on. The number of pairs consisting of a silver ion and an immediately adjacent silver ion (a first-order pair) was calculated as $(n_1 + n_2)NqX_1^2$, where N is Avogadro's number and X_1 is the concentration of silver ions. Similarly, the number of first order M^+M^+ pairs, where M^+ represents an alkali metal ion, were $(n_1 + n_2)NqX_2^2$, and the number of first-order M^+Ag^+ pairs, $(n_1 + n_2)NqX_1X_2$. Related expressions were obtained for the higher-order pairs. All were summed as

$$\varepsilon = \Sigma \, qu + \Sigma \, q'u' + \Sigma \, q''u'' + \cdots \tag{5.21}$$

where u represents intermolecular pair potential. Total lattice energy U_{total} was then given by $(n_1 + n_2)(X_1^2\varepsilon_1 + X_2^2\varepsilon_2 + 2X_1X_2\varepsilon_{12})$. ε_1 is the potential energy involved in making a hole to accommodate a solute molecule in the solvent, and ε_2 is that in removing a molecule of the solute from its pure liquid. The potential energy gained in filling the hole is $2\varepsilon_{12}$. The corresponding energies for the pure

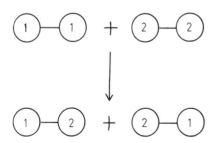

FIGURE 5.5 Diagrammatic representation of the quasi-crystalline concept of solution.

components are $n_1\varepsilon_1$ and $n_2\varepsilon_2$. The energy of mixing is therefore given by

$$\Delta U^m = \frac{-n_1 n_2}{n_1 + n_2}(2\varepsilon_{12} - \varepsilon_1 - \varepsilon_2) \tag{5.22}$$

The negative sign is introduced because work done represents loss of energy by the system. Similarly, partial energies of mixing are given by

$$\Delta \overline{U}_1^m = n_2^2(2\varepsilon_{12} - \varepsilon_1 - \varepsilon_2) \tag{5.23}$$

and

$$\Delta \overline{U}_2^m = n_1^2(2\varepsilon_{12} - \varepsilon_1 - \varepsilon_2) \tag{5.24}$$

These expressions apply equally well to nonelectrolyte solutions.

C. The Radial Distribution Function Model

Hildebrand and Wood [4] evolved an expression for the energy of mixing by consideration of the radial distribution curve. If the molar volumes of the components of a binary liquid system are different, there will be three different distribution functions covering the possible pairs, 1-1, 1-2, and 2-2. If there are $n_1 + n_2$ moles, there will be $n_1 N$ molecules of 1 capable of forming the center of a radial distribution, and each will be surrounded by $n_1 Ng(r)_{11}(4\pi r^2 \delta r)/(n_1 V_1 + n_2 V_2)$ of its own kind, giving a total of such pairs of

$$\frac{(1/2)n_1 N n_1 Ng(r)_{11}(4\pi r^2 \delta r)}{n_1 V_1 + n_2 V_2} = \frac{n_1 N^2 g(r)_{11}(2\pi r^2 \delta r)}{n_1 V_1 + n_2 V_2}$$

The number is halved to avoid counting the pairs twice. The following can be derived for pure component 1:

$$\text{Total potential energy at all radii} = U_1^{0-\infty} \tag{5.25}$$

$$= \frac{2\pi N^2 n_1}{n_1 V_1 + n_2 V_2} \int_{r=0}^{r=\infty} U_1 g(r)_{11} r^2 \, dr$$

$(n_1 V_1 + n_2 V_2)$ represents the total volume of the mixture. Similar expressions are obtained for the other components. Therefore, for the mixture,

$$\Delta U_{total}^{o-\infty} = \frac{2\pi N^2}{n_1 V_1 + n_2 V_2} \left[n_1^2 \int_{r=0}^{r=\infty} \Delta U_1 g(r)_{11} r^2 \, dr \right. \tag{5.26}$$

$$+ n_2^2 \int_{r=0}^{r=\infty} \Delta U_2 g(r)_{22} r^2 \, dr$$

$$\left. + 2n_1 n_2 \int_{r=0}^{r=\infty} \Delta U_{12} g(r)_{12} r^2 \, dr \right]$$

The partial molar energy of mixing of component 2 is obtained, as before, by differentiating with respect to n_2 at constant n_1, giving

$$\left(\frac{d \, \Delta U_2}{dn_2} \right)_{n_1} = 2\pi N^2 \left(\frac{n_1 V_1}{n_1 V_1 + n_2 V_2} \right)^2 V_2 \left[\frac{2}{V_1 V_2} \int_{r=0}^{r=\infty} \right. \tag{5.27}$$

$$\Delta U_{12} g(r)_{12} r^2 \, dr - \frac{1}{V_1^2} \int_{r=0}^{r=\infty} \Delta U_1 g(r)_{11} r^2 \, dr$$

$$\left. - \frac{1}{V_2^2} \int_{r=0}^{r=\infty} \Delta U_2 g(r)_{22} r^2 \, dr \right]$$

Substitution of $\Delta U_1^{o-\infty}$ from Eq. (5.25) and $\Delta U_2^{o-\infty}$ and $\Delta U_{12}^{o-\infty}$ from related expressions into Eq. (5.27) gives

$$\left(\frac{d \, \Delta \overline{U}_2}{dn_2} \right)_{n_1} = \phi_1^2 V_2 \left(\frac{2\Delta U_{12}^{o-\infty}}{V_1 V_2} - \frac{\Delta U_1^{o-\infty}}{V_1^2} - \frac{\Delta U_2^{o-\infty}}{V_2^2} \right) \tag{5.28}$$

D. Scatchard's Model

Scatchard [5] derived a similar model by calculating the total energy of a mixture, assuming that the mutual energy between two molecules depends only on the distance between them and that the molecular distribution is completely random. He expressed the energy of a mole of liquid (ΔU_1) as

$$\Delta U_1 = \Delta U_1^o - c \tag{5.29}$$

where ΔU_1^o is the energy under perfect gas conditions. Since ΔU_1^o is dependent only on temperature, it was considered additive and is ignored. c is the cohesive energy of the liquid, approximately equal to the energy of vaporization, ΔU^v. For a mixture, the total energy (ΔU_{total}) was given as

$$\Delta U_{total} = \frac{\text{total cohesive energy}}{\text{volume}} \tag{5.30}$$

Scatchard used the cohesive energy density (c), the energy of attraction per cubic centimeter, to express the energy of the mixture, thus:

$$\Delta U_{total} = \frac{c_1 X_1^2 V_1^2 + 2c_{12} X_1 X_2 V_1 V_2 + c_2 X_2^2 V_2^2}{X_1 V_1 + X_2 V_2} \tag{5.31}$$

$$\Delta U_1 = c_1 V_1 \qquad \text{and} \qquad \Delta U_2 = c_2 V_2$$

Hence the energy of mixing ΔU^m expressed by

$$-\Delta U^m = \Delta U_{total} + \Delta U_1 X_1 + \Delta U_2 X_2 \tag{5.32}$$

[the signs in Eq. (5.32) are reversed with respect to Eq. (5.13) because c represents energy of attraction] can be written in the form

$$-\Delta U^m = \frac{(c_1 X_1 V_1 + c_2 X_2 V_2)(X_1 V_1 + X_2 V_2) - c_1 X_1^2 V_1^2}{X_1 V_1 + X_2 V_2} \tag{5.33}$$

$$- \frac{2c_{12} X_1 X_2 V_1 V_2 - c_2 X_2^2 V_2^2}{X_1 V_1 + X_2 V_2}$$

which leads through

$$-\Delta U^m = \frac{c_1 X_1 V_1 X_2 V_2 + c_2 X_2 V_2 X_1 V_1 - 2c_{12} X_1 V_1 X_2 V_2}{X_1 V_1 + X_2 V_2} \tag{5.34}$$

to

$$\Delta U^m = -(c_1 + c_2 - 2c_{12}) \frac{X_1 X_2 V_1 V_2}{X_1 V_1 + X_2 V_2} \tag{5.35}$$

E. The Geometric Mean Assumption

One would surmise intuitively that the energy of a pair of unlike molecules would be the mean of the energies of the two equivalent like pairs. The application of this assumption to cohesive energy density in Eq. (5.35) gives $c_{12} = (c_1 c_2)^{1/2}$, and the equation simplifies to

$$\Delta U^m = -[(c_1)^{1/2} - (c_2)^{1/2}]^2 \phi_1 \phi_2 \tag{5.36}$$

The geometric mean is used, rather than the arithmetic mean, for the following reasons:

1. Forces of intermolecular attraction would be expected to behave in the same way as gravitational and electrostatic energies between point masses.
2. The geometric mean relationship has been confirmed experimentally [6,7].
3. If the unlike pair potential were the arithmetic mean of the two like pair potentials, the terms would cancel, giving a zero energy of mixing. This is contrary to experience.

F. Comparison of Equations Defining Energy of Mixing

Application of the geometric mean assumption to Eq. (5.28) derived from the radial distribution function model, gives

$$\Delta \overline{U}_2^m = \phi_1^2 V_2 \left[\left(\frac{\Delta U_1^{o-\infty}}{V_1^2} \right)^{1/2} - \left(\frac{\Delta U_2^{o-\infty}}{V_2^2} \right)^{1/2} \right]^2 \tag{5.37}$$

Scatchard's cohesive energy density is defined as the energy of attraction per cubic centimeter, so that the energy of attraction per mole will be $-\Delta U^{o-\infty} = cV$; therefore, integration of Eq. (5.36), followed by substitution of $-\Delta U^{o-\infty}/V$ for c, gives Eq. (5.37).

Hildebrand and Salstrom [3] described the mole fraction term X_1^2 as the probability that a given pair of ions is 1–1, while X_2^2 and X_1X_2 are the equivalent probabilities for 2–2 and 1–2 pairs, respectively. Such probabilities can be expressed in terms of $2\pi r^2 g(r)\delta r$, as in the radial distribution function model, but here $g(r)$ represents the radial distribution of a rigid, close-packed structure. Equation (5.22) can therefore be written in the form of Eqs. (5.27) and (5.37).

Application of the geometric mean assumption to Eq. (5.20) derived from van der Waals equation, gives

$$\Delta \overline{U}_2^m = \phi_1^2 V_2 \left[\left(\frac{a_1}{V_1} \right)^{1/2} - \left(\frac{a_2}{V_2} \right)^{1/2} \right]^2 \tag{5.38}$$

There is thus agreement between the three models.

Hildebrand and Scott considered that the vapor in equilibrium with its liquid is nearly ideal at ordinary temperatures, so that the energy per mole ($\Delta U^{o-\infty}$) can be equated with the energy of vaporization ΔU^v. The function δ defined by

$$\delta = \left(\frac{\Delta U^v}{V} \right)^{1/2} = \left(\frac{\Delta H^v - RT}{V} \right)^{1/2} \tag{5.39}$$

has been designated as the solubility parameter, so that Eq. (5.38) becomes

$$\Delta \overline{U}_2^m = \phi_1^2 V_2 (\delta_1 - \delta_2)^2 \tag{5.40}$$

The net free energy of mixing (ΔA^m) of a solute (2) in a solvent (1) is given by the van't Hoff isotherm,

$$\Delta A^m = -RT \ln f_2 \tag{5.41}$$

Since

$$\Delta A = \Delta U - T \Delta S \tag{5.42}$$

combination of Eqs. (5.41) and (5.42) gives the following for regular solutions:

$$\ln f_2 = - \frac{\Delta U}{RT} \tag{5.43}$$

where ΔS is ideal.

TABLE 5.1 Selected Solubility Parameters

Compound	Solubility parameter (Hildebrand's)		
	Hildebrand et al. [8]	Hoy [9]	Hansen and Beerbower [51][a]
Acetone	–	9.62	9.76
Benzene	9.2	9.16	9.06
Carbon di-sulfide	10.0	9.92	10.00
Carbon tetra-chloride	8.6	8.55	8.71
Chloroform	9.2	9.16	9.26
Cyclohexane	8.2	8.19	8.20
Diethyl ether	7.4	7.53	7.66
Ethyl acetate	–	8.91	8.85
Ethyl bromide	8.9	8.91	9.33
n-Heptane	7.4	7.50	7.5
n-Hexane	7.3	7.27	7.3
Naphthalene	9.9	–	9.89
n-Octane	7.5	7.54	7.6
1-Octanol	–	10.30	10.25

[a] Calculated from $\delta^2 = \delta_d^2 + \delta_p^2 + \delta_H^2$ (see page 219).

Ideal binary mixtures of liquids are miscible in all proportions (i.e., mole fraction solubility = 1); therefore, for a saturated solution of a liquid solute in a liquid solvent, which is a regular solution,

$$-\ln X_2 = \frac{V_2 \phi_1^2 (\delta_1 - \delta_2)^2}{RT} \tag{5.44}$$

Equation (5.44) shows the importance of the solubility parameter. The nearer δ_1 approaches δ_2, the greater will be the solubility. Furthermore, according to this treatment, when $\delta_1 = \delta_2$, the solution becomes ideal. The following applies to regular solutions of solids in liquids:

$$-\ln X_2 = \frac{\Delta H^f}{R} \frac{T_m - T}{T_m T} + \frac{V_2 \phi_1^2 (\delta_1 - \delta_2)^2}{RT} \tag{5.45}$$

The first term on the right-hand side is the expression derived for ideal solubility [Eq. (4.6)]. The second term therefore represents the energy, in excess of ideal, necessary to maintain the solute in solution. Also, since a = fX, the second term is equal to ln f_2, where f_2 is the activity coefficient. -RT ln f_2 is also termed the excess free energy of mixing, ΔG^E (since the entropy of mixing is zero in regular solutions). When ΔS^m is not ideal, as in nonregular solutions, it becomes part of ln f_2. This will be amplified later.

A selection of solubility parameters is given in Table 5.1; more comprehensive lists are given in the literature [8–10]. Solubility parameters were originally expressed in calories$^{1/2}$ cm$^{-3/2}$, awkward units, which have subsequently been contracted to a specific unit, the hildebrand. With the advent of SI units, one would expect solubility parameters to be expressed in J$^{1/2}$ m$^{-3/2}$, N$^{1/2}$ m^{-1}, or MPa, but none of these appears to have been adopted. In line with what seems to be accepted custom, solubility parameters will be quoted here in hildebrands, and the unit contracted to H.

III. THE TWO-DIMENSIONAL APPROACH TO REGULAR SOLUBILITY

The quasi-crystalline concept of solution involves the formation of a cavity in the solvent to accommodate a solute molecule, and the work done is assessed in terms of cohesive energy density. An alternative approach is to consider the energy associated with the loss of solvent-solvent and solute-solute interfaces and the creation of a new solute-solvent interface. This treatment gives rise to

$$-RT \ln X_2 = A_2 (\gamma_1 - \gamma_2)^2 \tag{5.46}$$

which has the same form as the regular solution expression [Eq. (5.44)], but cohesive energy density is replaced by surface tension (γ) and the volume fraction by the surface area of a solute molecule (A_2). It is assumed that the interfacial tension is the geometric mean of the two surface tensions. This is of doubtful validity, but no more so than when dealing with cohesive energy densities.

The work required to create a cavity in the solvent with a surface area (A_2) equivalent to that of one molecule of solute is equal to the product of the surface energy and the surface area. Since surface energy is numerically equal to surface tension, the work required $= (WC)_1 = \gamma_1 A_2$. Similarly, $(WC)_2 = \gamma_2 A_2$ units of energy are necessary to remove a solute molecule from bulk. The interaction of solute and solvent involves the disappearance of the newly created solute and solvent surfaces and the formation of a solute-solvent interface, giving a net work of adhesion (WA) of $(\gamma_{12} - \gamma_1 - \gamma_2)A_2$. The total work required is therefore $(WC)_1 + (WC)_2 + (WA) = -\gamma_{12}A_2$, which if equated to free energy of mixing yields

$$RT \ln X_2 = \gamma_{12}A_2 \qquad (5.47)$$

This equation assumes that mixing is random. The treatment has the advantage that interfacial tensions are readily measurable, whereas δ_{12} is not. It is, however, limited to mixtures of liquids whose polarities are sufficiently different for them to form an interface. The strength of the concept therefore lies in systems that deviate considerably from Raoult's law, in contrast to regular solution theory, which works best with liquids having similar polarities. The two approaches are therefore complementary and cover a wide range of solutes and solvents. The two-dimensional concept is thus most applicable to systems that are too polar in nature to fit regular solution relationships, and will therefore be considered in detail elsewhere.

For solid solutes, Eq. (5.47) must be expanded to

$$-\ln X_2 = \frac{\Delta H^f}{R} \frac{T_m - T}{T_m T} + \frac{\gamma_{12}A_2}{RT} \qquad (5.48)$$

to allow for the energy required to liquefy the solute. In such cases, interfacial tension should apply to the supercooled liquid solute.

Unfortunately, bulk interfacial tensions obtained experimentally are not a precise measure of intermolecular interfacial tension, which involves curved surfaces. Curvature correction factors (C), defined by

$$C = \frac{\gamma_{12}^m}{\gamma_{12}} \qquad (5.49)$$

are necessary to convert bulk values (γ_{12}) to microscopic values (γ_{12}^m) and these vary with the system under scrutiny. Factors for a series of alkyl-p-aminobenzoates in 22 pure and mixed solvents ranged from 0.39 to 0.59, with the majority lying between 0.50 and 0.55 [11].

Contributions of substituent groups to molecular surface are available in the literature [12], but these vary according to the method of calculation.

Example

Calculate the approximate mole fraction solubility of n-hexane in water at 25°C, using the following information.

Interfacial tension between n-hexane and water = 5.1×10^{-2} N m^{-1}

Surface area of a molecule of n-hexane = 3.19 nm^2

Avogadro's number = 6.02×10^{23} R = 8.315 J deg^{-1} mol^{-1}

Given that the observed solubility is 6.1×10^{-10} (mole fraction), calculate the curvature correction.

Solution:

$$-RT \ln X_2 = \gamma_{12} A_2$$

$$-\ln X_2 = \frac{3.19 \times 6.02 \times 10^{23} \times 5.1 \times 10^{-2}}{(10^{-9})^2 \times 8.315 \times 298} = 39.53$$

$$X_2 = 6.8 \times 10^{-18}$$

$$C = \frac{\ln X_{2(obs)}}{\ln X_{2(calc)}}$$

$$= \frac{21.22}{39.53}$$

$$= 0.54$$

IV. DETERMINATION OF SOLUBILITY PARAMETERS

A. From Heats of Vaporization

Heats of vaporization can be measured calorimetrically by differential scanning calorimetry (DSC) and differential thermal analysis (DTA) and introduced into Eq. (5.39) to calculate solubility parameters. The main disadvantage of the procedure is that material is lost by volatilization before the boiling point is reached, so that the observed heat capacity of the liquid will be higher than the true value, and the calculated heat of vaporization will represent a lower mass of sample than that originally weighed. Sealed pans are unsuitable, because of the high pressure that builds up. A technique [13] in which a pinhole in the lid of the pan is covered with a steel ball, which is removed with a magnet at the boiling point, is difficult to perform, and still loses some sample by pre-boiling-point volatilization. These losses can be corrected by analysis of the effluent.

The American Petroleum Institute Project 44 [14] is a reliable source of heats of vaporization. The *Handbook of Chemistry and Physics* [15] gives rounded-off figures which agree with those of Timmermann [16], who also gives the sources of his results.

B. From Vapor Pressures

Heats of vaporization may be obtained from the Clausius-Clapyron equation,

$$\frac{d \ln p}{dT} = \frac{\Delta H^V}{RT^2} \tag{5.50}$$

The procedure depends on the vapor obeying the perfect gas laws and is therefore accurate at low vapor pressures only. Ideal behavior can be checked by plotting ln p against 1/T, which should be rectilinear. Integration of Eq. (5.50) yields

$$\ln p_1 - \ln p_2 = \frac{\Delta H^V}{R}\left(\frac{1}{T_1} - \frac{1}{T_2}\right) \tag{5.51}$$

from which heat of vaporization can be calculated. Vapor pressures can often be obtained from the literature (e.g., Timmermans [16]). The isotenisoscope technique of Smith and Menzies [17,18] is a useful experimental method of determining vapor pressures.

Example

Solid iodine has vapor pressures of 41.3 and 207.9 Pa at 25 and 50°C, respectively. Use this information to estimate its solubility parameter. Gas constant = 1.98 cal mol^{-1} deg^{-1}; molar volume of iodine = 59 cm^3.

Solution:

Substituting in Eq. (5.51) yields

$$\ln \frac{207.9}{41.3} = \frac{\Delta H^V}{1.98}\left(\frac{1}{298} - \frac{1}{323}\right)$$

$$\Delta H^V = \frac{3.201}{2.597 \times 10^{-4}}$$

$$= 12.32 \text{ kcal mol}^{-1}$$

$$\delta = \left(\frac{\Delta H^V - RT}{V} \right)^{1/2}$$

$$= \left(\frac{12,320 - 1.98 \times 298}{59} \right)^{1/2}$$

$$\delta = 14.1 \text{ H}$$

When conditions are such that the vapor does not behave ideally, the more precise form of the Clausius-Clapyron equation must be used:

$$\frac{d \ln p}{dT} = \frac{\Delta H^V}{P(V_g - V_L)T^2} \tag{5.52}$$

where V_g and V_L are volumes of gas and liquid, respectively. Hoy [9] substituted for $P(V_g - V_L)$ from

$$P(V_g - V_L) = \frac{RT}{M} \sqrt{1 - \frac{PT_c^3}{P_c T^3}} \tag{5.53}$$

in Eq. (5.52) and obtained

$$\Delta H^V = \frac{d \ln p}{dT} \frac{RT^2}{MP} \sqrt{1 - \frac{PT_c^3}{P_c T^3}} \tag{5.54}$$

where M is molecular weight and P_c and T_c are critical pressure and temperature, from which reliable heats of vaporization could be calculated. Combination of Eqs. (5.53) and (5.54) with Antoine's equation,

$$\log p = \frac{-B}{T + C} + A \tag{5.55}$$

leads to

$$\delta = \left[\frac{RT}{M} \sqrt{1 - \frac{PT_c^3}{P_c T^3}} \frac{2.303BT^2}{(T + C)^2} \right]^{1/2} \tag{5.56}$$

A, B, and C are Antoine's constants [19].

Conditions in the region of critical are usually considerably removed from those at which solubility parameters are required. Hoy [9] circumvented this problem by using the empirically derived expression

$$\Delta H^V = \Delta H^o \exp\ (-mT) \qquad\qquad (5.57)$$

where ΔH^o is the heat of vaporization at a standard temperature and m is a constant. This allowed him to extrapolate from critical regions to the temperature of interest. He published an extensive list of solubility parameters determined in this way. Some of these are reproduced in Table 5.1. Ng [20] obtained heats of vaporization at temperatures at which vapor pressures were too low to measure, by calculating heats of vaporization at a series of elevated temperatures, using Eq. (5.57).

Example

The vapor pressures of *t*-butylcyclohexane at elevated temperatures are as follows:

Temperature, T (°K)	357.0	369.2	382.3	399.2	420.1	443.1	445.1
Vapor pressure, p (mmHg)	48.0	77.5	124.8	217.4	402.8	732.4	768.6

Given that the molar volume of *t*-butylcyclohexane is 173 $cm^3\ mol^{-1}$ at 25°C calculate its solubility parameter. R = 1.987 cal $mol^{-1}\ deg^{-1}$.

Solution:

$$\log\frac{p_1}{p_2} = \frac{\Delta H^V}{2.303R}\ \ \frac{1}{T_2} - \frac{1}{T_1}$$

Therefore, for the first two pairs of results,

$$\log\frac{77.5}{48.0} = \frac{\Delta H^V}{2.303 \times 1.987}\ \ \frac{1}{369.2} - \frac{1}{357.0}$$

$$\Delta H^V = \frac{0.2081 \times 2.303 \times 1.987}{9.256 \times 10^{-5}} = 10,286\ \text{cal mol}^{-1}$$

Results for the other temperatures, together with log enthalpies, are as follows:

ΔH^V	10,286	10,202	9961	9834	9617	9455
log ΔH^V	4.021	4.009	3.998	3.993	3.983	3.976

$$\Delta H^V = H^O \exp(-mT)$$

Therefore, taking logs, we have

$$\log \Delta H^V = \log H^O - mT$$

so that a plot of log ΔH^V against T will have a slope of -m and can be extrapolated to 298 K.

Linear regression of T against log ΔH^V yields

$$\log \Delta H^V = 4.1762 - 4.4154 \times 10^{-4} T$$

giving for T = 298 K,

$$\log \Delta H^V = 4.1762 - 4.4154 \times 10^{-4} \times 298 = 4.0446$$

Therefore,

$$\Delta H^V_{298} = 11,082 \text{ cal mol}^{-1}$$

$$\delta = \left(\frac{\Delta H^V - RT}{V} \right)^{1/2} = \left(\frac{11,082 - 1.987 \times 298}{173} \right)^{1/2} = 7.79 \text{ H}$$

C. From Boiling Points

Equation (5.58) has been derived empirically as a means of determining heats of vaporization, in cal mol^{-1}, of saturated hydrocarbons [8]. T_b represents boiling point in degrees Kelvin. The equation has been used extensively and has not always been limited to saturated hydrocarbons. It is frequently referred to as Hildebrand's rule.

$$\Delta H^V = 23.7T_b + 0.02T_b^2 - 2950 \tag{5.58}$$

Some solubility parameters calculated from this equation are compared in Table 5.1 with those obtained by other methods. It can be seen that predictions are usually quite good for saturated hydrocarbons.

D. From Refractive Indices

The intermolecular energy between molecules with low or zero dipole moments is dependent mainly on dispersion forces. The intermolecular pair potential energy (u) arising from dispersion forces between two like molecules is given by

$$u = -\frac{3\alpha^2 I}{4r^6} \tag{5.59}$$

where I is the ionization potential, α electron polarizability, and r intermolecular distance. Keller and others [21] suggested that since I varies only slightly from molecule to molecule, then

$$u \propto -\frac{\alpha^2}{r^6} \tag{5.60}$$

and

$$\delta \propto \frac{\alpha}{V} \tag{5.61}$$

α/V is related to refractive index (n) through the Lorenz-Lorenz equation

$$\frac{\alpha}{V} = \frac{0.75\pi N(n^2 - 1)}{n^2 + 2} \tag{5.62}$$

which leads to

$$\delta = \frac{C(n^2 - 1)}{n^2 + 2} \tag{5.63}$$

where C is a constant.

Keller et al. [21] plotted the solubility parameters of 96 hydrocarbons against their Lorenz-Lorenz functions and obtained a rectilinear plot with the 43 normal and branched alkanes, 13 cycloalkanes, and 12 alkenes and alkynes, giving a proportionality constant of C = 30.7. The remaining 28 hydrocarbons were aromatic; their results followed a smooth curve, which deviated from the rectilinear aliphatic plot but could be merged with it to give an overall uniform plot for all the 96 compounds, fitting the polynomial

$$\delta = -2.24 + 53x - 58x^2 + 22x^3 \tag{5.64}$$

where $x = (n^2 - 1)/(n^2 + 2)$. The authors warned that the relationship applied in principle only to hydrocarbons, but found that it could be extended to some nonhydrocarbons, such as carbon tetrachloride and carbon disulfide, which were expected to exhibit negligible polar interactions. A standard deviation of 0.2 H was claimed for the hydrocarbons, extending to 0.4 H when the other compounds were included. They concluded that the method was suitable only for measuring solubility parameters of lower molecular weight aliphatic and alicyclic hydrocarbons, but recommended it for determining the dispersion components of three-dimensional solubility parameters. This application will be described later.

Keller et al. [21] calculated solubility parameters from the Hildebrand rule [Eq. (5.58)]. James et al. [22] investigated the method using solubility parameters calculated from vapor pressures and found excellent correlation between solubility parameter and Lorenz-Lorenz function with straight-chain saturated hydrocarbons, but when branched-chain hydrocarbons were included, considerable scatter resulted. Figure 5.6 illustrates this weakness.

E. Using Substituent Constants

Equation (5.36) can be written in the form

$$\Delta U^m = \phi_1 \phi_2 \left(\frac{U_1}{V_1} - \frac{U_2}{V_2} \right)^2 \tag{5.65}$$

where U represents cohesive energy density per mole and V is molar volume. Small [23] suggested that for a mixture of n_1 moles of liquid 1 and n_2 moles of liquid 2, this equation is equivalent to

$$\Delta U^m (n_1 V_1 + n_2 V_2) = n_1 (U_1 V_1) + n_2 (U_2 V_2) \tag{5.66}$$

which implies that UV is an additive property. He introduced the parameter, molar attraction constant (F), which he defined by

$$F = UV \tag{5.67}$$

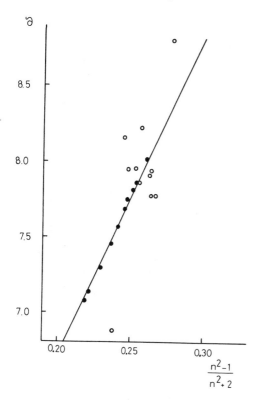

FIGURE 5.6 Relationship between solubility parameters and Lorentz-Lorentz functions of saturated hydrocarbons. ●, Normal alkanes; ○, other alkanes.

and which can be used through

$$\delta = \frac{\Sigma F}{V} \tag{5.68}$$

to calculate solubility parameters. Small [23] calculated a selection of molar attraction constants from the vapor pressures and molar volumes of a range of liquids. These are reproduced in Table 5.2.

The calculation of solubility parameters from Small's constants is simple; for example, for n-octane,

$$\delta = \frac{2 \times 214 + 6 \times 133}{164} = 7.48$$

TABLE 5.2 Molar Attraction Constants

Group	F ($cal^{1/2}$ $cm^{-3/2}$)		Group	F ($cal^{1/2}$ $cm^{-3/2}$)	
	Small [23]	Rheineck and Lin [24]		Small [23]	Rheineck and Lin [24]
CH_3	214	198	H	80–100	–
$-CH_2-$	133	140	OH	–	444
$CH_2=$	190	–	O (ether)	70	–
$CH-$	28	59	CHO	355–375[a]	347
$-CH(CH_3)_2$	456[a]	455	CO (ketone)	275	–
$-CH=$	111	–	COOH	390–410[a]	661
$-C-$	-93	–	COO (ester)	310	–
$C=$	19	–	CH_3COO	524[a]	540
$CHC-$	285	–	CN	410	–

Group			Group		
-C=C-	222	-	Cl (mean)	260	243
-CH=CH$_2$-	301[a]	298	Cl (single)	270	243
Phenyl	735	730	Cl (as in CCl$_2$)	260	243
Cyclohexyl	-	785	Cl (as in CCl$_3$)	250	243
Phenylene (o, m, p)	658	-	Br (single)	340	-
Naphthyl	1,146	-	I (single)	425	-
Five-membered ring	105–115	-	CF$_2$ (n-hydrocarbons)	150	-
Six-membered ring	95–105	-	CF$_3$ (n-hydrocarbons)	270	-
Conjugation	20–30	-	S (sulfides)	225	-
NO$_3$ (nitrates)	440	-	SH (thiols)	315	-
NO$_2$ (aliphatic nitro)	440	-	PO$_4$ (organic phosphates)	500	-
NH$_2$	-	233			

[a]Calculated by Rheineck and Lin from Small's values.

TABLE 5.3 Solubility Parameters Calculated from Group Numbers

Compound	Molar volume[a] (cc)	Measured[a]	Solubility parameter			
			Calculated			
			Small [23]	Hoy [9]	Rheineck[a] and Lin[b]	Fedors[c]
n-Hexane	132	7.3	7.27	7.26	7.18	7.29
n-Octane	164	7.5	7.48	7.44	7.49	7.55
Benzene	89	9.2	9.27	9.15	9.97	9.19
Toluene	107	8.9	8.87	9.00	8.68	9.14
Chloroform	81	9.2	9.60	10.4	11.3	8.77
Methyl chloride	55[d]	9.7[d]	8.74	8.82	8.01	8.22
Ethyl chloride	74	8.3	8.34	8.38	8.10	8.30

Propyl chloride	88[d]	8.5[d]	8.52	8.54	8.16	8.34
Chlorobenzene	102	9.5	9.85	9.56	10.2	9.95
Naphthalene	123	9.9	10.0	10.2	–	10.4
i-Octanol	158[d]	10.3[d]	–	–	10.3	10.3
Diethyl ether	105	7.4	7.28	7.71	–	7.25
Acetone	74	9.9[d]	9.50	9.39	–	9.07
Ethyl acetate	98.5	8.1	8.84	9.03	8.71	8.74

[a]Taken from Hildebrand et al. [8] unless otherwise stated.
[b]Molar volumes calculated using the method of Rheineck and Lin [24].
[c]Molar volumes calculated using the method of Fedors [26].
[d]Taken from Barton [10].

179

which agrees well with the observed values (Table 5.1); 164 is the experimental molar volume of *n*-octane [8]. Small claimed that the system was particularly reliable for hydrocarbons and admitted that for other compounds the additivity is not as strong. Some calculated results are shown in Table 5.3. Predictions appear to be good for aromatic and other hydrocarbons, but at best only approximate for the other compounds. The failure to predict solubility parameters for chlorinated hydrocarbons was attributed to steric factors. Examination of the values for chloroform and the alkyl chlorides in Table 5.3 offers support for this observation.

High-powered computers were not available in 1953, when Small published his results. Using sophisticated calculating equipment, Hoy [9] was able to reexamine Small's molar attraction constants over a broader range of compounds, using multiple regression analysis, and published a new set of values. These are reproduced in Table 5.4. With these constants the calculation is slightly different from Small's, in that the base value of 135.1 must be added to the energy term for all compounds. The solubility parameter of *n*-octane is now given by

$$\delta = \frac{2 \times 148.3 + 6 \times 131.5 + 135.1}{164} = 7.44$$

Solubility parameters calculated by Hoy's procedure are given in Table 5.3.

Rheineck and Lin [24] found that plots of solubility parameter against carbon number for various homologous series were curved and varied in form from one series to another. In contrast, both ΔU and V gave a series of parallel straight lines, each homologous series having a characteristic intercept. They therefore separated the two properties and assigned group contributions for molar volumes and molar cohesive energy densities. These are reproduced in Table 5.5. The solubility parameter for *n*-octane given by this procedure is calculated as follows:

$$\delta = \left[\frac{2 \times 990 + 6 \times 1230}{2 \times 34.0 + 6 \times 16.5} \right]^{1/2} = 7.49$$

With some series, a correction was necessary for the number of carbon atoms in the alkyl chain; these were rectilinearly related to the chain length and are given in Table 5.5. Applying the procedure to *n*-octanol yields

$$\delta = \left[\frac{990 + 7 \times 1230 + 7830 - 8 \times 80}{34.0 + 7 \times 16.5 + 8.7} \right]^{1/2} = 10.30$$

TABLE 5.4 Hoy's Molar Attraction Constants

Group	Molar attraction $[(\text{cal cc})^{1/2} \text{ mol}^{-1}]$	Group	Molar attraction $[(\text{cal cc})^{1/2} \text{ mol}^{-1}]$
$-CH_3$	148.3	$-S-$	209.42
$-CH_2-$	131.5	Cl_2	342.67
$>CH-$	85.99	Cl primary	205.06
$\underset{|}{-\overset{|}{C}-}$	32.03	Cl secondary	208.27
		Cl aromatic	161.0
$CH_2=$	126.54	Br	257.88
$-CH=$	121.53	Br aromatic	205.60
$>C=$	84.51	F	41.33
$-CH=$ aromatic	117.12	Structural features	
$-C=$ aromatic	98.12	Conjugation	23.26
$-O-$ (ether, acetal)	114.98	Cis	-7.13
$-O-$ epoxide	176.20	Trans	-13.50
$-COO-$	326.58	Four-membered ring	77.76
$>C=O$	262.96	Five-membered ring	20.99
$-CHO$	292.64	Six-membered ring	-23.44
$(CO)_2O$	567.29	Ortho substitution	9.69
$-OH\rightarrow$	225.84	Meta substitution	6.6

TABLE 5.4 (Continued)

Group	Molar attraction [(cal cc)$^{1/2}$ mol^{-1}]	Group	Molar attraction [(cal cc)$^{1/2}$ mol^{-1}]
—H acidic dimer	-50.47	Para substitution	40.33
OH aromatic	170.99		22.56
NH$_2$	226.56		
—NH—	180.03		
—N—	61.08		62.5
C≡N	354.56		
NCO	358.66	Base value	135.1

TABLE 5.5 Molar Attraction Constants and Group Contributions to Molar Volume

Group	Contribution to molar volume (ml mol^{-1})	Molar attraction constant (cal mol^{-1})	Correction for chain length (cal mol^{-1} number of carbon atoms^{-1})
CH	-0.5	970	0
CH$_2$	16.5	1230	0
CH$_3$	34.0	990	0
OH	8.7	7830	-80
NH$_2$	19.0	2570	-90
Cl	24.0	2790	-60
CHO	26.0	4340	-170
COOH	27.0	7830	+220
CH$_3$CO	42.5	–	–
CH=CH$_2$	44.0	2000	0
CH$_2$COO	50.5	5550	-100
CH(CH$_3$)$_2$	67.5	2950	0
Phenyl	75.0	7450	-220
Cyclohexyl	95.0	7040	-220

Source: Ref. 24.

The solubility parameter calculations described above assume that the solute is molecularly dispersed in solution. Hoy [9] suggested that for solutes, such as acetic acid, which dimerize in organic solvents, the solubility parameter should be corrected by multiplying by $1/(2)^{1/2}$. Similarly, he considered that allowance should be made for intramolecular hydrogen bonding and quoted a molar attraction constant for hydrogen-bonded hydroxyl of 225.84 for this purpose.

Jayasri and Yaseen [25] made a statistical evaluation of published solubility parameters. They ignored values considered to be in doubt and combined the remainder to predict the most probable results. Their calculations involved least squares linear correlation of δ with $1/V$, a relationship which they considered better than direct correlation of solubility parameter with molar volume.

Fedors [26] approached the problem in the same way as Rheineck and Lin, by treating energy of mixing and molar volume separately. Substituent constants are given in Table 5.6. These are summed and the solubility parameter calculated as the square root of the sum of the energy of mixing substituent constants divided by the sum of the molar volume substituent constants. Thus for:

1-Octanol, $CH_3(CH_2)_7OH$

	$\Delta\Delta U$	ΔV
CH_3	1125	33.5
$(CH_2)_7$	8260	112.7
OH	7120	10.0
	16505	156.2

$$\delta = \sqrt{\frac{16505}{156.2}} = 10.28 \ H$$

Observed solubility parameter = 10.3 H

Fedor's approach to cyclic compounds was to open the rings, treat the resultant structure as an open-chain compound, and then apply a correction for ring closure; for example:

Naphthalene,

The rings are opened to give

$$=CH-C-CH=CH-CH=$$
$$\|$$
$$=CH-CH=CH-C-CH=$$

from which the solubility parameter is calculated as follows:

	$\Delta\Delta U$	ΔV
$(-CH=)_8$	8,240	108.0
$(-C=)_2$	2,060	-11.0
2 × six-membered rings	500	32.0
5 conjugated carbons	2,000	-11.0
	12,800	118.0

TABLE 5.6 Fedor's Substituent Constants

Group	ΔΔU (cal mol⁻¹)	ΔV (cm³ mol⁻¹)	Group	ΔΔU (cal mol⁻¹)	ΔV (cm³ mol⁻¹)
CH_3	1,125	33.5	CH_2	1,180	16.1
CH	820	-1.0	C	350	-19.2
$H_2C=$	1,030	28.5	$-CH=$	1,030	13.5
$C\equiv$	1,030	-5.5	$HC\equiv$	920	27.4
$-C=$	1,690	6.5	Ring closure (five or more atoms)	250	16
Ring closure (three or four atoms)	750	18	Conjugation (each double bond in ring)	400	-2.2
Halogen attached to C=)	-20% of ΔΔU of halogen	4.0	CO_3 (carbonate)	4,200	22.0
$COOH$	6,600	28.5	COO	4,300	18.0
CO	4,150	10.8	CHO	5,100	22.3
$(COO)_2$ (oxalate)	6,400	37.3	C_2O_3 (anhydride)	7,300	30.0
$HCOO$ (formate)	4,300	32.5	$CONH_2$	10,000	17.5
$CONH$	8,000	9.5	CON	7,050	-7.7
$HCON$	6,600	11.3	$HCONH$	10,500	27.0
$COCl$	5,000	38.0	NH_2	3,000	19.2
			N	1,000	-9.0

TABLE 5.6 (Continued)

Group	ΔΔU (cal mol⁻¹)	ΔV (cm³ mol⁻¹)	Group	ΔΔU (cal mol⁻¹)	ΔV (cm³ mol⁻¹)
NH	2,000	4.5	CN	6,100	24.0
—N=	2,800	5.0	NO$_2$ (aromatic)	3,670	32.0
NO$_2$ (aliphatic)	7,000	24.0	NO$_2$ (nitrite)	2,800	33.5
NO$_3$	5,000	33.5	NCO	6,800	35.0
SCN	4,800	37.0	NF	1,210	24.5
NF$_2$	1,830	33.1	OH	7,120	10.0
O	800	3.8	PO$_4$	5,000	28.0
OH (Disubstituted or on adjacent C atoms)	5,220	13.9	SH	3,450	28.0
			S$_2$	5,700	23.0
PO$_3$	3,400	22.7	SO$_4$	6,800	31.6
S	3,380	12	F (disubstituted)	850	20.0
SO$_3$	4,500	27.6	F (trisubstituted)	550	22.0
F	1,000	18.0	Cl	2,760	24.0

CF$_2$ (perfluoro compounds)	1,020	23.0	Cl (disubstituted)	2,300	26.0
			Cl (trisubstituted)	1,800	27.3
CF$_3$ (perfluoro compounds)	1,020	57.5	I	4,550	31.5
Br	3,700	30.0	I (disubstitued)	4,000	33.3
Br (disubstituted)	2,950	31.0	I (trisubstituted)	3,900	37.0
Br (trisubstituted)	2,550	32.4	Ga	3,300	-2.0
B	3,300	-2.0	Tl	3,300	-2.0
Al	3,300	-2.0	Ge	1,930	-1.5
In	3,300	-2.0	Pb	4,100	2.5
Si	810	0.0	As	3,100	7.0
Sn	2,700	1.5	Bi	5,100	9.5
P	2,250	-1.0	Te	4,800	17.4
Sb	3,900	8.9	Cd	4,250	6.5
Se	4,100	16.0			
Zn	3,460	2.5			
Hg	5,450	7.5			

Source: Ref. 26.

$$\delta = \sqrt{\frac{12,800}{118.0}} = 10.42 \text{ H}$$

Observed solubility parameter = 9.9 H

The four methods of calculating solubility parameters are compared in Table 5.3. Sometimes, as with *n*-hexane and *n*-octane, all methods give good predictions, whereas with others, such as ethyl acetate, all predictions are disappointing. With most of the compounds in Table 5.3, the quality of the prediction varies from one method to another, and none of the methods gives the best predictions overall. It is therefore recommended that all methods be used to estimate new solubility parameters, and that the most appropriate figure be selected after scrutiny of the four results.

The substituent constant approach can be used for calculating solubility parameters of simple compounds, but it is more useful for complex molecules when the solubility parameter of a closely related compound is known. The accuracy of the method obviously decreases with increasing molecular complexity.

F. From Solubilities

The solubility parameter of a solute can be determined by measuring its solubilities in a series of solvents or solvent blends and plotting solubility against solubility parameter of solvent. Chertkoff and Martin [27] determined the solubility parameter of benzoic acid by this procedure, using a series of binary mixtures of *n*-hexane, ethyl acetate, ethanol, and water as solvents. An approximately parabolic plot was obtained, giving a plateau region from about 10.2 to 11.8 H, and similar results were obtained with other solvent mixtures. Later work [28] pinpointed the solubility parameter at 11.2 H. Precise results can be obtained by plotting a first derivative curve and observing where it crosses the zero axis.

Example

The solubilities of testosterone propionate in a series of toluene-nitrobenzene blends, together with the corresponding solvent solubility parameters, are given below. Prepare a first derivative plot and thereby calculate the solubility parameter of the solute.

Mole fraction solubility	0.199	0.214	0.225	0.231	0.234	0.234	0.230	0.227
Solvent blend solubility parameter	8.9	9.02	9.15	9.27	9.41	9.55	9.86	10.0

Solution:

For the first two pairs of results:

Mean solubility parameter = $\dfrac{8.9 + 9.02}{2}$ = 8.96

Solubility parameter increment = $\Delta \delta_1$ = 9.02 − 8.9 = 0.12

Mole fraction solubility increment = ΔX_2 = 0.214 − 0.199 = 0.015

$\dfrac{\Delta X_2}{\Delta \delta_1} = \dfrac{0.015}{0.12} = 0.125$

Similarly:

Mean solubility parameter	9.09	9.21	9.34	9.48	9.71	9.93
$\Delta X_2 / \Delta \delta_1$	0.085	0.050	0.021	0.000	-0.013	-0.021

A plot of mean solubility against $\Delta X_2 / \Delta \delta_1$ yields Fig. 5.7. The line crosses the ordinate at about 9.48, indicating a solubility parameter of 9.5 H.

James and Roberts [29] determined the solubility parameters of some testosterone esters by plotting log solubility against solvent solubility parameter, using a range of different solvents, and obtained two intersecting straight lines, from which the solute solubility parameter could be located precisely. It appears, however, that their choice of solvents was fortunate, since when the work was repeated with a larger range of solvents [22], the plot showed considereable scatter which could not be resolved into any simple relationship.

When solvent blends are used, determinations should be made using more than one pair of solvents, since a specific solute-solvent interaction could give rise to a misleading result. This is illustrated in Fig. 5.8, which shows solubility-solubility parameter plots for testosterone propionate in three different sets of binary solvent mixtures. The plots are entirely different, and it has been suggested that the fact that testosterone propionate forms some 1:2 complexes with 1,2-dichloroethane through its 3-keto carbonyl, and only 1:1 complexes with the other solvents [30], could be significant.

Solubility parameters can also be determined from solubilities by substitution into Eq. (5.44) or (5.45). Again, determinations should be carried out with more than one solvent. Anomalous

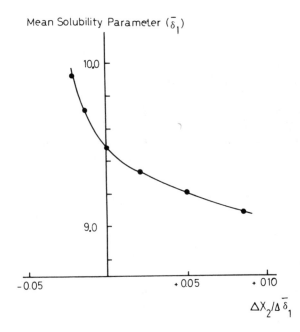

Mean Solubility Parameter $(\bar{\delta}_1)$

FIGURE 5.7 Solubilities of testosterone propionate in nitrobenzene-toluene blends, second derivative plot.

results are possible even with apparently inert solvents; for example, the method gave solubility parameters for testosterone propionate between 9.9 and 10.0 H in normal paraffins and 10.4 H in cyclohexane [22]. The disagreement was shown to be due to differences in molecular geometry.

Cavé et al. [31] described a multiple regression method of interpreting solubility-solubility parameter plots which do not give a sharp maximum. If the regular solubility equation (5.45) is expanded to give

$$-\ln X_2 = \frac{\Delta H^f}{R} \left(\frac{1}{T} - \frac{1}{T_m} \right) + \frac{V_2 \phi_1^2}{RT} (\delta_1^2 - 2\delta_1 \delta_2 + \delta_2^2) \qquad (5.69)$$

it can be rearranged to give

$$\frac{1}{\phi_1^2} \left[\ln X_2 + \frac{\Delta H^f}{R} \left(\frac{1}{T} - \frac{1}{T_m} \right) \right] = -\frac{V_2}{RT} \delta_2^2 + \frac{2V_2}{RT} \delta_1 \delta_2 \qquad (5.70)$$
$$-\frac{V_2}{RT} \delta_1^2$$

This can be expressed in the general form

$$z = a + b\delta_1 + c\delta_1^2 \tag{5.71}$$

where

$$z = \frac{1}{\phi_1^2} \left[\ln X_2 + \frac{\Delta H^f}{R} \left(\frac{1}{T} - \frac{1}{T_m} \right) \right] \tag{5.72}$$

$$a = -\frac{V_2}{RT} \delta_2^2 \tag{5.73}$$

$$b = \frac{2V_2}{RT} \delta_2 \tag{5.74}$$

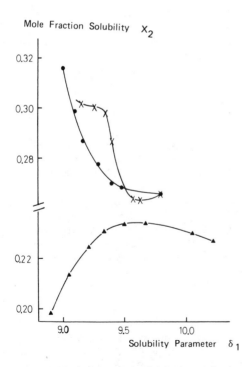

FIGURE 5.8 Solubilities of testosterone propionate in solvent blends. x, Nitrobenzene-toluene; ▲, 1,2-dichloroethane-*cis*-1,2-dichloro-ethylene; ●, 1,2-dichloroethane-*trans*-1,2-dichloroethylene.

and

$$c = -\frac{V_2}{RT} \tag{5.75}$$

Values of z and δ_1 for a range of solvents or solvent blends can be inserted into Eq. (5.71), and a, b, and c evaluated by multiple regression analysis. δ_2 is then calculated as $-2a/b$.

G. From Dielectric Constants

Attempted correlations between dielectric constants and solubilities have been described in Chapter 3. In those investigations, the solubilities of a given solute in a series of solvent blends were found to go through a maximum at a dielectric constant characteristic of the solute. Similar plots have been obtained when solubilities were plotted against solvent solubility parameter, and the use of such plots to determine solute solubility parameters is described in the preceding section. This resemblance was noted by Paruta et al. [32], who followed the observation through by suggesting that dielectric constants, which are known for most solvents and are also easily determined experimentally, could be used to predict solubility parameters. Their results are shown in Fig. 5.9. Most of the solvents, particularly those with high solubility parameters, closely follow

$$\delta = 0.22\varepsilon + 7.5 \tag{5.76}$$

where ε represents dielectric constant, but there were several solvents that deviated considerably from the equation. It was pointed out that the best correlation occurred, fortuitously, with the solvents of pharmaceutical interest; those that deviated were nonpolar solvents, which are of less pharmaceutical significance.

A more critical assessment [33] found that dielectric constants and solubility parameters were related, provided that the solvent systems were restricted to liquids exhibiting similar bonding characteristics. The procedure failed when there was a wide variation in the chemical nature of the solvents.

H. By Chromatography

Thermodynamic parameters of both mobile and stationary phases have been determined by gas-liquid chromatography (GLC) [34]. The method has the advantage that the solution can be considered as infinitely dilute. The quantity of mobile phase that is dissolved is

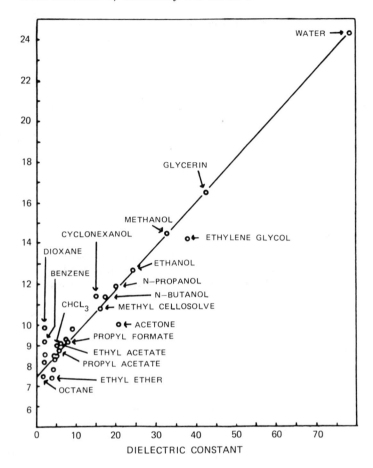

FIGURE 5.9 Plot of solubility parameters of common solvents against their respective dielectric constants. (From Ref. 32.)

expressed as the specific retention volume (V_g), the volume of vapor absorbed by 1 g of stationary phase, corrected to standard operating conditions. It is calculated from [35]

$$V_g = \frac{t_R F}{w_L} J_2^3 \frac{760}{P_o}$$

(5.77)

where t_R is retention time, F the flow rate at normal temperature and pressure, and P_o the outlet pressure in mmHg. J_2^3 is a correction to the flow rate for the pressure gradient along the column the inlet pressure P_i being greater than P_o, and can be calculated from [36]

$$J_2^3 = \frac{3[(P_i/P_o)^2 - 1]}{2[(P_i/P_o)^3 - 1]} \tag{5.78}$$

Since V_g is proportional to concentration, the enthalpy of solution (ΔH^S) can be determined from

$$\ln \frac{V_{g(1)}}{V_{g(2)}} = - \frac{\Delta H^S}{R} \left(\frac{1}{T_1} - \frac{1}{T_2} \right) \tag{5.79}$$

by determining specific retention volumes ($V_{g(1)}$, $V_{g(2)}$) at two temperatures, T_1 and T_2. DiPaola-Baranyi et al. [34] obtained enthalpies of solution of a range of hydrocarbons by determining specific retention volumes at a series of temperatures and plotting $\ln V_g$ against $1/T$.

Partial enthalpy of mixing of the solute ($\Delta \bar{H}_2^m$)* can be obtained by a similar treatment of the solute activity coefficient (f_2):

$$\Delta \bar{H}_2^m = \frac{d \ln f_2}{d(1/T)} \tag{5.80}$$

It is the enthalpy required to overcome nonideal interactions in the solution and as expressed above, represents the solution of a liquid. In contrast, the energy of solution obtained by GLC represents solution of a vapor in a liquid. The difference between ΔH^S and $\Delta \bar{H}_2^m$ is therefore equal to the enthalpy of vaporization (ΔH_2^v) of the solute. This is expressed in

$$\Delta H_2^v = \Delta \bar{H}_2^m - \Delta H^S \tag{5.81}$$

---

*The terminology of inverse chromatography refers to the compound injected to the column as the solvent and symbolizes parameters relating to it with the subscript 1. The stationary phase, although it is actually the solvent, is given the subscript 2. The convention is not used here but is common in the chromatography literature. The mobile phase is frequently called the probe molecule, to lessen the confusion.

which provides a means of calculating solubility parameters, using Eq. (5.39). DiPaola-Baranyi [34] quoted $\Delta \overline{H}_2^m = 2676$ cal mol^{-1} and $\Delta H^S = -6117$ cal mol^{-1} for n-octane in polymethyl acrylate at 100°C, which on substitution in Eq. (5.81) yields $\Delta H_2^V = 8.79$ kcal mol^{-1}, in good agreement with an experimental value of 8.69 kcal mol^{-1} at 100.5°C. Solute activity coefficients were calculated [34] from*

$$\ln f_2 = \ln \frac{273R}{P_2^o V_g M_1} - \frac{P_2^o(B_{22} - V_2)}{RT} \qquad (5.82)$$

where P_2^o is the saturated vapor pressure and V_2 the molar volume of the liquid solute, and M_1 is the molecular weight of the stationary phase. B_{22} is the second virial coefficient, which was obtained from Eq. (2.6) [38].

Some specimen calculations are now given to demonstrate the arithmetic of the procedure.

Example

Calculation of Specific Retention Volume (V_g) [35] using Silicone 702 as stationary phase at 56.2°C given the following information.

---

*Patterson et al. [37] pointed out that Eq. (5.82) contains the molecular weight of the stationary phase, which is frequently unknown, and suggested that the weight fraction activity coefficient (a_2/w_2) is a better parameter. a_2 is the activity of the solute and w_2 is defined as the weight of solute divided by the weight of solvent. The weight fraction activity coefficient is therefore the rational activity coefficient (f_2), multiplied by the ratio of solvent to solute molecular weight (M_1/M_2). Thus

$$\ln \frac{a_2}{w_2} = \ln f_2 + \ln \frac{M_1}{M_2}$$

and substitution in Eq. (5.82) yields

$$\ln \frac{a_2}{w_a} = \ln \frac{273R}{P_2^o V_g M_1} + \frac{P_2^o}{RT}(B_{22} - V_2) \qquad (5.83)$$

1. The chart recorder showed that 58.2 min had elapsed from the time of injection to the peak maximum for methyl propionate, with a corresonding value of 2.7 min for an unreactive gas (hydrogen).

    Corrected retention time (t_R) = 58.2 − 2.7 = 55.5 min

2. The flow rate was 11.0 ml of nitrogen per minute at STP, giving an uncorrected retention volume of 55.5 × 11.0 = 610.5 ml.

3. The pressure at the inlet of the column (P_i) was 123 cm mercury; at the outlet (P_o) it was 78.1 cm, and the atmospheric pressure was 76 cm. The correction factor for the pressure drop across the column is therefore,

$$J_2^3 = \frac{3(123.0/78.1)^2 - 1}{2(123.0/78.1)^3 - 1} = 0.765$$

and the pressure drop across the flow meter = 76.0/78.1.

4. The weight of stationary phase was 2.82 g.

$$V_g = \frac{610.5 \times 0.765 \times 76.0}{78.1 \times 2.82} = 161 \text{ ml}$$

Example

Calculation of Enthalpy of Solution (ΔH^S). The specific retention volumes of a hydrocarbon during GLC determinations were 563 ml at 90°C and 362 ml at 110°C. Enthalpy of solution over this range is therefore given by

$$\ln 563 - \ln 362 = \frac{-\Delta H^S}{1.98}\left(\frac{1}{363} - \frac{1}{383}\right)$$

$$\Delta H^S = \frac{-1.98(6.333 - 5.892)}{(2.75 - 2.61) \times 10^{-3}}$$

$$= -6237 \text{ cal mol}^{-1}$$

Example

Calculation of Enthalpy of Mixing (ΔH_2^m). The activity coefficients of *n*-octane in polymethyl acrylate at three temperatures are given in the following table.

T (K)	$1/T \times 10^3$	$f = \dfrac{a_2}{w_2}$	ln f
363	2.755	47.15	3.8533
373	2.681	42.58	3.7541
383	2.611	39.41	3.6740

Reciprocals of temperature and natural logarithms of activity coefficients are given in the second and fourth columns, respectively. Linear regression of $1/T$ (= X) against ln f (= Y) gives a slope of

$$\frac{d \ln f}{d(1/T)} = 1.18 \times 10^3$$

Therefore,

$$\Delta H_2^m = 1.98 \times 1.18 = 2.34 \text{ kcal mol}^{-1}$$

If there is no volume change on mixing, and the resulting solution is dilute, $\Delta \bar{H}_2^m = \Delta \bar{U}_2^m$ and ϕ_1^2 can be approximated to unity. Equation (5.40) then becomes

$$\Delta \bar{H}_2^m = V_2 (\delta_1 - \delta_2)^2 \qquad (5.84)$$

Expansion and rearrangement gives

$$\delta_2^2 - \frac{\Delta \bar{H}_2^m}{V_2} = (2\delta_1)\delta_2 - \delta_1^2 \qquad (5.85)$$

so that a plot of $\delta_2^2 - \Delta \bar{H}_2^m / V_2$ against δ_2 should give a straight line of slope $2\delta_1$ and intercept δ_1^2, providing a method for measuring the solubility parameters of nonvolatile compounds. DiPaola-Baranyi [34] applied this procedure to hydrocarbons as probe molecules, using polystyrene and polymethyl acrylate as stationary phase, and obtained two reasonable rectilinear plots. Solubility parameters calculated from the slopes agreed well with those obtained from the intercepts and were of the anticipated order of magnitude.

Excess thermodynamic parameters of mixing represent energy in excess of that involved in the formation of ideal solutions. Since $\Delta A = \Delta U - T \Delta S$, and the entropy of mixing of a regular solution is, by definition, equal to that of an ideal solution, $\Delta \bar{A}^E = \Delta \bar{U}^E$, and provided that there is no volume change on mixing, these parameters are also equal to $\Delta \bar{G}^E$ and $\Delta \bar{H}^m$. $\Delta \bar{G}^E$ may therefore be substituted for $\Delta \bar{H}_2^m$ in Eq. (5.85) to give

$$\Delta \bar{G}_2^E = V_2 (\delta_1 - \delta_2)^2 \tag{5.86}$$

DiPaola-Baranyi et al. [34] calculated excess Gibbs free energies from

$$\Delta \bar{G}_2^E = RT \ln \frac{a_2}{w_2} \tag{5.87}$$

and plotted $\delta_2 - (\Delta \bar{G}_2^E / V_2)$ against δ_2 using hydrocarbons as probe molecules. They again obtained reasonable rectilinear plots and calculated solubility parameters from the slopes and intercepts.

In a third approach [34], the Flory treatment was combined with Hildebrand theory to give

$$\chi = \frac{V_2}{RT} (\delta_1 - \delta_2)^2 \tag{5.88}$$

where χ is the reduced residual chemical potential [39]. Rearrangement gives an equation in χ analogous to Eq. (5.85), so that a plot of $(\delta_2^2 / RT) - (\chi / V_2)$ against δ_2 should yield a straight line with slope $2\delta_1 / RT$ and intercept δ_1^2 / RT. Good straight lines were obtained, as shown in Fig. 5.10. Results obtained from Eqs. (5.84), (5.86), and (5.88) are compared in Table 5.7. Agreement between results is only fair, but they are sufficiently interesting to warrant a more rigorous assessment of the procedure, particularly with non-volatile pharmaceutical solids suspended on an inert matrix as stationary phase. It could be argued that the procedure is an expensive variation on the solubility method of determining solubility parameters, but it does have the added advantages that it can be used with solvents in which solubilities are low and that the answer obtained applies to infinitely dilute solutions.

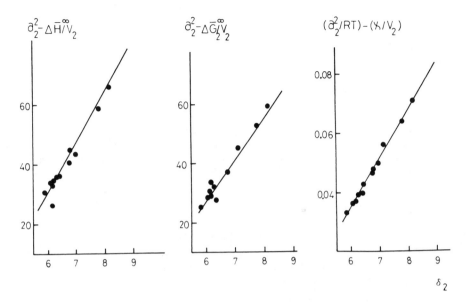

FIGURE 5.10 Estimation of solubility parameters from chromatographic data. (Abstracted from Ref. 34.)

TABLE 5.7 Solubility Parameters of Gas Chromatography Stationary Phases

	Solubility parameter		
	Eq. (5.88)	Eq. (5.86)	Eq. (5.84)
Polystyrene at 193°C			
slope	7.6 ± 0.2	7.1 ± 0.5	8.0 ± 0.6
intercept	7.6 ± 0.2	7.6 ± 0.4	8.2 ± 0.4
Polymethyl acrylate at 100°C			
slope	8.5 ± 0.3	8.4 ± 0.4	10.4 ± 0.6
intercept	8.8 ± 0.2	9.1 ± 0.4	10.5 ± 0.4

Source: Ref. 34.

I. From Surface Tensions

Surface free energy (γ) is related to energy of vaporization by [8]

$$\gamma = \frac{K'(\Delta H^V - RT)}{V^{2/3} N^{1/3}} \tag{5.89}$$

K' is a constant, ΔH^V the enthalpy of vaporization, V the molar volume, and N is Avogadro's number.

Hansen [40] divided solubility parameters into three components (page 219), and Beerbower [41] rewrote Hansen's equation in the form

$$\Delta H^V - RT = A + B + C \tag{5.90}$$

where A, B, and C are the contributions to cohesive energy density of London, Keesom, and hydrogen bonding forces, respectively, and are equal to the corresponding three-dimensional parameters (see Section II.A in Chapter 6) multiplied by molar volume. He linked the expression to Eq. (5.89) to give

$$\gamma = \frac{K(A + B + C)}{V^{2/3}} \tag{5.91}$$

where $K = K'/N^{1/3}$. Computer evaluation of Eq. (5.91), using results from 100 liquids, gave $K = 0.07147$, so that

$$\gamma = \frac{0.07147(\Delta H^V - RT)}{V^{2/3}} \tag{5.92}$$

giving

$$\delta = \left(\frac{\Delta H^V - RT}{V}\right)^{1/2} = \left(\frac{\gamma}{V^{1/3}}\right)^{1/2} \left(\frac{1}{K}\right)^{1/2} \tag{5.93}$$

$$= 3.74 \left(\frac{\gamma}{V^{1/3}}\right)^{1/2}$$

Equation (5.93) was claimed to apply to "regular" liquids, electron donors, and electron acceptors, but not to donor-acceptor-containing groups such as OH and COOH. The constant 3.74 assumes that the three types of forces are omnidirectional; more precise correlations were anticipated by Beerbower if B were multiplied by 0.643 and

TABLE 5.8 Solubility Parameters Calculated from Surface Tensions

Compound	Surface tension (dyn cm^{-1})	Molar volume (cm^3)	Solubility parameter (H)
Benzene	28.9	89	9.51
Carbon tetra- chloride	27.0	97	9.07
Chloroform	27.1	81	9.37
Bromoform	41.5	88	11.42
n-Hexane	18.4	132	7.11
Carbon disulfide	32.3	61	10.71

C by 0.620. Becher [42] confirmed the constant 3.74, using both geometrical and thermodynamic arguments.

Neither Beerbower nor Becher gave examples of solubility parameters calculated from Eq. (5.93). Results calculated for a limited range of liquids, given in Table 5.8, show poor agreement with solubility parameters obtained by other methods.

Roberts and Thomas [43] used surface tensions to determine the solubility parameter of o-hydroxypropylcellulose. They reasoned that the poorer the solvent for a given solute, the greater would be the tendency of the solute to move to the air-solvent interface, so that the difference between the surface tensions of solvent and solution should be minimal when solvent solubility parameters were equal. Fig. 5.11 shows the plots obtained with 0.75% w/v solutions in acetone-water and dimethylformamide-tetrahydrofuran blends. A solubility parameter of 10.9 H was obtained with the former, and 10.6 with the latter.

J. From the Kauri Butanol Value

The kauri butanol test is a standard method for assessing the solvent power of liquids. It measures the volume of a 20% solution of a standard kauri resin in n-butanol, necessary to produce a cloud point in the liquid. Kauri butanol (KB) values are claimed to be linearly related to solubility parameter, for example [10],

$$\delta = 6.31 + 0.029(KB) \tag{5.94}$$

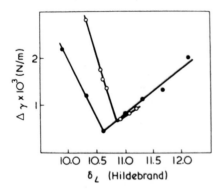

FIGURE 5.11 Differences ($\Delta \gamma$) between the surface tensions of o-hydroxypropyl cellulose solutions and solvent surface tensions as a function of solvent solubility parameters. ○, Acetone-water mixtures; ●, dimethylformamide-tetrahydrofuran mixtures. (From Ref. 43.)

K. From Viscosities

The specific viscosity (η_{sp}) of a solution is the relative increase in viscosity of the solution (η) over that of the pure solvent (η_0) and is defined by

$$\eta_{sp} = \frac{\eta - \eta_0}{\eta_0} \qquad (5.95)$$

A plot of specific viscosity over concentration of solute in percentage w/v against percentage w/v intercepts the viscosity axis at the intrinsic viscosity, which represents the specific viscosity at infinite dilution. The limiting viscosity number (LVN) is the same parameter, except that the concentrations are expressed in grams per milliliter. Roberts and Thomas [43] plotted LVN for solutions of o-hydroxypropylcellulose in various solvents and solvent blends against solubility parameter, and found that the limiting viscosity numbers passed through two minima, one corresponding with a solubility parameter of 10.65 H. This agreed with 10.2 H calculated by Small's method [23] and with 10.6 to 10.9 H from surface tensions.

L. From HLB Values

Little [44] derived the following from experimental data relating HLB values (page 116) of 15 detergents with their solubility parameters.

$$\delta = \frac{118.8}{54 - HLB} + 6.0 \tag{5.96}$$

Correlation of observed and calculated solubility parameters gives

$$\delta_{calculated} = 1.025\delta_{observed} - 0.237 \qquad\qquad \tag{5.97}$$

n	r	s
15	0.994	0.296

which indicates for the results quoted that Eq. (5.96) provides a means of predicting solubility parameters of anionic and nonionic surfactants when their HLB values are known.

V. DETERMINATION OF VOLUME FRACTIONS

For dilute solutions it is often sufficient to assume that ϕ_1 equals 1. For more precise work, the process of successive approximations can be used. In this procedure, ϕ_1 is first approximated to 1, and X_2 calculated using either Eq. (5.44) for liquids or Eq. (5.45) for solids. An approximate value of ϕ_1 can then be estimated from

$$\phi_1 = \frac{(1 - X_2)V_1}{(1 - X_2)V_1 + X_2 V_2} \tag{5.98}$$

using the value of X_2 obtained in the previous calculation. The process is repeated using the new value of X_2, and continued with successive estimates of X_2 until a constant value of ϕ_1 is obtained.

Example

The ideal mole fraction solubility of naphthalene at 20°C is 0.261. Calculate its regular solubility in carbon tetrachloride at the same temperature.

	Carbon tetrachloride	Naphthalene
Solubility parameters (H)	8.6	9.9
Molar volumes (cm^3)	97	123

Solution:

First approximation: call ϕ_1 unity. Substitution in the equation

$$-\ln X_2 = -\ln a_2 + \frac{\phi_1^2 V_2 (\delta_1 - \delta_2)^2}{RT}$$

gives

$$-\ln X_2 = -\ln 0.261 + \frac{123(8.6 - 9.9)^2}{293 \times 1.987}$$

$$= 1.700$$

$$\ln X_2 = -1.700$$

giving

$$X_2 = 0.183$$

Second approximation: call X_2 0.183. Substitution in Eq. (5.98) gives

$$\phi_1 = \frac{(1 - 0.183)97}{(1 - 0.183)97 + (0.183 \times 123)}$$

$$= 0.779$$

$$-\ln X_2 = -\ln 0.261 + \frac{0.779 \times 123(8.6 - 9.9)^2}{293 \times 1.987}$$

$$= 1.343 + 0.217$$

$$\ln X_2 = -1.560 \quad \text{or} \quad X_2 = 0.210$$

Third approximation: call X_2 0.210, giving, by the same process as before, X_2 = 0.214.

Fourth approximation: call X_2 0.214, giving X_2 = 0.214.

The answer is now a constant, so the regular solubility can be fixed at 0.214.

When comparing observed and calculated solubilities, one may use a value of ϕ_1 calculated from the observed solubility.

VI. DETERMINATION OF MOLAR VOLUMES

The molar volumes (V) of many liquids are available in the literature. Hildebrand et al. [8] contains a useful list. Densities (ρ) are quoted more frequently than molar volumes and can be used to calculate apparent molar volumes from

$$V = \frac{\text{molecular weight}}{\rho} \tag{5.99}$$

Densities of liquids are also comparatively easy to measure, when the information is not available. Bauer and Lewin [45] describe the various methods.

Molar volumes of compounds that normally occur in the solid state are rarely found in the literature. Approximate molar volumes (that of the supercooled liquid is required) can be calculated from the lattice spacings of the solid, if they are known, or from the density of the solid. Density may be determined by flotation. Crystals are immersed in a series of liquids in which the material is insoluble and the density taken as that of the liquid in which it remains suspended. Blends of liquids or solid in liquid solutions may be used as suspending media. The technique may be extended to the determination of densities of liquids or liquid-in-liquid solutions. Alternatively, the density of a liquid can be measured by weighing in a graduated capillary tube. The partial molar volume of a solute ($\overline{V}_2$) can be calculated from this information, using

$$\frac{X_1 M_1 + X_2 M_2}{\text{density of solution}} = X_1 \overline{V}_1 + X_2 \overline{V}_2 = V^{mix} \tag{5.100}$$

where M_1 and M_2 represent molecular weights.

Cavé et al. [31] determined the densities of 10 solutions of butyl-p-hydroxybenzoate in n-propanol and obtained apparent molar volumes (V^{mix}) of each solution from Eq. (5.100). Regression of X_2 against V^{mix} in the form of

$$V^{mix} = \alpha + \beta X_2 + \gamma X_2^2 \tag{5.101}$$

gave $\alpha = 76.451$, $\beta = 99.007$, and $\gamma = 9.2823$. As an example, a solution containing 0.1094 mole fraction of butyl p-hydroxybenzoate ($M_2 = 194$) in n-propanol ($M_1 = 60$) was found to have a density of 0.8532, giving

$$V^{mix} = \frac{60(1 - 0.1094) + 0.1094 \times 194}{0.8532} = 87.51$$

Acree and Carstensen [46] used the following

$$\overline{V}_1 = V^{mix} + X_2 \frac{\delta V^{mix}}{\delta X_1} \tag{5.102}$$

$$\overline{V}_2 = V^{mix} - X_1 \frac{\delta V^{mix}}{\delta X_1} \tag{5.103}$$

Substitution for V^{mix} from Eq. (5.101), and differentiation yielded

$$\overline{V}_1 = \alpha - \gamma X_2^2 \qquad\qquad (5.104)$$

and

$$\overline{V}_2 = \alpha + \beta + \gamma X_2 (1 + X_1) \qquad\qquad (5.105)$$

from which the partial molar volumes could be calculated. Thus for the example above,

$$\overline{V}_1 = 76.451 - 9.2823 \times 0.1094 = 75.4$$

and

$$\overline{V}_2 = 76.451 + 99.007 + 9.2823 \times 0.1094(1 + 0.8906) = 177.4$$

VII.   EFFECT OF TEMPERATURE ON SOLUBILITY PARAMETERS

The solubility parameters of hydrocarbons are considered by Barton [10] to decrease by about 0.01 H for each degree rise in temperature. The information reproduced in Table 5.9 shows that for a limited range of nonpolar solvents, enthalpies of vaporization (ΔH^V) decrease and molar volumes (V) increase with increasing temperature, giving resultant solubility parameters that decrease with increasing temperature. Regression of δ against T confirms the increment of 0.01 H for these liquids. DiPaola-Baranyi and Guillet [34] determined the solubility parameters of 20 aromatic and aliphatic hydrocarbons at 298, 373, and 466 K, using a gas chromatographic technique. Their results gave a mean increment of 0.011 H.

Benson [47] expressed the configurational energy (ΔU^c) of a liquid as a power series in density (ρ),

$$\Delta U^c = -B_1 \rho^{6/3} + B_2 \rho^{8/3} - B_3 \rho^{10/3} + B_4 \rho^{12/3} \qquad (5.106)$$

where the B's are constants. For the intermolecular distances occurring in liquids, it was considered that the last three terms could be dropped and the approximate energy of vaporization (ΔU^V) given by

$$\Delta U^V = (\Delta U^c_L - \Delta U^c_g) = A(\rho_1^2 - \rho_g^2) \qquad (5.107)$$

TABLE 5.9 Enthalpies of Vaporization, Molar Volumes, and Solubility Parameters of Some Nonpolar Liquids at Various Temperatures

Solvent	T K	ΔH_v (cal mol^{-1})	V (cm^3)	δ (cal$^{1/2}$ cm$^{-3/2}$)
Benzene	298	8092	89.5	9.15
	333	7616	93.5	8.62
	373	7077	98.0	8.04
Carbon disulfide	273	6807	59.0	10.29
	294	6687	60.0	10.03
	311	6531	61.5	9.80
	322	6429	62.2	9.70
Carbon tetra- chloride	277	7964	94.5	8.85
	294	7810	96.5	8.65
	311	7639	98.5	8.44
	322	7510	100.0	8.30
Cyclohexane	298	7895	109.0	8.19
	354	7204	116.5	7.47
Toluene	298	9085	107.0	8.91
	384	7998	116.5	7.87
n-Hexane	273	7663	124.0	7.57
	298	7525	128.0	7.36
	342	6923	136.0	6.78

A is a constant and the subscripts represent liquid and gas, respectively. Since the density of the vapor is negligible in comparison with that of the liquid, and $V = 1/\rho$, Eq. (5.107) reduces to

$$\Delta U^V = \frac{A}{V^2} \tag{5.108}$$

This is reminiscent of van der Waals correction for cohesive energy. However, regression analysis of the results in Table 5.9 gave exponents in V of 0.6 to 1.1, suggesting that Eq. (5.108) has little predictive value and that the direct relationship between δ and T suggested by Barton [10] is more realistic.

Activity coefficients are dependent on differences between pairs of solubility parameters. If solubility parameters vary rectilinearly with temperature, all with a slope of 0.01 H $\deg^{-1}$, any effect of temperature on δ will approximately cancel out. Hildebrand et al. [8] describe temperature corrections as "virtually worthless, even if done carefully" and suggest that it is sufficient to use solubility parameters corresponding to one convenient temperature.

Hoy [9] empirically evolved the relationship

$$\Delta H^V = \Delta H^O \exp(-mt) \tag{5.109}$$

in which m is a constant and ΔH^O is the enthalpy of vaporization at some standard temperature. The rationale is described elsewhere (page 174).

VIII. INTERNAL PRESSURE

It has been shown in Section III of Chapter 2 that two types of intermolecular forces exist in liquids. There is an attractive force, represented by a trough in the plot of intermolecular energy against intermolecular distance, and a repulsive force, which comes into play when the molecules are close together. The internal pressure of a liquid is the algebraic sum of the two forces, but at low pressures and high temperatures, when the liquid is expanded, the repulsive force is small and the internal pressure is approximately equal to the attractive component. The energy associated with this attractive force is the energy of vaporization, which is generally used as a measure of internal energy, because experimentally determined values are more readily available. However, the two properties are not strictly the same. Internal pressure (π) is the change in internal energy with volume at constant temperature ($\delta U/\delta V)_T$, and is defined by the thermodynamic equation of state

$$\pi = \left(\frac{\delta U}{\delta V}\right)_T = T \left(\frac{\delta P}{\delta T}\right)_V - P \tag{5.110}$$

where P is the external pressure and is negligible for liquids. Internal pressure is calculated from the variation in pressure with temperature at constant volume. Experimental procedures for measuring internal pressure are described by Barton [48], Smith and Hildebrand [49], and Bagley et al. [50].

REFERENCES

1. J. A. V. Butler, D. W. Thomson, and W. H. Maclennan, The free energy of the normal aliphatic alcohols in aqueous solution: Part I. The partial vapour pressures of aqueous solutions of methyl, n-propyl and n-butyl alcohols, *J. Chem. Soc.*, 674—686 (1933).
2. J. H. Hildebrand and C. A. Jenks, Solubility: IV. Solubility relations of naphthalene and iodine in the various solvents, including a method for estimating solubility data, *J. Am. Chem. Soc.*, 42, 2180—2189 (1920).
3. J. H. Hildebrand and E. J. Salstrom, Thermodynamic properties of liquid solutions of silver bromide with alkali bromides. *J. Am. Chem. Soc.*, 54, 4257—4261 (1932).
4. J. H. Hildebrand and S. E. Wood, The derivation of equations for regular solutions, *J. Chem. Phys.*, 1, 817—822 (1933).
5. G. Scatchard, Equilibria in non-electrolyte solutions in relation to the vapor pressures and densities of the components, *Chem. Rev.*, 8, 321—333 (1931).
6. W. Westwater, H. W. Frantz, and J. H. Hildebrand, The internal pressure of pure and mixed liquids, *Phys. Rev. 31*, 135—144 (1928).
7. J. H. Hildebrand and J. M. Carter, A study of van der Waals forces between tetrahalide molecules, *J. Am. Chem. Soc.*, 54, 3592—3603 (1932).
8. J. H. Hildebrand, J. M. Prausnitz, and R. L. Scott, *Regular and Related Solutions*, Van Nostrand Reinhold, New York, 1970.
9. K. L. Hoy, New values of the solubility parameters from vapor pressure data, *J. Paint Technol.*, 42, 76--118 (1970).
10. A. F. M. Barton, Solubility parameters, *Chem. Rev.*, 75, 731—753 (1975).
11. S. H. Yalkowsky, S. C. Valvani, and G. L. Amidon, Solubility of non-electrolytes in polar solvents: IV. Non-polar drugs in mixed solvents, *J. Pharm. Sci.*, 65, 1488—1494 (1976).

12. S. C. Valvani, S. H. Yalkowsky, and G. L. Amidon, Solubility of non-electrolytes in polar solvents: VI. Refinements in molecular surface area computations, *J. Phys. Chem.*, *80*, 829–835 (1976).

13. J. L. McNaughton and C. T. Mortimer, Differential scanning calorimetry, in *IRS, Physical Chemistry Series 2*, Vol. 10, Butterworths, London, 1975, pp. 1–44.

14. F. D. Rossini, D. D. Wagman, W. H. Evans, S. Levine, and I. Jaffe, *Selected Values of Physical and Thermodynamic Properties of Hydrocarbons and Related Compounds*, American Petroleum Institute Research Project 44, Carnegie Press, Pittsburgh, Pa., 1952.

15. R. C. Weast, *Handbook of Chemistry and Physics*, Chemical Rubber Company, Cleveland, 1970.

16. J. Timmermans, *Physical Constants of Pure Organic Compounds*, Vols. 1 and 2, Elsevier, Amsterdam, 1950.

17. A. Smith and A. W. Menzies, Studies in vapor pressure: III. A static method for determining vapor pressures of solids and liquids, *J Am. Chem. Soc.*, *32*, 1412–1434 (1910).

18. G. W. Thomson, in *Techniques of Chemistry*, Vol. 1, Part 1 (A. Weissberger, ed.), Interscience, New York, 1959, pp. 401-522.

19. G. W. Thomson, The Antoine equation for vapor pressure data, *Chem. Rev. 38*, 1–39 (1946).

20. C. T. Ng, The influence of structure on the solubility profiles and biological activities of some androgens, Ph.D. thesis, University of Wales, 1974.

21. R. A. Keller, B. L. Karger, and Ll. R. Snyder, Use of the solubility parameter in predicting chromatographic retention and eluotropic strength, in *Gas Chromatography* (R. Stock, ed.), Institute of Petroleum, London, 1970, pp. 125–140.

22. K. C. James, C. T. Ng, and P. R. Noyce, Solubilities of testosterone propionate and related esters in organic solvents, *J. Pharm. Sci.*, *65*, 656–659 (1976).

23. P. A. Small, Some factors affecting the solubility of polymers, *J. Appl. Chem.*, *3*, 71–80 (1953).

24. A. E. Rheineck and K. F. Lin, Solubility parameter calculations based on group contributions, *J. Paint Technol.*, *39*, 511–514. (1968).

25. A. Jayasri and M. Yaseen, Solubility parameter values suggested using the reported and calculated values of organic compounds, *J. Oil Colour Chem. Assoc.*, *63*, 61–69 (1980).

26. R. F. Fedors, A method for estimating both the solubility parameters and molar volumes of liquids, *Polym. Eng. Sci.*, *14*, 147–154 (1974).

27. M. J. Chertkoff and A. N. Martin, The solubility of benzoic acid in mixed solvents, *J. Pharm. Sci.*, *49*, 444–447 (1960).

28. F. A. Restaino and A. N. Martin, Solubility of benzoic acid and related compounds in a series of n-alkanols, *J. Pharm. Sci.*, *53*, 636–639 (1964).

29. K. C. James and M. Roberts, The solubilities of the lower testosterone esters, *J. Pharm. Pharmacol.*, *20*, 709–714 (1968).

30. K. C. James and P. R. Noyce, An infra red study of solute-solvent interactions of testosterone propionate, *J. Pharm. Pharmacol.*, *22* (Suppl.), 109S–113S (1970).

31. G. Cavé, R. Kothari, F. Puisieux, A. N. Martin, and J. T. Carstensen, Solubility parameters from maxima in solubility/solvent plots, *Int. J. Pharm.*, *5*, 267–272 (1980).

32. A. N. Paruta, B. J. Sciarrone, and N. G. Lordi, Correlation between solubility parameters and dielectric constants, *J. Pharm. Sci.*, *51*, 704–705 (1962).

33. W. G. Gorman and G. D. Hall, Dielectric constant correlations with solubility and solubility parameters, *J. Pharm. Sci.*, *53*, 1017–1020 (1964).

34. G. DiPaola-Baranyi and J. E. Guillet, Estimation of polymer solubility parameters by gas chromatography, *Macromolecules*, *11*, 228–235 (1978).

35. A. B. Littlewood, C. S. G. Phillips, and D. T. Price, The chromatography of gases and vapours: Part V. Partition analysis with columns of silicone 702 and of tritolyl phosphate, *J. Chem. Soc.*, 1480–1489 (1955).

36. A. T. James and A. J. P. Martin, Gas-liquid partition chromatography: the separation and micro-estimation of volatile fatty acids from formic acid to dodecanoic acid, *Biochem. J.*, *50*, 679–690 (1952).

37. D. Patterson, Y. B. Tewari, H. P. Schreiber, and J. E. Guillet, Applications of gas-liquid chromatography to the thermodynamics of polymer solutions, *Macromolecules*, *4*, 356–359 (1971).

38. M. L. McGlassen and D. J. B. Potter, An apparatus for the measurement of the second virial coefficients of vapours; the second virial coefficients of some n-alkanes and of some mixtures of n-alkanes, *Proc. R. Soc. London*, *267A*, 478–500 (1962).

39. B. E. Eichinger and P. J. Flory, Thermodynamics of polymer solutions: Part I. Natural rubber and benzene, *Trans. Faraday Soc.*, *64*, 2035–2052 (1968).

40. C. M. Hansen, The universality of the solubility parameter, *Ind. Eng. Chem. Prod. Res. Dev.*, *8*, 2–11 (1969).

41. A. Beerbower, Surface free energy: a new relationship to bulk energies, *J. Colloid Interface Sci.*, *35*, 126–132 (1970).

42. P. Becher, The calculation of cohesive energy density from the surface tension of liquids, *J. Colloid Interface Sci.*, *38*, 291–293 (1972).

43. G. A. F. Roberts and I. M. Thomas, Determination of the solubility parameter of *o*-hydroxypropyl cellulose, *Polymer*, *19*, 459–461 (1978).

44. R. C. Little, Correlation of surfactant hydrophile-lipophile balance (HLB) with solubility parameter, *J. Colloid Interface Sci.*, *65*, 587–588 (1978).

45. N. Bauer and S. Z. Lewin, Determination of density, in *Physical Methods of Organic Chemistry*, Part I (A. Weissberger, ed.), Interscience, New York, 1959, pp. 131–190.

46. W. E. Acree and J. T. Carstensen, Comment on solubility parameters from maxima in solubility/solvent plots, *Int. J. Pharm.*, *8*, 69–70 (1981).

47. S. W. Benson, Intermolecular forces and energies of vaporization of liquids, *J. Chem. Phys.*, *15*, 367–373 (1947).

48. A. F. M. Barton, Internal pressure. A fundamental liquid property, *J. Chem. Educ.*, *48*, 156–162 (1971).

49. E. B. Smith and J. H. Hildebrand, Liquid isochores and derived functions of n-C_7F_{16}, c-$C_6F_{11}CF_3$, c-$C_4Cl_2F_6$, n-2,2,3-$C_4Cl_3F_7$, $CCl_2F.CCl_2F$ and CCl_4, *J. Chem. Phys.*, *31*, 145–147 (1959).

50. E. B. Bagley, T. P. Nelson, and J. M. Scagliano, Three dimensional solubility parameters and their relationship to internal pressure measurements in polar and hydrogen bonding solvents, *J. Paint Technol.*, *43*(555), 35–42 (1971).

51. C. M. Hansen and A. Beerbower, Solubility parameters, in *Encyclopedia of Chemical Technology*, Suppl. Vol., Wiley, New York, 1971, pp. 889–910.

6

"Nearly Regular" Solutions

I. ENTROPY OF MIXING

Ideal solutions have been defined in Chapter 4 as dispersions of molecules in which unlike molecules have the same affinity for each other as they do for their own kind. It is therefore assumed that there is nothing to prevent the molecules from arranging themselves in a completely random fashion as far as contact permits, and the position of any molecule within the distribution will be entirely a matter of chance. If, however, the concentration of solute molecules surrounding each solute molecule is greater, on average, than the concentration of solvent molecules, the distribution is not random and the solution is not ideal. Similarly, a preference of solute for solvent, or solvent for solvent, or any other orderly pattern in the molecular array, eliminates the system from ideal status.

Since entropy is a measure of disorder, it can be used as a criterion of ideality by specifying that the entropy of mixing in an ideal solution is equal to or greater than that involved in any other solution process. In a regular solution, the differences between solvent-solvent, solute-solvent, and solute-solute intermolecular forces are sufficiently small for thermal motion to keep the molecules randomly dispersed. A regular solution can therefore be defined as one involving no entropy change when a small amount of one of its components is transferred to it from an ideal solution of the same composition, the total volume remaining unchanged. Deviations from regular solution behavior may thus be assessed by observing the entropy change involved in forming the solution.

The entropy of mixing (ΔS^m) of an ideal solution can be calculated by considering the number of possible configurations in a random distribution. The following equation was obtained by this means [1].

$$\Delta S^m = -R(X_1 \ln X_1 + X_2 \ln X_2) \tag{6.1}$$

Differentiation with respect to X yields

$$\Delta \bar{S}_1^m = -R \ln X_1 \tag{6.2}$$

and

$$\Delta \bar{S}_2^m = -R \ln X_2 \tag{6.3}$$

which give the partial entropies of mixing, $\Delta \bar{S}_1^m$ and $\Delta \bar{S}_2^m$. These expressions apply to spherical molecules of similar shape and size. When these properties vary significantly from solute to solvent, the distribution will be influenced in favor of the most economical way in which the molecules can fit together. The equations have, however, been shown to apply to mixtures of elongated molecules that differ in chain length, such as the normal paraffins [2,3]. Flory [4] and Huggins [5], independently derived the following equation for linear molecules with segments occupying different sites in a lattice of small molecules:

$$\Delta S^m = -R(X_1 \ln \phi_1 + X_2 \ln \phi_2) \tag{6.4}$$

Differentiation gives the partial entropy of mixing, for example,

$$\Delta \bar{S}_2^m = -R \ln \phi_2 + \phi_1 \left(1 - \frac{V_2}{V_1}\right) \tag{6.5}$$

V represents molar volume and ϕ volume fraction.

These equations are useful in calculating entropies of mixing of high-polymer solutions which deviate from Raoult's law and yet are formed with negligible heat of mixing. The nonideality of these systems is a consequence of the entropy of mixing. When $V_2 = V_1$, Eq. (6.5) reduces to Eq. (6.3).

The heat change occurring when a solute is dissolved in a solvent is expressed quantitatively by the van't Hoff isochore,

$$\frac{d \ln a_2}{dT} = \frac{\Delta H}{RT^2} \tag{6.6}$$

ΔH is the heat or enthalpy of solution and a_2 the activity of the solute. For ideal solutions ΔH is synonymous with the heat of fusion of the solute, and for regular solutions, with the heat of fusion plus the heat of mixing. Integration of Eq. (6.6) gives

$$\ln a_2 = \frac{-\Delta H}{R} \frac{1}{T} + \text{constant} \tag{6.7}$$

so that a plot of $\ln a_2$ against $1/T$ should be rectilinear with a slope of $-\Delta H/R$.

The expression

$$\frac{d \ln a}{da} = \frac{1}{a}$$

is a standard mathematical form and may be used to rewrite the van't Hoff isochore, as follows:

$$\frac{d \ln a_2}{dT} = \frac{\Delta H}{RT} \frac{1}{T} = \frac{\Delta H}{RT} \frac{d \ln T}{dT} \tag{6.8}$$

which yields the following equation for saturated ideal solutions:

$$R \frac{d \ln a_2}{d \ln T} = \frac{\Delta H^f}{T} \tag{6.9}$$

Heat of fusion increases with temperature because the heat capacity of the supercooled liquid is greater than that of the solid. The increase is roughly equivalent to the increase in temperature, so that $\Delta H^f/T$ is reasonably constant; for example, $\Delta H^f/T$ for iodine decreases only 2.8% in moving from 25°C to 50°C. Plots of $\log a_2$ against $\log T$ are in fact rectilinear, provided that the saturated solution is not too concentrated. The free energy of solution of a saturated solution is zero, because solution and solute in excess are in equilibrium; therefore,

$$\Delta G = \Delta H - T \Delta S = 0 \qquad (6.10)$$

leading to the equation

$$\Delta S = \frac{\Delta H^f}{T} \qquad (6.11)$$

For dilute nonideal solutions, $X_2 \cong a_2$; therefore,

$$R \frac{d \ln X_2}{d \ln T} = \Delta S \qquad (6.12)$$

Variation in solubility with temperature can therefore be expressed by plotting $\ln X_2$ against $\ln T$, just the same as the usual procedure of plotting $\ln X_2$ against $1/T$. The slope of the former gives the entropy of mixing and that of the latter gives the heat of mixing.

The entropies of mixing of real solutions can vary considerably from the ideal value. If the solute complexes with the solvent, the entropy of mixing will be lower than ideal because the intermolecular arrangement of the solution will be more ordered than the isolated individual components. However, as the solution becomes more dilute, the entropy of solution will approach ideal, since the solute molecules will be so far apart that even if complexation did not occur, each molecule would be surrounded entirely by solvent molecules. The entropy of solution will also be low if the solute associates in solution, because the system will be more ordered than an ideal solution.

Solute-solvent interactions can be investigated by comparing the entropy of mixing, calculated from Eq. (6.12) with the entropy of solution obtained with Eq. (6.3). Figure 6.1 is an example. $R \ln X_2$ is plotted against $R(d \ln X_2/d \ln T)$ for solutions of testosterone propionate in a range of solvents. The solvents that are known to complex with testosterone propionate form a cluster in the bottom left of the graph and have entropies of solution lower than the entropy of fusion of the pure solute. In contrast, the saturated hydrocarbon solvents give a straight line, indicating that the results of the two derivations of entropy are linearly related when the solvent does not interact with the solute. Extrapolation to $-R \ln X_2 = 0$ gives the entropy of fusion of the solute.

One would anticipate that marked differences in molar volume between solute and solvent could give rise to low entropies of mixing.

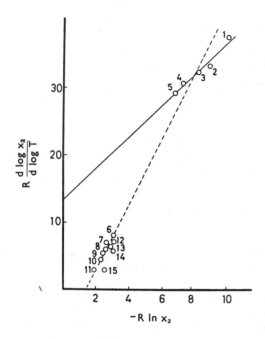

$$R \frac{d \log x_2}{d \log T}$$

$-R \ln x_2$

FIGURE 6.1 Entropies of solution of testosterone propionate at 40°C. 1, *n*-pentane; 2, *n*-hexane; 3, cyclopentane; 4, cyclohexane; 5, decalin; 6, carbon tetrachloride; 7, nitrobenzene; 8, benzene; 9, 1,2-dichloroethane; 10, *cis*- and *trans*-1,2-dichloroethylene; 11, chloroform; 12, carbon disulfide; 13, tetralin; 14, toluene; 15, chlorobenzene. ----, Regression on all points, ———, regression on saturated hydrocarbons only. (From Ref. 6.)

If, for example, a low molecular weight solute were dissolved in a high molecular weight solvent, solute molecules would be expected to locate themselves preferentially in the interstices between the solvent molecules, with a resulting increase in order and decrease in entropy. This is, in fact, suggested by the Flory-Huggins equation [Eq. (6.5)], which incorporates the ratio of solute and solvent molar volumes. Figure 6.1 indicates that no such effect applies to the systems it represents, since there is no correlation between the molar volumes of the hydrocarbon solvents and the order in which they appear on the plot. Hildebrand et al. [7] obtained similar results for iodine (molar volume = 59) in a series of solvents with molar volumes ranging from 104 to 540. In a similar way, one would intuitively expect differences in molecular shape to give rise to preferred orientations in the molecular distribution. This appears to have a greater effect on entropy of mixing than molecular size and will be discussed later.

Fung and Higuchi [8] examined the solubilities of a range of polar solutes in nonpolar solvents and found that deviations from ideal solubility could be accounted for by the entropy of mixing, calculated from the Flory-Huggins equation [Eq. (6.5)].

II. EXTENSIONS OF REGULAR SOLUTION THEORY

Hildebrand theory implies that a regular solution will be formed when the solute and solvent have similar internal pressures. However, experience has shown that this assumption does not always apply. The internal pressure of a molecule represents a balance between London, Keesom, and hydrogen-bonding forces, and similarity of internal pressures does not demand that the balance is also similar. A consequence of this is that situations which fit regular solution theory with any precision almost invariably involve low-polarity molecules which interact mainly through London forces. The properties of solutions containing strongly interacting molecules, such as alcohols and water, strongly deviate from regular solution theory, but there are intermediate systems whose properties are similar to those of regular solutions. Extensive attempts have been made to modify the existing relationships so that the properties of the intermediate group can be predicted. These have followed two lines of investigation, the three-dimensional solubility parameter approach and the extended regular solution theory treatment.

A. Three-Dimensional Solubility Parameters

In this approach, London, Debye, Keesom, and hydrogen-bonding forces are considered separately and allocated separate solubility parameters. The concept began with Blanks and Prausnitz [9], who divided classical solubility parameters into polar (τ) and nonpolar (λ) components. Thus for a nonpolar solute,

$$c_{22} = \frac{\Delta U_2^V}{V_2} = \lambda_2 \qquad (6.13)$$

and for a polar solute,

$$c_{22} = \frac{\Delta U_2^V}{V_2} = \lambda_2 + \tau_2 \qquad (6.14)$$

ΔU_2^V is the energy of vaporization. The two components were separated by using the homomorph concept, that is, by placing λ_2 equal to the solubility parameter of a nonpolar molecule having similar shape and molar volume. The difference between the energies of vaporization of homomorph and original compound is then equal to τ_2.

Polar effects, however, rarely occur in the absence of simultaneous hydrogen bonding, and the Blanks-Prausnitz approach was therefore limited in its scope. Crowley et al. [10] introduced a hydrogen-bonding parameter based on the shift of the OD stretching vibrational band in methanol-D, on changing from benzene to the particular compound. Gordy [11,12] had measured these shifts by adding small quantities of methanol-D to solutions of the compounds in benzene. Some results, reproduced in Table 6.1, show that the proton-attracting power decreases in the order amino > ether > ketone > ester. The shifts were too large for comparison with conventional solubility parameters, so Crowley et al. [10] used one-tenth of the observed shift for their hydrogen-bonding parameters. As with Blanks and Prausnitz [9], combinations of only two parameters, in this case Hildebrand's solubility parameter and the hydrogen-bonding parameter, could not explain all situations.

Hansen [13] rationalized this procedure by assuming that the total energy of vaporization (ΔU^V) was the sum of ΔU_d^V, ΔU_p^V, and ΔU_H^V, the energies required to overcome dispersion forces and polar forces and to break hydrogen bonds, respectively. Dividing all terms by molar volume gives

$$\delta^2 = \delta_d^2 + \delta_p^2 + \delta_H^2 \tag{6.15}$$

Activity coefficients (f) would then be predicted by

$$-\ln f_2 = \frac{V_2 \phi_1^2}{RT} [(\Delta \delta_p)^2 + (\Delta \delta_d)^2 + (\Delta \delta_H)^2] \tag{6.16}$$

where Δ represents the difference between solute and solvent, but the equation does not appear to have shown much success. The concept does, however, provide a means of selecting suitable solvents for a particular solute, although even in this application there are frequent exceptions.

The three-dimensional solubility approach can be criticized in several respects.

1. The methods for deriving the solubility parameters are sometimes crude and usually open to criticism. Fitting the best

TABLE 6.1 OD Stretching Frequencies and Shifts
of Deuteromethanol in Various Solvents

Solvent	Frequency (cm^{-1})	Shift (cm^{-1})
Benzene	2681	—
Bromobenzene	2681	0
Pure liquid	2494	187
Nitrobenzene	2653	28
o-Nitrotoluene	3632	49
Ethyl acetate	2597	84
Amyl acetate	2591	90
n-Buteraldehyde	2567	117
Benzaldehyde	2597	84
Methyl ethyl ketone	2604	77
Acetone	2584	97
Dioxan	2584	97
Diethyl ether	2551	130
Isopropyl ether	2558	123
Methyl cyanide	2618	63
Benzyl cyanide	2604	77
Monoamylamine	2532	149
Di-n-propylamine	2481	200
Monobutylamine	2513	168
Di-n-butylamine	2475	206
Tributylamine	2463	218
Pyridine	2500	181
Piperidine	2439	242
Quinoline	2427	254
α-Picoline	2488	193
Nicotine	2488	193
n-Butyl ether	2571	110

Source: Ref. 12.

values to the observed solubilities involves large margins of error, and the selection of homomorphs can be highly subjective.

2. Some methods of allocating parameters, such as by refractive index, are based on properties of the pure liquid, whereas others involve an arbitrarily chosen combination of liquids. The solubility method involves a solute and a variety of solvents, or solvent blends, each imparting its own solute-solvent interaction, but usually characterized by a parameter measured on the pure solvents. The answer gives the parameter for the most appropriate solvent but gives no indication of the escaping tendency of the solute. The same criticism can be leveled at the classical solubility parameter approach, but in the three-dimensional approach the error is magnified threefold.

3. Solvent blends cannot logically be allocated parameters by weighted molar volume averaging, in the same way as with classical solubility parameters.

In the earlier work with three-dimensional solubility parameters, solubility profiles were shown in the form of three-dimensional diagrams which were difficult to construct and to understand. Teas [14] simplified the approach by using triangular diagrams. He split Eq. (6.16) into force functions (f), defined for dispersion forces, for example, by

$$f_d = \frac{\delta_d^2}{\delta^2} \tag{6.17}$$

so that for chloroform, for which $\delta_d = 8.65$, $\delta_p = 1.50$, and $\delta_H = 2.80$,

$$f_d = \frac{8.65^2}{8.65^2 + 1.50^2 + 2.80^2} = \frac{74.82}{84.91} = 0.88$$

$$f_p = \frac{1.50^2}{84.91} = 0.03$$

$$f_H = \frac{2.80^2}{84.91} = 0.09$$

This gives the point on the triangular diagram shown in Fig. 6.2.

For most solvents, the force function for dispersion tends to be considerably greater than the other two, so that the coordinates

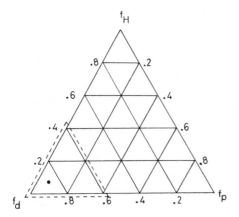

FIGURE 6.2 Triangular diagram representation of three-dimensional solubility parameters.

tend to concentrate in the bottom left-hand corner of the diagram. This can be rectified by taking only a portion of the triangle; for example, the area enclosed by the dashed line in Fig. 6.2 is sufficient to indicate the coordinates of chloroform and could be enlarged to the size of the full diagram, thus giving a larger, but restricted scale.

Figure 6.3 illustrates how easy these diagrams are to interpret. Combinations of parameters within the enclosed area represent suitable solvents for the solute under examination.

1. Determination of Dispersion Solubility Parameters.

a. The homomorph method. A homomorph is a nonpolar molecule having approximately the same size and shape as the polar molecule it represents. Normal alkanes can be used as homomorphs for straight-chain compounds. Blanks and Prausnitz [9] constructed Fig. 6.4 for this purpose, using experimental values for n-alkanes. Comparisons must be made at corresponding states, so a family of plots were presented, each representing a different reduced temperature (T_R). If, for example, the dispersion solubility parameter at 25°C for chloroform, which has a critical temperature of 536 K, is required,

$$T_R = \frac{298}{536} = 0.56$$

The 0.55 plot in Fig. 6.4 (which is nearest and sufficiently close to 0.56) is therefore traced to the molar volume of chloroform (81 cc

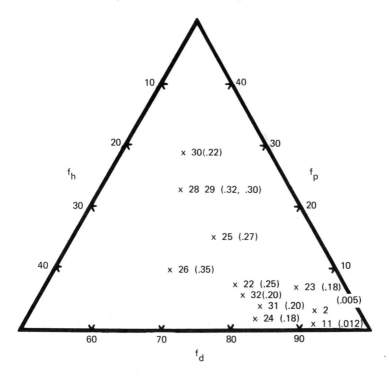

FIGURE 6.3 Triangular solubility plot for testosterone propionate.
2, n-hexane; 11, cyclohexane; 22, benzene; 23, carbon disulfide;
24, carbon tetrachloride; 25, chlorobenzene; 26, chloroform; 28, *trans*-
dichloro-ethylane; 29, *cis*-dichloroethylene; 30, nitrobenzene; 31,
tetralin; 32, toluene. Figures in parenthesis are mole fraction solubilities. (From Ref. 15.)

mol^{-1}), which corresponds to a heat of vaporization of 4.85 kcal mol^{-1},
equivalent to a dispersion parameter of $4.85/81 - 7.74$ $cal^{1/2}$ $cm^{-3/2}$.

The homomorph for a nonlinear molecule is the nonpolar molecule
most resembling it in shape and molar volume at the same reduced
temperature. Thus cyclohexane can be used as homomorph for dioxane and 2-ethyl propane for methylisopropyl ether. Nonpolar
compounds such as carbon disulfide and carbon tetrachloride were
initially assigned dispersion parameters equal to the Hildebrand solubility parameter, on the grounds that interaction energy resulted
from dispersion forces only. Other components have since been detected, however; carbon tetrachloride, for example, has been allocated a hydrogen-bonding parameter of 0.03 [16]. Similarly, the
assumption that δ_p and δ_H are zero is no longer applied to aromatic
hydrocarbons, which are now known to have both hydrogen-bonding

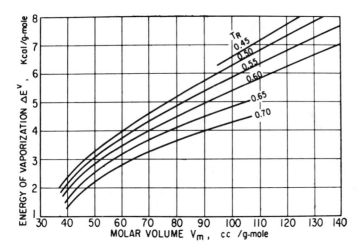

FIGURE 6.4 Energies of vaporization for hydrocarbons. (From Ref. 9.)

and polar components. The homomorph principle is therefore somewhat arbitrary with respect to nonlinear molecules.

  b. From refractive index. A more objective method is based on the Lorenz-Lorenz equation, which was initially used, with limited success, to calculate Hildebrand solubility parameters (see Section IV. D in Chapter 5). In this work [17] it was found that the Hildebrand solubility parameters (δ) of aliphatic and alicyclic hydrocarbons complied with

$$\delta = 30.7 \left(\frac{n^2 - 1}{n^2 + 2} \right) \tag{6.18}$$

provided that the Lorenz-Lorenz function $(n^2 - 1)/(n^2 + 2)$ did not exceed 0.28. Correlation of δ with the Lorenz-Lorenz function beyond this limit gave a smooth curve, incorporating aromatic hydrocarbons and other nonpolar or slightly polar compounds and empirically fitting

$$\delta = -2.24 + 53x - 58x^2 + 22x^3 \tag{6.19}$$

where $x = (n^2 - 1)/(n^2 + 2)$. The plot is reproduced in Fig. 6.5. It was pointed out [17] that the refractive indices had been obtained with the pure liquids. Therefore, since the compounds on which Eq. (6.19) was based had either zero or negligible polar interactions in their pure liquid state, the equation could be used to calculate

dispersion parameters. Good agreement was in fact obtained between dispersion parameters calculated from Eq. (6.19) and from
the homomorph procedure.

Example

Calculate the dispersion parameter of ethyl acetate, given that the
refractive index at 25°C is 1.3701.

Solution:

$$x = \frac{n^2 - 1}{n^2 + 2} = \frac{1.3701^2 - 1}{1.3701^2 + 2} = 0.2262$$

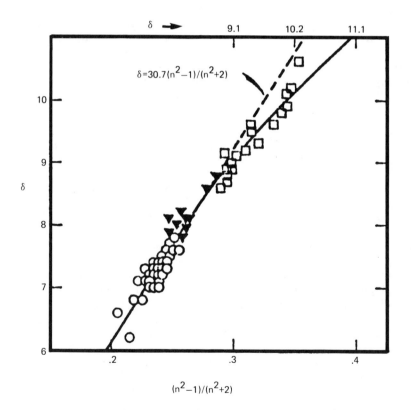

$$\delta = 30.7(n^2 - 1)/(n^2 + 2)$$

$$(n^2 - 1)/(n^2 + 2)$$

FIGURE 6.5 Relationships between hydrocarbon solubility parameters
and refractive index. ○: alkanes, alkenes, alkynes; ▲: cycloalkanes;
□: aromatics. (From Ref. 17.)

$$\delta_d = -2.24 + 53 \times 0.2262 - 58 \times 0.2262^2 + 22 \times 0.2262^3$$

$$= 7.04 \text{ cal}^{1/2} \text{ cm}^{-3/2} \quad (H)$$

2. Determination of Polar Solubility Parameters. Polar parameters of compounds having no hydrogen-bonding capability can be calculated from

$$\delta^2 = \delta_d^2 + \delta_p^2 \tag{6.20}$$

δ is obtained from $(\Delta U^V/V)^{1/2}$ and δ_d either from the Lorenz-Lorenz function or through a homomorph.

A similar procedure can be used for hydrogen-bonding compounds by assuming that $(\delta^2 - \delta_d^2)^{1/2}$ represents a combined parameter embracing both hydrogen-bonding and polar forces. Hansen [18] separated the combined parameter into polar and hydrogen-bonding parameters by a process of trial and error in which he laboriously processed a large number of solubility results and established values of δ_p and δ_H that best fit the data. He later confirmed his calculations [19] using the following modification of an equation derived for calculation of the contribution of permanent dipoles to the cohesive energy of a liquid:

$$\delta_d^2 = \frac{12,108}{V^2} \frac{\varepsilon - 1}{2\varepsilon + n^2} (n^2 + 2)\mu^2 \text{ cal cm}^{-3} \tag{6.21}$$

where V is molar volume, ε dielectric constant, n the refractive index to the D line of sodium and μ the dipole moment in debye units. Corrections were necessary for molecules in which the centers of the dipole and the molecule did not coincide. Calculated values for 65 solvents agreed well with "trial-and-error results," confirming Hansen's original observations.

Hansen and Beerbower [16] derived partial polar parameters for a range of polar substituent groups. These are reproduced in Table 6.2 and are to be used independently of the nature of any nonpolar substituents. Thus ethyl chloride, which has a molar volume of 74 $\text{cm}^3 \text{ mol}^{-1}$, gives a polar parameter of $\delta_p = 300/74 = 4.05$, where 300 is the contribution of Cl, in reasonable agreement with the experimental value of 4.4. The ethyl group gives a contribution of zero.

B. The Extended Solubility Parameter Approach

The principal weakness of the heat-of-mixing expression given by Eqs. (5.44) and (5.45) is that the cohesive energy density between

TABLE 6.2 Group Contributions to Polar and Hydrogen-Bonding Solubility Parameters

Group	Polar parameter, $V\delta_p$ [(cal cc)$^{1/2}$ mol^{-1}]	Hydrogen-bonding parameter, $V\delta^2_H$ (cal mol^{-1})	
		Aliphatic	Aromatic
—F	225 ± 25	0	0
—Cl	300 ± 100	100 ± 20	100 ± 20
Cl₂	175 ± 25	165 ± 10	180 ± 10
—Br	300 ± 25	500 ± 100	500 ± 100
—I	325 ± 25	1000 ± 200	
—O—	200 ± 50	1150 ± 300	1250 ± 300
>CO	390 ± 15	800 ± 250	400 ± 125
—COO—	250 ± 25	1250 ± 150	800 ± 150
—CN	525 ± 50	500 ± 200	550 ± 200
—NO₂	500 ± 50	400 ± 50	400 ± 50
—NH₂	300 ± 100	1350 ± 200	2250 ± 200
>NH	100 ± 15	750 ± 200	
—OH	250 ± 30	4650 ± 400	4650 ± 500
(—OH)ₙ	n(170 ± 25)	n(4650 ± 400)	n(4650 ± 500)
—COOH	220 ± 10	2750 ± 250	2250 ± 250

Source: Ref. 16.

solute and solvent is not necessarily equal to the geometric mean of the individual solute and solvent cohesive energy densities. An empirical geometric mean coefficient (l_{12}) has been introduced in Eq. (5.45) to correct for this difference.

$$-\ln X_2 = -\ln a_2 + \frac{\phi_1^2 V_2}{RT} [(\delta_1 - \delta_2)^2 + 2l_{12}\delta_1\delta_2] \qquad (6.22)$$

Equation (5.45) has also been expressed in the form

$$\ln f_2 = A(\delta_1^2 + \delta_2^2 - w_{12}) \qquad (6.23)$$

in which f_2 is the solute activity coefficient and A is $\phi_1^2 V_2/RT$. w_{12} is an interaction parameter which accurately quantifies the cohesive energy density between solute and solvent. Comparison of the two equations indicates that the parameters are related according to

$$w_{12} = 2(1 - l_{12})\delta_1\delta_2 \qquad (6.24)$$

Examination of Eqs. (6.22) to (6.24) suggests three types of situation.

1. When $w_{12} = 2\delta_1\delta_2$: The enthalpy of solution is then pre-
    dicted by Eq. (5.45), and the solution can be described as
    regular.
2. When $w_{12} > 2\delta_1\delta_2$: An example of this situation occurs
    when a proton-donating (protic) liquid, such as chloroform,
    is mixed with a proton-accepting (protolytic) liquid, such as
    acetone. The liquids are able to hydrogen bond with each
    other but not with their own kind. The calculated regular
    solubility will then be less than the observed value, because
    the true enthalpy of mixing is lower than the calculated
    enthalpy of mixing.
3. When $w_{12} < 2\delta_1\delta_2$: This occurs when like molecules asso-
    ciate and unlike molecules do not. Typical examples are
    solutions of hydroxy compounds in hydrocarbons, or of non-
    polar solutes in water. In this case, the calculated regular
    solubility exceeds the experimental solubility.

The interaction parameter w_{12} has not been evaluated theoretically. Martin and Carstensen [20] assumed that when a range
of similar solvents are used to dissolve a given solute, w_{12} is directly proportional to $\delta_1\delta_2$, as

$$w_{12} = 2K\delta_1\delta_2 \tag{6.25}$$

where K is the proportionality constant. Equation (6.25) leads to

$$\frac{\log f_2}{A} = \delta_2^2 - 2K\delta_1\delta_2 + \delta_1^2 \tag{6.26}$$

which is a power series in δ_1. Martin used power series of this type, sometimes extended as far as the fourth power of δ_1, and obtained good agreement with the observed solubilities of theophylline [21], caffeine [22], and testosterone and testosterone propionate [23]. The procedure can be used to estimate the solubilities of missing members of a related group of compounds by interpolation or extrapolation, and could possibly be extended from one system to a closely related system.

An interesting feature of this approach is that molecular interactions can be expressed in terms of the constant K. When K = 1, the solution is regular, although it is possible that the value of K is an artifact and that solvating and self-associating effects have canceled each other out. When K < 1, the solubility is less than regu­lar, and the solute or solvent, or both, can be considered to be self-associated. An intermediate situation exists when K > 1 but is less than $(\delta_1^2 - \delta_2^2)/\delta_1\delta_2$, or, in other words, the solubility is less than ideal. It is probable that solute-solvent association is occurring, but it is partially counterbalanced by some self-association. Finally, when K > 1, and the solubility exceeds ideal, association of a specific nature exists between solute and solvent. Figure 6.6 illustrates the principles of this argument. It also shows how the foregoing criteria can be expressed in terms of activity coefficient (a) or l_{12}.

Hydrogen bonding between testosterone propionate and polar solvents can be assessed in terms of the 3-keto stretching frequency shift of the steroid. James et al. [15] related these shifts to the geometric mean coefficient (l_{12}), indicating that deviations from regular solution behavior of these systems were a consequence of the hydrogen bonding causing a higher solute-solvent cohesive energy density than that predicted by the geometric mean. Their results, reproduced in Fig. 6.7, indicate that infrared shifts could provide a basis for evaluation of l_{12}.

Errors arising from the failure of the geometric mean assumption also arise in low-polarity mixtures and result from differences in molecular geometry, which hinders intimate molecular contact. Shape is a more critical factor than size. The shapes of saturated hydrocarbons can be expressed in terms of a branching ratio (r), defined by

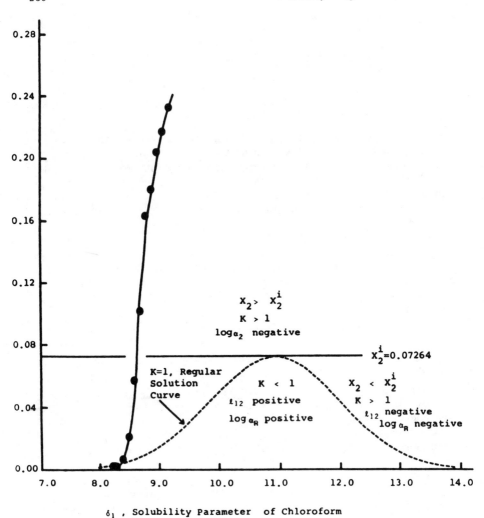

δ_1 , Solubility Parameter of Chloroform
and Cyclohexane Mixtures

FIGURE 6.6 Mole fraction solubilities of testosterone in cyclohexane-chloroform mixtures. (From Ref. 23.)

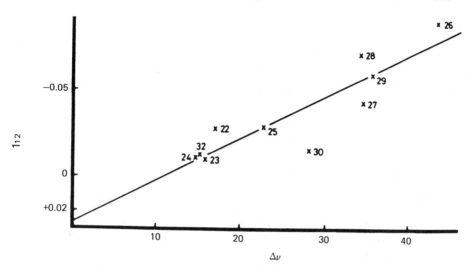

FIGURE 6.7 Relationship between carbonyl stretching frequency shift and l_{12}. Coding as for Fig. 6.3, plus 27, 1,2-dichloroethane. (From Ref. 15.)

$$r = \frac{\text{number of methyl groups}}{\text{total number of carbon atoms}} \qquad (6.27)$$

and have been shown to follow the same order as l_{12} for the solubilities of benzene in a series of hydrocarbons [7]. l_{12} can be evaluated by substituting the experimental solubility into Eq. (6.22). James et al. [15] have demonstrated a linear relationship between r and l_{12} for the solubilities of androstanolone propionate and testosterone propionate in a range of hydrocarbons. They considered that since ascent of steroid ester homologous series involved only minor changes in molecular structure, l_{12} for one ester could be used to estimate solubilities of neighboring esters in the series. This procedure was successful in predicting solubilities of some androstanolone, nandrolone, and testosterone esters.

Unlike the irregularities arising from solute-solvent interaction, the foregoing effects give a lower calculated cohesive energy density than the observed value, so that l_{12} is positive and is assumed to occur because solvent and solute molecules are unable to approach each other as closely as their own kind. Since attractive forces fall off in proportion to the sixth power of distance of separation, failure of unlike molecules to approach each other as closely as anticipated will give rise to a marked discrepancy between calculated and true solute-solvent cohesive energy densities.

REFERENCES

1. O. Stern, The entropy of solid solutions, *Ann. Phys.*, *49*, 823–841 (1916).
2. J. H. Hildebrand, The validity of Raoult's law for paraffin molecules of very different length, *J. Am. Chem. Soc.*, *59*, 794–798 (1937).
3. J. H. Hildebrand and J. W. Sweny, The entropy of solution of hexane with hexadecane, *J. Phys. Chem.*, *43*, 297–300 (1939).
4. P. J. Flory, Thermodynamics of high polymer solutions, *J. Chem. Phys.*, *9*, 660–661 (1941).
5. M. L. Huggins, Solutions of long chain compounds, *J. Chem. Phys.*, *9*, 440 (1941).
6. D. B. Bowen and K. C. James, The effect of temperature on the solubilities of testosterone propionate in low polarity solvents, *J. Pharm. Pharmacol.*, *22*, 104S–108S (1970).
7. J. H. Hildebrand, J. M. Prausnitz, and R. L. Scott, *Regular and Related Solutions*, Van Nostrand Reinhold, New York, 1970.
8. H. L. Fung and T. Higuchi, Molecular interactions and solubility of polar non-electrolytes in non-polar solvents, *J. Pharm. Sci.*, *60*, 1782–1788 (1971).
9. R. F. Blanks and J. M. Prausnitz, Thermodynamics of polymer solubility in polar and non-polar systems, *Ind. Eng. Chem.*, *Fundam.*, *3*, 1–8 (1964).
10. J. D. Crowley, G. S. Teague, and J. W. Lowe, A three dimensional approach to solubility, *J. Paint Technol.*, *38*, 269–280 (1966).
11. W. Gordy, Spectroscopic comparison of the proton attracting properties of liquids, *J. Chem. Phys.*, *7*, 93–99 (1939).
12. W. Gordy and S. C. Stanford, Spectroscopic evidence for hydrogen bonds: comparison of proton attracting properties of liquids, III, *J. Chem. Phys.*, *9*, 204–214 (1941).
13. C. M. Hansen, The universality of the solubility parameter, *Ind. Eng. Chem.*, *Prod. Res. Dev.*, *8*, 2–11 (1969).
14. J. P. Teas, Graphic analysis of resin solubilities, *J. Paint Technol.*, *40*, 19–25 (1968).
15. K. C. James, C. T. Ng, and P. R. Noyce, Solubilities of testosterone propionate and related esters in organic solvents, *J. Pharm. Sci.*, *65*, 656–659 (1976).
16. C. M. Hansen and A. Beerbower, Solubility parameters, in *Encyclopedia of Chemical Technology*, Suppl. Vol., Wiley, New York, 1971, 889–910.
17. R. A. Keller, B. L. Karger, and L. R. Snyder, Use of the solubility parameter in predicting chromatographic retention and eluotropic strength, in *Gas Chromatography* (R. Stock, ed.), Institute of Petroleum, London, 1970, pp. 125–140.

18. C. M. Hansen, The three-dimensional solubility parameter—key to paint-component affinities: I. Solvents, plasticizers, polymers and resins, *J. Paint Technol.*, *39*, 104–117 (1967).
19. C. M. Hansen and K. Skaarup, Three-dimensional solubility parameter—key to paint component affinities: III. Independent calculation of the parameter components, *J. Paint Technol.*, *39*, 511–514 (1967).
20. A. Martin and J. Carstensen, Extended solubility approach: solubility parameters for crystalline solid compounds, *J. Pharm. Sci.*, *70*, 170–172 (1981).
21. A. Martin, J. Newburger, and A. Adjei, Extended Hildebrand solubility approach: II. Solubility of theophylline in polar binary solvents, *J. Pharm. Sci.*, *69*, 487–491 (1980).
22. A. Adjei, J. Newburger, and A. Martin, Extended Hildebrand approach: III. Solubility of caffeine in dioxane-water mixtures, *J. Pharm. Sci.*, *69*, 659–661 (1980).
23. A. N. Martin, P. L. Wu, A. Adjei, M. Mehdizadeh, K. C. James, and C. Metzler, Extended Hildebrand solubility approach: testosterone and testosterone propionate in binary solvents, *J. Pharm. Sci.*, *71*, 1334–1340 (1982).

7

Solute-Solute and
Solvent-Solvent Associations

The molecules of associated liquids contain both electron-donating and electron-accepting centers which are capable of donor-acceptor interactions with centers on neighboring molecules. Thus water is known to exist in the form of a flickering, three-dimensional network held together by hydrogen bonds between electron-donating oxygen atoms and electron-accepting hydrogen atoms. Alcohols behave similarly, forming chains of hydrogen-bonded molecules. These structures persist in solutions in which the associated liquid is the solvent, and in concentrated solutions in which it is the solute. Association of solute molecules decreases with dilution, and in very dilute solutions the molecules become completely dispersed. Simpler associated species also exist in solution; for example, it is well known that benzoic acid dimerizes when dissolved in organic solvents. Solute-solute and solvent-solvent association both influence the properties of solutions, and their behavior can be regarded from two viewpoints, the chemical interpretation and the physical interpretation.

I. CHEMICAL INTERPRETATION

The partial pressures of the components of an ideal binary liquid mixture can be calculated by Raoult's law (page 128). If the molecules of A are associated in a binary mixture of liquids A and B, positive deviation from Raoult's law will be observed. If it is assumed that dimerization occurs,

$$2A = A_2 \tag{7.1}$$

then according to Eq. (7.1), the concentrations of A and A_2 will be $X_A(1 - \alpha)$ and $\alpha X_A/2$, respectively. α is the degree of association and X_A is the mole fraction of liquid A in the mixture. Application of the law of mass action gives

$$K = \frac{X_A \alpha}{2(1 - \alpha)^2 X_A^{\ 2}} \tag{7.2}$$

where K is the association constant for the dimerization process. Expansion and rearrangement of Eq. (7.2) gives

$$2KX_A \alpha^2 - (4KX_A + 1)\alpha + 2KX_A = 0 \tag{7.3}$$

leading to

$$\alpha = \frac{(4KX_A + 1) \pm (8KX_A + 1)^{1/2}}{4KX_A} \tag{7.4}$$

which provides a method for calculating the degree of association. At equilibrium the total number of A and A_2 species in the solution will be $X_A(1 - \alpha+\alpha/2)$ or $X_A(1 - \alpha/2)$; therefore, in pure liquid consisting of $A + A_2$, $X_A = 1$, and the observed saturated vapor pressure ($p^o_{A(obs)}$) will be given by

$$p^o_{A(obs)} = p^o_A \left[1 - \frac{4KX_A + 1}{8KX_A} \pm \frac{(8KX_A + 1)^{1/2}}{8KX_A} \right] \tag{7.5}$$

where p_A^o is the saturated vapor pressure that would be obtained if the liquid were completely dissociated into individual molecules. If K is given the arbitrary value of 1, Eq. (7.5) solves to

$$p_{A(obs)}^o = \text{either } 0.00 \text{ or } 0.75 \; p_A^o$$

The real root of Eq. (7.5) is obviously 0.75, which was obtained by using the positive sign. In this and all subsequent calculations using Eq. (7.5), the negative sign yielded an imaginary root.

The significance of the foregoing calculation is that the measured saturated vapor pressure of liquid A will be less than would be anticipated from Raoult's law and that the discrepancy is due to dimerization of molecules of A. If increasing amounts of liquid B, which is assumed to be molecularly dispersed are added, as the concentration of liquid A in the solution decreases, so also does the degree of dimerization (α). A consequence of this is that the saturated vapor pressure will be greater relative to that predicted by Raoult's law. For example, if $X_A = 0.5$ and $K = 1$, substitution into

$$\bar{P}_A = p_{A(obs)}^o \; \frac{X_A \left[1 - \dfrac{4KX_A + 1}{8KX_A} + \dfrac{(8KX_A + 1)^{1/2}}{8KX_A} \right]}{X_A \left[1 - \dfrac{4KX_A + 1}{8KX_A} + \dfrac{(8KX_A + 1)^{1/2}}{8KX_A} \right] + X_B} \qquad (7.6)$$

yields $\bar{P}_A = 0.447 p_{A(obs)}^o$, where $\bar{P}_A$ is the partial vapor pressure of the $X_A = 0.5$ solution. This represents $0.447 \times 100/0.75 = 59.6\%$ of the observed saturated vapor pressure, compared with 50% if the liquids obeyed Raoult's law. The process of association therefore gives rise to positive deviation from Raoult's law. The deviation increases with increasing K and with the mean number of molecules in the complexes.

Although these factors undoubtedly contribute to the degree of deviation from Raoult's law, and were at one time accepted as the sole cause, the chemical interpretation is currently being subjected to a great deal of crticism. The main point of argument is that even with high values of K and large numbers of molecules forming associates, calculations of the type shown above are unable to match the experimental deviations.

II. PHYSICAL INTERPRETATION

In Chapter 6 it was suggested that when complexation occurred between solute and solvent, an unusually high cohesive energy must

operate between their molecules. The result of this was that the
geometric mean was an underestimate of the cohesive energy density, and the observed solubility was greater than that calculated
by regular solution theory. A similar argument can be advanced
for the behavior of solutions in which one of the components associates. The fact that its molecules associate implies that the component has a high cohesive energy density, with the result that
the geometric mean is too high an estimate of the cohesive energy
between solute and solvent [i.e., $u_{12} < (u_1 u_2)^{1/2}$] and that the
calculated solubility is higher than the observed value.

The physical interpretation of association can be expressed
through the extended solubility parameter approach in the form [1]

$$\log X_2 = \log X_2^i - A(\delta_1^2 + \delta_2^2 - 2K\delta_1\delta_2) \tag{7.7}$$

where X_2 and X_2^i are the observed and ideal mole fraction solubilities
of solute, respectively, and δ_1 and δ_2 are solubility parameters of
solvent and solute. A is an abbreviation of the expression $V_2\phi_1^2/$
2.303 RT, the components of which are assumed to be constant in the
present context. K is a factor that assesses the way in which the
geometric mean is operating. Thus, if K = 1, the geometric mean
precisely predicts the solute-solvent cohesive energy density, and
the equation reduces to that for a regular solution. If K < 1, the
geometric mean is an overestimate of the solute-solvent cohesive energy density, and the observed solubility is less than regular. Thus,
when solute-solute or solvent-solvent association occurs, δ_1 or δ_2,
or both, are large and yield a large geometric mean to represent
what is, in fact, a low cohesive energy between unlike molecules.
Hildebrand et al. [2] used the symbol l_{12} to represent the difference between the geometric mean and the true cohesive energy density. $(1 - l_{12})$ is therefore equivalent to K in Eq. (7.7).

The concept can be illustrated by Fig. 6.6, which shows the
plots of ideal and regular solubilities of a solute having a solubility
parameter of 11 H, over a solvent solubility parameter range of 8
to 14 H. Any solubilities lying on or near the regular solubility
line represent systems in which the K in Eq. (7.7) is equal to 1
and are regular solutions. If the solubility lies below the regular
solution line, K is less than 1, or put in another way, l_{12} is positive. This is considered to apply to systems in which like molecules
have associated. This area in Fig. 6.6 is probably not the sole
preserve of associated solutes and solvents; steroid esters have been
found to have subregular solubilities in saturated hydrocarbons,
even though other tests indicated that the solutions behaved regularly. The behavior in this case was attributed to steric effects and is
described elsewhere (page 217).

Martin et al. [1] considered that when the observed solubility exceeded ideal, solute-solvent complexation occurred, showing up in Eq. (7.7) as a positive value of K, which is sufficiently large to make $2K\delta_1\delta_2$ greater than $\delta_1^2 + \delta_2^2$, thereby giving an activity coefficient greater than 1. The most interesting region of Fig. 6.6 is that lying between the regular and ideal plots. Here K is greater than 1 but not great enough to make the activity coefficient term of Eq. (7.7) negative. This region was considered to represent systems in which solute-solute and/or solvent-solvent association occur concurrently, creating a balance between opposing tendencies. Martin et al. [1] suggested that a balance of this sort could place an observed solubility on the regular solution line, even though the actual solution is not regular.

III. EXPERIMENTAL METHODS

A. Colligative Properties

Vapor pressure, osmotic pressure, depression of freezing point, and elevation of boiling point all depend on the total number of molecules and associates in solution, and therefore provide a means of measuring the mean number of molecules per associate and of calculating association constants. The techniques are applicable only to very dilute solutions, which are systems in which association is at its least. Nonionic species can be expected to follow Henry's law up to at least several mole percent [3].

A problem with freezing- and boiling-point techniques is that they require the use of a standard solute which is known to remain in the monomeric state in solution in the particular solvent, for the calculation of the cryoscopic or ebullioscopic constants. That the standard is, in fact, in the monomeric state could be difficult to prove.

Tucker and Christian [4] have described an apparatus for determining association of solutes in solution. The vapor pressure of the solvent is first determined alone, and then an accurately measured volume of solute is added and the pressure redetermined. Fugacities (f_2) were found to be related to solute mole fraction (X_2) by an equation of the form

$$f_2 = aX_2 - bX_2^2 \tag{7.8}$$

so that differentiation of f_2 with respect to X_2 and placing X_2 equal to zero gave the Henry's law constant at infinite dilution (K_H^∞). The concentration of monomer $(X_{2,\text{monomer}})$ was then calculated from $X_{2,\text{monomer}} = f_2/K_H^\infty$. The total mole fraction of solute in the various aggregates was then given by $X_2 - X_{2,monomer}$, from which mass action equations involving the various association equilibria could be tested by least squares procedures.

Example

The fugacities of benzene (f_B) in aqueous solutions have been shown to follow the equation [4]

$$f_B = 3.527 \times 10^5 X_B - 3.07 \times 10^7 X_B^2$$

where X_B is the total mole fraction of benzene. Calculate the equilibrium constants for self-association of benzene in this solvent at (a) $X_B = 10^{-4}$ and (b) $X_B = 3 \times 10^{-4}$, assuming that the process is exclusively dimerization.

Solution:

$$\text{Henry's constant } (K_H) = \frac{f_B}{X_B}$$

Therefore, the infinite dilution Henry's constant (K_H^∞) is obtained by differentiating the equation and placing X_B equal to zero:

$$\frac{d}{dX_B}(3.527 \times 10^5 X_B - 3.07 \times 10^7 X_B^2) = 3.527 \times 10^5 - 3.07$$
$$\times 2 \times 10^7 X_B$$

When $X_B = 0$, $K_H^\infty = 3.527 \times 10^5$.
    (a) When $X_B = 10^{-4}$,

$$f_B = 3.527 \times 10^5 \times 10^{-4} - 3.07 \times 10^7 \times 10^{-8} = 34.96$$

$$X_{B(monomer)} = \frac{f_B}{K_H^\infty} = \frac{34.96}{3.527 \times 10^5} = 9.91 \times 10^{-5}$$

giving*

---

*This is the quantity of benzene in the dimer; therefore, $[B_2]$ is half this value.

$$X_{B(dimer)} = X_B - 9.91 \times 10^{-5} = 10^{-4} - 9.91 \times 10^{-5}$$
$$= 9.00 \times 10^{-7}$$

Substitution yields

$$K = \frac{[B_2]}{[B]^2}$$

$$= \frac{0.5 \times 9 \times 10^{-7}}{(9.91 \times 10^{-5})^2} = 45.8$$

(b) Similarly, when $X_B = 3 \times 10^{-4}$,

$$K = 45.9$$

B. Distribution

The distribution law states that if a solute is distributed between two immiscible solvents, or the conjugate solutions produced by two partially miscible solvents in equilibrium with each other, the ratio of the activities in the two solutions will be constant. The constant is termed the *partition* or *distribution coefficient,* and provided that the solutions are dilute, can be approximated to

$$\frac{c_o}{c_w} = K_d \tag{7.9}$$

in which K_d is the formal partition coefficient and c_o and c_w the total concentrations of solute in the two solutions, which will be assumed to be oil (O) and water (W). Expressed in this way, the law applies only if the solute is present in the same form in the two solutions. If, however, the solute is associated in one solvent and not in the other, the distribution law will apply only to the molecularly dispersed solute species, and the true partition coefficient $K_{p,1}$, will be given by

$$K_{p,1} = \frac{\text{monomer concentration in oil phase}}{\text{monomer concentration in water phase}} \tag{7.10}$$

The failure of associating solutes to obey the distribution law, as expressed by Eq. (7.9), can be turned to advantage and used to calculate association constants. The methodology will be described in detail in Chapter 9.

C. Infrared Spectrophotometry

As explained in Chapter 8, donor-acceptor interaction between an
atom in a particular molecule and a neighboring molecule has the
effect of decreasing the stretching frequency of the bond joining
that atom to the remainder of the molecule to which it belongs.   The
mechanism obviously applies also when the two participating molecules are identical.   Transitions of this type can be detected by
infrared spectrophotometry.   A typical spectrum, of the hydroxyl
stretching region of testosterone in chloroform solution, is reproduced in Fig. 7.1.   There is a sharp, fairly symmetrical absorption
band near 3600 cm^{-1} and a broader peak at about 3450 cm^{-1}.   Only
the 3600-cm^{-1} peak was detectable in dilute solutions, but as the
testosterone concentration was increased, the 3450-cm^{-1} band began
to appear, and the two bands increased in intensity to a similar
extent with increasing concentration.   The higher-frequency peak
represents the monomer, and the other, the association of hydroxy
groups with groups on neighboring molecules.

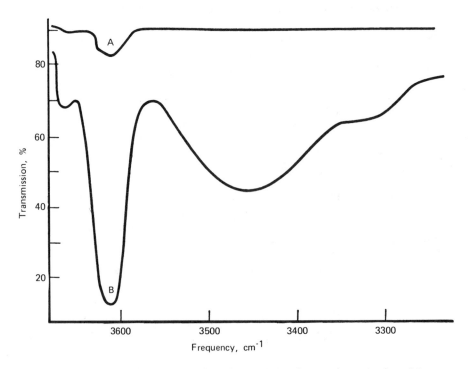

FIGURE 7.1 Hydroxyl stretching spectrum of testosterone in chloroform.   (A) dilute solution; (B) concentrated solution.   (From Ref.
8.)

TABLE 7.1 Hydroxyl Stretching Frequencies of Some Monomeric and Associated 3-Keto-17-hydroxy Steroids

Steroid	Monomer frequency (cm^{-1})	N-mer frequency (cm^{-1})	Frequency shift (cm^{-1})
	Solvent:	carbon tetrachloride	
Androstanolone	3625	3490	135
Testosterone	3625	3485	140
Dehydrotestosterone	3623	3475	148
Methylandrostanolone	3623	3490	133
Methyltestosterone	3623	3485	138
Methandienone	3624	3475	149
Nandrolone	3626	3485	141
	Solvent:	benzene	
Androstanolone	3591	3485	106
Testosterone	3592	3480	112
Dehydrotestosterone	3591	3465	126
Methylandrostanolone	3590	3485	105
Methyltestosterone	3591	3480	111
Methandienone	3591	3475	116
Nandrolone	3592	3480	112

Source: Ref. 6.

The strength of the interaction is a function of the frequency shift between monomer and associated peaks. This is illustrated by Table 7.1, which gives the hydroxyl stretching frequency shifts of some 3-keto-17-hydroxy steroids in carbon tetrachloride and in benzene. The interaction occurs between the 3-keto, which functions as an electron donor, and the 17-hydroxy, which is the electron-acceptor. The basicity, and therefore the electron-donating power of the 3-keto group, would be expected to increase with the degree of β unsaturation, and this is in fact the case. Androstanolene (XXI) and methylandrostanolone (XXII), which are saturated ketones, give the smallest shifts, and dehydrotestosterone (XXVI) and methandienone (XXVII), which are β,β-unsaturated ketones, give the greatest,

(XXI)   R = H   Androstanolone
(XXII)   R = CH$_3$ Methylandrostanolone

(XXIII)   R = H; R' = CH$_3$ Testosterone
(XXIV)   R = R' = H   Nandrolone
(XXV)   R = R' = CH$_3$ Methyltestosterone

(XXVI)   R = H   Dehydrotestosterone
(XXVII)   R = CH$_3$ Methandienone

while testosterone (XXIII), nandrolone (XXIV), and methyltestosterone (XXV), which have only one β double bond, occupy an intermediate position. Not all transitions are amenable to this treatment; for
example, the carbonyl stretching frequencies accompanying the results shown in Table 7.1 exhibited no measurable shift [6]

The hydroxyl stretching monomer peaks are sharp and narrow, so that peak area is proportional to peak height, which is therefore proportional to monomer concentration. Fletcher and Heller [7] investigated the self-association of 1-octanol and 1-butanol in *n*-decane, using the first overtone of the hydroxyl stretching region. A similar spectrum to Fig. 7.1 was found, and at low concentrations, when self-association would be expected to be small, there was a Beer's law relationship between the absorbance of the monomer peak and the total alcohol concentration. An extinction coefficient (ε_1) for the monomer could therefore be evaluated. If association is considered to involve a series of equilibria exemplified by

$$nS_1 \overset{K_{1,n}}{\rightleftharpoons} S_n \qquad (7.11)$$

where S_1 represents monomer and S_n represents n-mer, the concentration of each n-mer will be governed by

$$K_{1,n} = \frac{S_n}{S_1^n} \qquad (7.12)$$

Total concentatration of alcohol ($[S]_{(tot)}$) is given in

$$[S]_{(tot)} = [S_1] + 2[S_2] + 3[S_3] + \cdots + n[S_n] \qquad (7.13)$$

and the concentration of each n-mer is governed by Eq. (7.12). Rearrangement and substitution for $[S_1]$ from $[S_1] = a_1/\varepsilon_1$, where a_1 is the absorbance of the monomer peak, gives

$$[S]_{(tot)} = \frac{a_1}{\varepsilon_1} + \frac{2K_{1,2}a_1^2}{(\varepsilon_1)^2} + \frac{3K_{1,3}a_1^3}{(\varepsilon_1)^3} + \cdots + \frac{nK_{1,n}a_1^n}{(\varepsilon_1)^n} \qquad (7.14)$$

Fletcher and Heller [7] solved this power series by inserting experimental values of $[S]_{(tot)}$ and a_1, and fitting a regression line in which the difference between the sums of squares of observed and calculated values was minimal. The program was arranged so that negative association constants could be eliminated on the grounds that this indicated that there was no equilibrium for such n-mers. It revealed that association was predominently in the form of tetramer.

The simplest situation occurs when the compound dimerizes [n = 2 in Eq. (7.11)], and the absorbing groups on both molecules take part in the association process. 3,4-Disubstituted-5-hydroxyfuran-2-ones behave in this way [8], the hydroxyl group of each molecule in the dimer interacts with an electron-donating group on the other, to form a cyclic dimer. At low solute concentrations, self-association is negligible and the monomer hydroxyl stretching absorbance (E) obeys Beer's law, the plot of total solute concentration $[S]_{(tot)}$ against absorbance taking the form of a straight line arising from the origin. The following applies to this concentration range:

$$[S]_{tot} = \frac{E}{\varepsilon_o} \qquad (7.15)$$

where ε_o is the limiting molecular extinction coefficient, defined as the molecular extinction coefficient at infinite dilution. Association sets in at higher concentrations, and some of the dissolved solute will contribute to the absorbance of the dimer absorption band rather than the monomer band. Beer's law is no longer obeyed and the plot converges toward the concentration axis. $[S]_{tot}$ is now expressed as E/ε, where ε, the apparent molecular extinction coefficient of the monomer stretching absorbance, is the coefficient operating at the specific solute concentration and varies with the magnitude of $[S]_{tot}$. The association constant (K_{12}) is given by

$$K_{12} = \frac{[S_2]}{[S]^2} = \frac{[S]_{tot} - [S]}{[S]^2} = \frac{E/\varepsilon - E/\varepsilon_o}{(E/\varepsilon_o)^2} \qquad (7.16)$$

Some of the E's cancel. Multiplication of numerator and denominator by ε, and substitution for $E = \varepsilon[S]_{tot}$ yields

$$K_{12} = \frac{1 - \varepsilon/\varepsilon_o}{[S]_{tot}(\varepsilon/\varepsilon_o)^2} \qquad (7.17)$$

which provides a means of calculating dimerization constants.

A combination of partitioning and spectrophotometry has been used to investigate the dimerization of trifluoroacetic acid in organic solvents [9]. A layer of solution was placed in a specially designed infrared absorption cell so that it was located below the radiation beam and the spectrophotometer recorded the absorption of the vapor only. The total pressure (P) of the vapor is given by

$$P = P_m + P_d = P_m + 2K_{1,2}P_m^2 \qquad (7.18)$$

in which P_m and P_d are the partial pressures of monomer and dimer, respectively. If E is the extinction of the monomer band, ε the molecular extinction coefficient, and d the pathlength, conversion of molar units to pressure will give

$$P = \frac{ERT}{\varepsilon d} + 2K_{1,2} \left(\frac{ERT}{\varepsilon d} \right)^2 \tag{7.19}$$

Henry's law states that

$$\bar{p} = K_H [S]_{tot} \tag{7.20}$$

where $\bar{p}$ is partial pressure and K_H is Henry's constant. $\bar{p}$ is equivalent to P in Eq. (7.19), and substitution from Eq. (7.20) gives

$$[S]_{tot} = \frac{ERT}{\varepsilon K_H d} + 2K_{1,2} \left(\frac{ERT}{\varepsilon K_H d} \right)^2 \tag{7.21}$$

or

$$\frac{[S]_{tot}}{E} = \frac{RT}{\varepsilon K_H d} + 2K_{1,2} \left(\frac{RT}{\varepsilon K_H d} \right)^2 \cdot E \tag{7.22}$$

which indicates that a plot of $[S]_{tot}/E$ against E will give a straight line. Henry's constant can be evaluated from the intercept and $K_{1,2}$ from the slope.

Free energies of dimerization were negative and gave an inverse rectilinear relationship to the free energies of transfer of monomer from vapor to solvent. The inference is that the solvent is competing with solute monomers for other solvent monomers, and highlights an experimental difficulty associated with studies of solute-solute interactions. The solute is usually poorly soluble in solvents that do not interfere with the dimerization process, so that solutions sufficiently concentrated for accurate measurements to be taken are in excess of solubility, while good solvents usually complex with the solute and thereby interfere with solute-solute association.

IV. HYDROPHOBIC INTERACTION

A substantial volume of evidence has accumulated over recent years suggesting that nonpolar molecules and groups tend to be attracted to each other in an aqueous environment. The most characteristic feature is that the process is accompanied by unusually high negative entropies of solution, which have led to the idea of a solvation sphere of water molecules surrounding the solute, in a more ordered state than in the bulk of the solvent. The phenomenon is described as hydrophobic bonding or hydrophobic interaction, and both these terms are frequently invoked in scientific discussions.

Efforts to confirm that lipid molecules associate in water have been largely contradictory. For example, the main evidence for the association of benzene in water comes indirectly from measurements with diphenyl, which predicted a free energy of dimerization of -4.75 kJ mol^{-1} [10]. In contrast, vapor pressure measurements on benzene solutions in water yielded a small positive value (0.41 kJ mol^{-1}) [4]. Similarly, the enthalpies of transfer of small hydrocarbons from nonpolar solvents to water vary from slightly negative to small positive values at around 298 K [11].

Present opinion is that attraction between hydrophobic groups plays little part in hydrophobic interaction, and that the driving force comes from the high cohesive energy of the water molecules, which excludes the hydrophobic species, forcing them to cluster together. The process causes disruption of the isotropic arrangement of water molecules. It has been suggested [12] that the hydrophobic species take up a configuration such that the hydrogen bonds between the water molecules are restored and the resultant orderly arrangement brings about a fall in entropy.

The concept of hydrophobic effect has received little support from studies of compounds consisting entirely of hydrophobic groups, mainly because the degree of interaction is small. However, when a compound having a strong hydrophobic component also contains one or more hydrophilic groups, hydrophobic interactions occur and are easily detected and assessed. The most obvious example is the self-association of surfactants into micelles. These are aggregations of usually about 100 molecules, in which the hydrophobic groups form a core with the hydrophilic groups pointing outward. They form stable, colloidal dispersions in water, giving the impression of enhanced solubility of the monomolecular species. Micelles are also formed by biological lipids in which the hydrophilic influence is small in comparison with the hydrophobic contribution. Association of hydrophobic groups, with hydrophilic groups orientated toward an aqueous environment, also leads to formation of vesicles and membranes. The conformation of proteins in their natural environment is also dependent on such considerations. Two monographs on hydrophobic interactions have appeared recently [11,13].

REFERENCES

1. A. N. Martin, P. L. Wu, A. Adjei, M. Mehdizadeh, K. C. James, and C. Metzler, Extended Hildebrand solubility approach: testosterone and testosterone propionate in binary solvents, *J. Pharm. Sci.*, *71*, 1334–1340 (1982).

2. J. H. Hildebrand, J. M. Prausnitz, and R. L. Scott, *Regular and Related Solutions*, van Nostrand Reinhold, New York, 1970.

3. S. D. Christian, A. A. Taha, and B. W. Gash, Molecular complexes of water in organic solvents and in the vapour phase, *Chem. Soc. Q. Rev.*, *24*, 30–36 (1970).

4. E. E. Tucker and S. D. Christian, A prototype hydrophobic interaction. The dimerization of benzene in water, *J. Phys. Chem.*, *83*, 426–427 (1979).

5. K. C. James and M. Ramgoolam, Complexation of some 3-keto-17-hydroxy steroids in polar solvents, *Spectrochim. Acta, 31A*, 1599–1604 (1975).

6. M. Ramgoolam, Effects of molecular interactions on the solubilities of some androgen alcohols, Ph.D. thesis, University of Wales, 1974.

7. A. N. Fletcher and C. A. Heller, Self association of alcohols in nonpolar solvents, *J. Phys. Chem.*, *71*, 3742–3756 (1967).

8. S. Kovac, E. Socaniova, E. Beska, and P. Rapos, Hydrogen-bonding in 3,4-disubstituted-5-hydroxyfuran-2(SH)-ones, *J. Chem. Soc. Perkin Trans. 2*, 105–107 (1973).

9. S. D. Christian and T. L. Stevens, Association of trifluoracetic acid in vapor and in organic solvents, *J. Phys. Chem.*, *76*, 2039–2044 (1972).

10. A. Ben-Naim, J. Wilf, and M. Yaacobi, Hydrophobic interactions in light and heavy water, *J. Phys. Chem.*, *77*, 95–102 (1973).

11. C. Tanford, *The Hydrophobic Effect: Formation of Micelles and Biological Membranes*, 2nd ed., Wiley-Interscience, New York, 1980.

12. H. S. Frank and M. W. Evans, Free volume and entropy in condensed systems: III. Entropy in binary liquid mixtures; partial molal entropy in dilute solutions; structure and thermodynamics in aqueous electrolytes, *J. Chem. Phys.*, *13*, 507–532 (1945).

13. A. Ben-Naim, *Hydrophobic Interactions*, Plenum Press, New York, 1980.

8

Solute-Solvent Complexation

I. THE ASSOCIATION PROCESS

In the experiments leading to the regular solution concept [1], Hildebrand and Jenks observed that plots of log solubility against 1/T for
violet colored solutions of iodine formed a regular family of curves
(page 156), but those which were red deviated from the general pattern. Hildebrand concluded [2] that the iodine was molecularly dispersed in the violet solutions, but was solvated in the red solutions.
   Iodine is a Lewis acid [3] and, as such, is able to accept a lone
pair of electrons from a Lewis base. Ethers and carbonyl compounds
are examples of Lewis bases, and solvate iodine by donating the lone
pairs of electrons on their oxygen atoms. This process is an example
of donor-acceptor complexation, a subject that has been reviewed by
Bent [4]. Compounds in which hydrogen and one or more electron-
withdrawing groups are linked to the same carbon atom, such as

chloroform and 1,2-dichloroethane, are also Lewis acids and are
capable of complexing with Lewis bases. In these compounds, hydrogen is the electron acceptor and forms a hydrogen bond with the
electron donor. Interactions involving hydrogen bonds are regarded
as a special type of donor-acceptor complexation. The term *electron
transfer complex* is usually confined to donor-acceptor complexes not
involving hydrogen bonds. Complexes vary in stability from weak,
cluster complexes that exist only in solution, to stable molecules
that can be isolated.

Interaction between like molecules was considered in Chapter 7.
Interaction between two solutes dissolved in an inert solvent can
potentiate an increase or a decrease in solubility, but when the complexing species are solute and solvent, enhanced solubility must always result. In this chapter emphasis is placed on complexation between solute and solvent and the influence of the process on solubility. Solute-solvent complexation can be expressed generally by

$$nS + mL \overset{K}{\rightleftharpoons} S_n L_m \tag{8.1}$$

where n is the number of molecules of substrate (S) and m the number of molecules of complexing agent (L) in the complex. In this
particular context, S is also solute, and L solvent. K is the stability constant; the greater its value, the greater the degree of
complexation. Frequently, more than one type of complex is formed
by a complexing system, differing from each other in the values of
n and m.

Liquids that interact to form complexes are invariably mutually
soluble in all proportions, but the resulting solutions are not ideal
except at extremes of concentration, when one component is in considerable excess and the behavior of the resulting dilute solution
approximates to ideal. Thus chloroform and diethyl ether are completely misible, but they exhibit negative deviation from Raoult's
law (page 150) because a hydrogen-bonded complex is formed between
the two molecules. When a solid solute complexes with a liquid solvent, there is a limit of solute concentration above which the mixture
ceases to be a homogeneous liquid. This represents the formal
solubility of the solute (complexed + uncomplexed).

The extended solubility parameter approach expresses solubility
in the form

$$\ln X_2 = \ln a_2 - A(\delta_1^2 + \delta_2^2 - w_{12}) \tag{8.2}$$

where w_{12} is the true solute-solvent cohesive energy density. Thus
if $w_{12} = 2\delta_1\delta_2$, the solution behaves regularly. The fact that two

species form a complex infers that they have a high affinity for each other, so that the cohesive energy density between solute and solvent is normally greater than $2\delta_1\delta_2$. The solution would therefore not behave regularly and the solubility would be greater than predicted by regular solution theory. Furthermore, if $w_{12} > (\delta_1^2 + \delta_2^2)$, the expression in parentheses in Eq. (8.2) will be negative and the solubility greater than ideal. Martin et al. [5] used this concept as a criterion of complexation, namely that when the observed solubility exceeded the predicted ideal solubility [Eq. (6.24)], strong solute-solvent complexation was occurring. The principle cannot be applied to solutions of liquids in liquids, since ideal solubilities in these systems are infinite and therefore cannot be exceeded. Complexation under these circumstances can be detected from vapor pressure measurements and the consequent negative deviation from Raoult's law.

The effects of complexation on the solubility of a solid can be represented by a phase solubility diagram. The general experimental method for constructing this involves adding quantities of solute in excess of its solubility to various concentrations of complexing agent dissolved in an inert solvent. The mixtures are brought to equilibrium at the required temperature and the saturated solutions analyzed for total concentration of the solute, irrespective of its molecular state. The phase diagram is constructed by plotting total molar concentration of solute against the molar concentration of complexing agent added.

Higuchi and Connors [6] classified phase diagrams into two groups, type A and type B. Type B plots apply to insoluble complexes and are not expected to fit situations in which a solvent is the complexing agent. Figure 8.1 shows the three general forms of type A diagrams. They have the same intercept at zero complexing agent concentrations (S_0), characteristic of the solute, and representing its solubility in the pure, inert solvent. Initially, the total quantity of solute in solution $[S]_t$ increases with complexing agent concentration $[L]_t$, but the plots differ at high complexing agent concentrations. If 1:1 complexation occurs, this initial portion will be rectilinear. Similar diagrams are obtained with higher complexes, provided that they are first order with respect to L (i.e., S_2L, S_3L, etc.). Type A_L diagrams continue rectilinearly, up to the solubility limit of the complexing agent in the inert solvent.

A type A_N plot, in which the effect of complexing agent appears to diminish as its concentration increases, is obtained when the solubility of the complex in the inert solvent is limited. The inflection marks the extent of solubility of the complex; increase in complexing agent concentration beyond this point may yield more molecules of complex, but they are precipitated, and the total apparent concentration of solute in solution remains constant. A similar plot occurs if the complexing agent associates with itself, as in

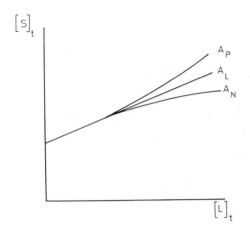

FIGURE 8.1   Phase solubility diagrams of type A systems.

$$2L \rightleftharpoons L_2 \tag{8.3}$$

$$S + L \rightleftharpoons SL \tag{8.4}$$

and the equilibrium constant of Eq. (8.4) is greater than that of
Eq. (8.3), Eq. (8.4) will predominate at first, but as the complexing agent concentration increases, Eq. (8.3) will become more important and relatively less solute will pass into solution as SL.

A change in the nature of the solvent with complexing agent
concentration is another factor that potentiates the formation of an
A_N phase diagram.   In the presence of large quantities of complexing agent, the solvent no longer behaves in the same way as in the
pure state, with the result that the complexation constants and the
quantity of uncomplexed solute in solution may change.   This situation could involve a rise instead of a fall in $[S]_t$ with increasing
complexing agent concentration.   The change in inert solvent concentration is an associated factor.   If the complexing agent is a
solid and its solution in the inert solvent is prepared on a weight-
in-volume basis, the amount of inert solvent required to produce
the necessary volume will remain reasonably independent of complexing agent concentration, provided that the concentration of complexing agent is low.   However, as the quantity of complexing agent is
increased, significant quantities of solvent will be displaced, and
less will be required to adjust to volume.   This means that less inert solvent is available to dissolve the uncomplexed solute, with a
resultant decrease in the value of S_0.   The solubility limits of solid
complexing agents are usually reached before their influence on the

volume of solvent begins to take hold. The effect is more marked
with liquid complexing agents, because the volumes of liquids are
usually additive and liquids are usually misible over a larger concentration range than solids in liquids. Experimenters therefore tend
to test liquid-liquid systems to higher complexing agent concentrations. Preparation of weight-in-weight mixtures does nothing to improve the situation.

Figure 8.2 is a typical experimental example and represents the
solubilities of testosterone in mixtures of octanol and cyclohexane.
The two solvents are misible in all proportions, so that the concentrations could be ranged from one pure solvent to the other. The
total testosterone in solution increases with octanol concentration in
an approximately rectilinear fashion, but closer inspection reveals
that the points follow a shallow sigmoidal form, and the tailing off
at high octanol contents could be due to the effect described above.

If complexes of higher order in L than 1 are formed (i.e., SL_2,
SL_3, etc.), the plot A_p of Fig. 8.1 will be obtained. Figure 8.3
is a combination of all type A plots and represents the total apparent solubilities of testosterone as solute in chloroform (as complexing agent)-cyclohexane mixtures. The initial portion of the plot is
interpreted as SL complexation, and the upward part of the curve
as involving SL_2 and SL_3 formation. The point at which the plot
levels off corresponds to a molar ratio of 1 of testosterone to 3 of

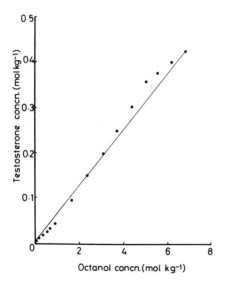

FIGURE 8.2 Solubilities of testosterone in cyclohexane-octanol mixtures at 25°C. (From Ref. 7.)

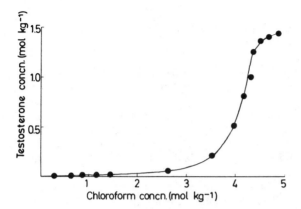

FIGURE 8.3   Solubilities of testosterone in chloroform-cyclohexane
mixtures at 25°C.   (From Ref. 7.)

chloroform.   The final horizontal portion of the plot is assumed to
be the limit of solubility of the 1:3 complex.   1:3 complexation between chloroform and testosterone has been established by other
methods [8,9].

The relevance of solute-solvent interaction to the general study
of solubility can be condensed to the statement that the process
appears to facilitate the solution of a quantity of solute in excess
of that predicted by regular solution theory.   The resulting system
is not a solution in the classical terms of a random dispersion of
solute molecules in solvent molecules, but from a practical point of
view, it usually has all the properties that are required of a solution.   Electron-donating and electron-accepting liquids are therefore
in greater demand as solvents than are inert fluids, such as hydrocarbons.   They are also valuable cosolvents, which can be blended
with nonpolar solvents to provide media with affinity for both hydrophilic and lipophilic materials.   The enhancement in solubility can be
explained in terms of an energy balance between the various molecular interactions occurring in the system, influenced in particular by
the high cohesive energy density between solute and solvent molecules.

Phase solubility diagrams are complicated by the presence of an
inert solvent which is necessary to maintain the system in the liquid
state.   With most of the systems examined by this technique, both
solute and complexing agent have been solids.   Even when the complexing agent is a liquid, there will be combinations of solute, complexing solvent, and complex for which the most stable form is the
solid state under the conditions operating, and although the product
is a stable solid solution, its appearance may be interpreted as insolubility.   However, when a solid phase separates in a phase

solubility exercise, it is usually the limited solubility of the complex in the inert solvent that is responsible. Thus, while the phase solubility technique gives valuable information, the inert solvent, upon which it relies, has no real place in a consideration of the effects of solute-solvent complexation on solubility. It is more relevant to think in terms of a mixture consisting entirely of solute and solvent. Under these circumstances two parameters of the equilibrium, the complexation or stability constant (K) and the stoichiometric quantities of the participants of the process (n and m), are the most important.

II. THE COMPLEXATION CONSTANT

If we consider solute-solvent interaction as the formation of only one complex species, represented in general form by Eq. (8.1), application of the law of mass action and rearrangement gives

$$[S_n L_m] = K[S]^n [L]^m \tag{8.5}$$

The quantity of complex produced is therefore directly proportional to the complexation constant (K). Complexation produces a more ordered system, with a consequent decrease in entropy; therefore, the higher the value of K, the greater the fall in entropy accompanying complexation. The van't Hoff equation

$$\Delta G = -RT \ln K \tag{8.6}$$

states that the higher the complexation constant, the lower will be the Gibbs free energy of complexation, so the net result of free energy and entropy will be a lowering of the enthalpy of complexation. It may therefore be concluded that the solute-solvent cohesive energy density will be a positive function of the complexation constant of the interaction between solute and solvent, and the greater the value of K, the greater will be the total solubility of S in L.

III. THE STOICHIOMETRIC PROPORTION

On a mole fraction basis, the sum of the analytical concentrations of S and L is unity (i.e., $X_{S(t)} + X_{L(t)} = 1$). If $X_{S_n L_m}$ is small, Eq. (8.5) can be written in the form of

$$X_{S_n L_m} = K X_{S(t)}^n (1 - X_{S(t)})^m \tag{8.7}$$

Differentiating $X_{S_n L_m}$ with respect to $X_{S(t)}$ and placing the result equal to zero yields the concentration of solute, $X_{S(max)}$, which corresponds to the maximum concentration of complex. This solves to

$$X_{S(max)} = \frac{n}{n + m} \qquad (8.8)$$

which indicates that the greater the value of m, the more complexing agent will be required to achieve the maximum concentration of complex. Usually, complexation involving values of n and/or m in excess of unity takes place in stages; for example,

$$S + L = SL \qquad (8.9)$$

$$SL + L = SL_2 \qquad (8.10)$$

$$SL_2 + L = SL_3 \qquad (8.11)$$

and so on.

IV. METHODS OF DETERMINING EQUILIBRIUM PARAMETERS

A. Electronic Absorption

The first investigation of solute-solvent interactions from electronic spectra was carried out on iodine solutions in aromatic solvents [10]. The original intention was to correlate the color of the solution with the degree of complexation, but the maxima in the visible region were small and their wavelengths occurred in a random fashion. The spectra are reproduced in Fig. 8.4. All the aromatic solvent solutions, except benzotrifluoride, gave an intense band around 300 nm, which was considered to be characteristic of iodine-aromatic complexes. Benzotrifluoride, which contains the strong, electron-attracting CF_3 group, gave no absorption band in this region. The concentration of the complex [SL] is therefore given by

$$[SL] = \frac{E}{\varepsilon} \qquad (8.12)$$

where ε is the molecular extinction coefficient at the maximum around 300 nm, given by

$$\varepsilon = \frac{E}{[S]_t} \qquad (8.13)$$

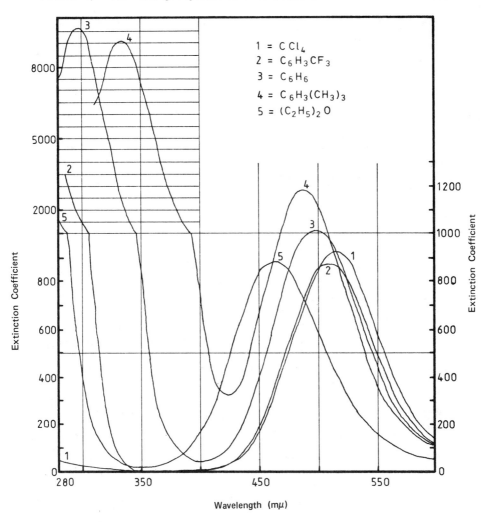

FIGURE 8.4 Electronic absorption of iodine in various solvents. (From Ref. 10.)

where E is the absorbance under the conditions operating and $[S]_t$ is the total molar concentration of iodine.

It was assumed that 1:1 complexation occurred, so that the following applies:

$$K = \frac{[SL]}{([S]_t - [SL])([L]_t - [SL])} \tag{8.14}$$

$[L]_t$ is the total aromatic solvent concentration, which is in large excess, so that $([L]_t - [SL])$ approximates to $[L]_t$, and substitution for $[SL]$ from Eq. (8.12) yields

$$\frac{[S]_t}{E} = \frac{1}{K\varepsilon} \frac{1}{[L]_t} + \frac{1}{\varepsilon} \tag{8.15}$$

This has the form of a rectilinear equation, so that the plot of $[S]_t/E$ against $1/[L]_t$ gives a straight line with intercept $1/\varepsilon$. Substitution of this value into the slope yielded K. The straight-line form of the plots confirmed that the complexes were 1:1 (m = n = 1), and the complexation constants (K) fell in the order anticipated for a complex in which π electrons of the aromatic ring were donated to the iodine molecules.

Example

The absorbances obtained with a range of benzene-carbon tetrachloride solutions of iodine at 297 nm are summarized in the first three columns of Table 8.1. Use this information to calculate the equilibrium constant for the 1:1 complexation of benzene with iodine.

	Benzene	Carbon tetrachloride
Density (kg m^{-3})	897	1632
Molecular weight	78	Not required

Solution:

Taking the results for 80% benzene as an example yields

$$[\text{benzene}] = \frac{800 \times 897}{1,000 \times 78} = 9.20 \text{ mol dm}^{-3}$$

TABLE 8.1 Spectrophotometric Data for Iodine in Benzene-Carbon Tetrachloride Mixtures at 297 nm

Benzene	$[I_2]$ (mol dm^{-3} × 10^5)	E	$[I_2]/E$ × 10^5	Benzene (mol dm^{-3})	$\dfrac{1}{[benzene]}$
100	3.26	0.317	10.3	11.5	0.0869
90	6.96	0.657	10.6	10.4	0.0966
80	10.4	0.949	11.0	9.20	0.109
60	10.4	0.827	12.6	6.90	0.145
20	17.4	0.699	24.9	2.30	0.435
8	43.5	0.853	51.0	0.920	1.09
4	21.8	0.234	93.0	0.460	2.18

Therefore,

$$\frac{1}{[benzene]} = 0.109 \ dm^3 \ mol^{-1}$$

$$\frac{[I_2]}{E} = \frac{10.4 \times 10^{-5}}{0.949} = 1.10 \times 10^{-4} \ dm^3 \ mol^{-1}$$

The results of similar calculations on the remaining results are given in the last three columns of Table 8.1.

Regression analysis of 1/[benzene] against $[I_2]/E$ gives

$$\frac{[I_2]}{E} = \frac{3.97 \times 10^{-4}}{[benzene]} + 7.02 \times 10^{-5} \qquad \begin{array}{cc} n & r \\ 7 & 1.000 \end{array}$$

Molecular extinction of complex $[SL] = \dfrac{1}{7.02 \times 10^{-5}}$

$$= 14,200$$

Complexation coefficient $(K) = \dfrac{1}{3.97 \times 10^{-4} \times 14,200}$

$$= 0.177 \ dm^3 \ mol^{-1}$$

The iodine-aromatic solvent systems examined by Benesi and Hildebrand enjoy the advantage that neither substrate nor complexing solvent absorb at the wavelength maximum of the complex. Higuchi et al. [11] examined the situation where all three species absorb at the chosen wavelength. They used the expression ΔE and $\Delta \epsilon$, where ΔE is the difference between the absorbance of the mixture, and the sum of the absorbances of S and L if they did not complex. $\Delta \epsilon$ is the corresponding term for molecular extinction coefficients. The two were shown to be related through

$$[SL] = \frac{\Delta E}{\Delta \epsilon} \tag{8.16}$$

Expansion and rearrangement of Eq. (8.14) gives

$$[SL] = \frac{[S_t][L_t] + [SL]^2}{(1/K) + [S_t] + [L_t]} \tag{8.17}$$

So that if it is assumed that $[SL]^2$ is small in comparison with $[S_t][L_t]$, then when $[SL]$ is substituted from Eq. (8.14) in Eq. (8.16) we have

$$\frac{[S_t][L_t]}{\Delta E} = \frac{[S_t] + [L_t]}{\Delta \varepsilon} + \frac{1}{K \, \Delta \varepsilon} \tag{8.18}$$

This is an equation of a straight line, so if $([S_t][L_t])/\Delta E$ is plotted against $[S_t] + [L_t]$, the slope will give $\Delta \varepsilon$, which on substitution into the intercept yields K. If $[SL]^2$ cannot be ignored, expansion of Eq. (8.17) will give a quadratic equation in $[SL]$, which can be solved by inserting the estimated value of K from the plot of Eq. (8.18).

Moriguchi and Kaneniwa [12] also started with Eqs. (8.16) and (8.17), and developed

$$\frac{[L_t]}{\Delta E} + \frac{\Delta E}{[S_t]\Delta \varepsilon^2} = \frac{1}{\Delta \varepsilon [S_t]} \left(\frac{1}{K} + [L_t] \right) + \frac{1}{\Delta \varepsilon} \tag{8.19}$$

They suggested that an estimate of $1/\Delta \varepsilon$ be first obtained, using the Benesi-Hildebrand equation [Eq. (8.15)], and this be substituted into $[L_t]/\Delta E + \Delta E/[S_t](\Delta \varepsilon)^2$, which was plotted aginst $1/[S_t]$ to get an improved value of $1/\Delta \varepsilon$. This step was repeated until a constant intercept was obtained. K was then calculated from Eq. (8.19).

The value of K obtained by any of the foregoing methods is dependent on the units used to express concentration. Benesi and Hildebrand [10] used mole fraction units to measure $[L_t] - [SL]$ and molarities for $[S_t]$ and $[SL]$ whose units canceled, leaving a dimensionless K. Kuntz et al. [13] discussed the choice of concentration units when using the Benesi-Hildebrand equation, and favored molarity. Molartities are used in the example in this section, giving an answer in liters mol^{-1}.

Other variations on the Benesi-Hildebrand equation have been published by Rose and Drago [14] and Kakemi et al. [15]. The Benesi-Hildebrand equation and variations thereon can be applied to any technique in which complex concentration is related to a physical property.

B. Infrared Absorption

When a chemical group complexes with an atom on a neighboring molecule, the properties of the bond joining the group to its parent molecule are changed. The associated changes in the infrared spectrum take the form of shifts to higher or lower frequencies, peak broadening, increase or decrease in absorption intensity, or the appearance of new peaks. Of these, the effect on the stretching vibrational frequency is the most important. Less energy is required to stretch a bond in which one of the atoms is complexed to another molecule than is required to stretch the corresponding free bond. The result

is that the vibrational frequency moves to a longer wavelength.
The difference is termed the frequency shift and is defined by

$$\text{Frequency shift} = \frac{\Delta \nu}{\nu} = \frac{\nu - \nu_0}{\nu} \tag{8.20}$$

ν_0 represents the frequency of the gaseous state and ν the frequency of the complexed species. It is not always possible to re-
cord a spectrum of the gaseous state, particularly if the substance
is a solid, in which case a solution in an inert solvent is normally
used as reference. Spectral modifications that occur when a compound goes into solution are collectively termed *solvent effects*.

The frequency shift is not a precise measure of the strength
of the interaction, but the two properties are loosely related, so
that shifts are frequently used to assess the strength of the interaction. Bellamy et al. [16] studied solvent effects by directly comparing the frequency shifts of two different solutes in the same
variety of solvents. If the shifts were dependent on the same properties, a straight line of slope 45° would be obtained when the shifts
of one solute were plotted against those of the other. Any complexing solvent that behaved differently with one solute compared
with the other solute would give a point off the line. If the two
solutes behaved differently in all the solvents, the plot would deviate from 45°. This procedure was used to establish whether the
17—OH group of androstanolone was complexing as an electron donor
or as an electron acceptor [8], by comparing its hydroxyl stretching frequency shifts with the carbonyl stretching frequency shifts
of cyclohexanone. The electron-accepting solvents gave a 45° plot,
indicating that the mode of interaction of the hydroxyl group was
the same as that of the carbonyl group, and therefore probably involved the oxygen atom. This is reproduced in Fig. 8.5. The
aromatic solvents gave a negative slope, suggesting that they behaved as electron donors with one solute and as electron acceptors
with the other. A variation on the Bellamy, Hallam, and Williams [16]
(BHW) plot is to plot the shift against a parameter that is a measure
of electron density; for example, a plot of frequency shift of the
17-hydroxy group of androstanolone against the Hammett σ functions
of the aromatic solvents had a negative slope, indicating that the
solvents were acting as electron donors [8]. The results are shown
in Fig. 8.6.

When the spectra of a series of mixtures taking part in the same
equilibrium, all having the same total concentration but with different proportions of starting materials are traced on the same chart,
there will be one point through which all the spectra will pass. A
typical example is shown in Fig. 8.7. It represents the ester carbonyl stretching region for testosterone propionate. The higher-

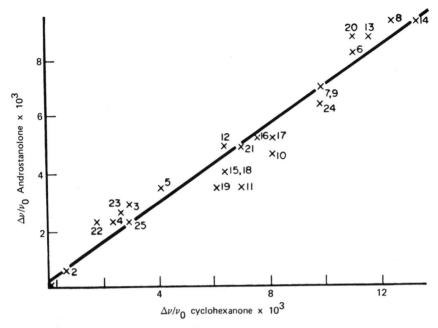

FIGURE 8.5 Correlation of relative carbonyl stretching shifts of
cyclohexanone and relative "monomer" hydroxyl shifts of androstanolone. 1, *n*-hexane; 2, cyclohexane; 3, carbon tetrachloride; 4, tetra-
chloroethylene; 5, carbon disulfide; 6, chloroform; 7, dichloromethane;
8, bromoform; 9, 1,2-dichloroethane; 10, *cis*-1,2-dichloroethylene;
11, *trans*-1,2-dichlorethylene; 12, trichlorethylene; 13, 1,1,2,2-
tetrachloroethane; 14, 1,1,2,2-tetrabromoethane; 15, benzene; 16,
bromobenzene; 17, chlorobenzene; 18, toluene; 19, xylene; 20, nitrobenzene; 21, anisole; 22, diethyl ether; 23, dioxane; 24, nitroethane;
25, tetrahydrofuran. (From Ref. 8.)

frequency band is for the uncomplexed ester, and the lower-frequency
band for the complexed ester. The steroid concentration was kept
constant and the solvent varied from 100% cyclohexane to 100% chloroform. The intersection is called an *isosbestic point* and its presence
indicates that the components are in equilibrium. If there are a
series of consecutive equilibria, as in Eqs. (8.9) to (8.11), each
will be characterized by its own isosbestic point, those for the
higher-order complexes appearing at progressively higher complexing agent concentrations and progressively lower frequencies. If
the pattern is reversed and the isosbestic points move to higher
frequencies with increasing complexing agent concentration, a sequence exemplified by

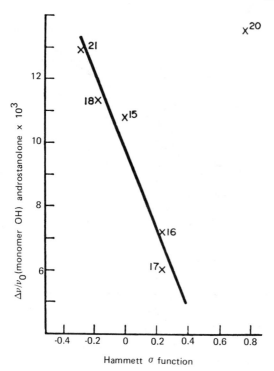

FIGURE 8.6 Correlation of relative "monomer" hydroxyl shifts of androstanolone with Hammett functions of solvents. Solvent code as for Fig. 8.5. (From Ref. 8.)

$$S + L = SL \qquad\qquad (8.21)$$

and

$$S + SL = S_2L \qquad\qquad (8.22)$$

would be anticipated. Isobestic points also occur in the electronic region. The significance of isobestic points in relation to electronic spectra is discussed by Cohen and Fischer [17].

A refinement of simple observation of isosbestic points is to plot the intensities of the absorption maxima against complexing agent concentrations. This procedure, termed *continuous variation*, is shown in Fig. 8.8, which has been developed from the results traced in Fig. 8.7. The chosen frequencies represent the two maxima and an inflection. Each plot extrapolates to a minimum at a solute-complexing agent molar ratio of 1:1, indicating 1:1 complexation.

Example

The ester carbonyl oxygen of testosterone propionate forms one or more hydrogen bonds with chloroform. The uncomplexed carbonyl stretching frequency, given by solutions of testosterone propionate in cyclohexane, occurs around 1745 cm^{-1}, while the maximum of the chloroform complex occurs at a lower frequency. A typical family of absorption curves is shown in Fig. 8.7. A series of synthetic mixtures were prepared by mixing the quantities of testosterone and chloroform, shown below, and adjusting to 2 ml with cyclohexane.

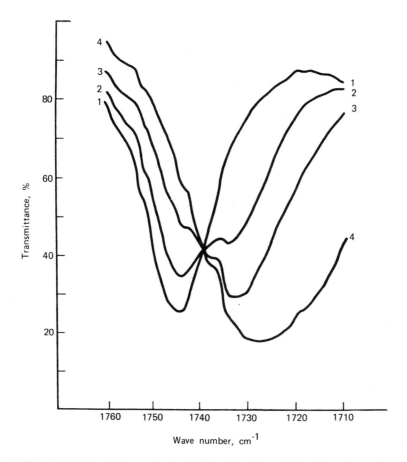

FIGURE 8.7 Carbonyl stretching bands of the 17-ester group of testosterone propionate in various cyclohexane-chloroform solvent blends. Molar ratios of chloroform to testosterone propionate, 1, 0; 2, 8.4; 3, 25.1; 4, 67.0. (From Ref. 9.)

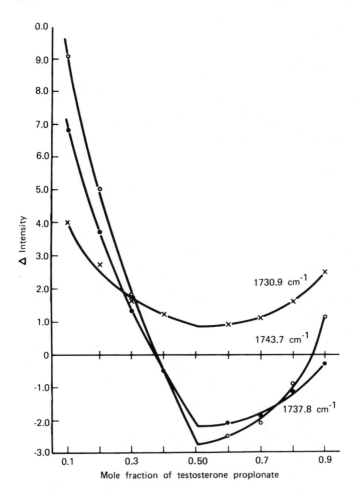

FIGURE 8.8 Determination of stoichiometric ratio of testosterone propionate-chloroform complex by continuous variation. (From Ref. 9.)

The percentage transmissions at 1743.7 cm^{-1} are also given in the table. Use this information to determine the ratio of ester carbonyl to chloroform in the combination. Molecular weights: testosterone propionate, 344.5; chloroform, 119.4.

Weight of steroid (mg)	Weight of chloroform (mg)	Percent of transmission at 1743.7 cm^{-1}
8.3	25.8	96.0
8.3	0	87.0
16.5	22.9	86.0
16.5	0	81.0
24.8	20.1	80.0
24.8	0	78.0
33.0	17.2	73.5
33.0	0	74.0
49.6	11.5	64.0
49.6	0	66.5
57.2	8.6	60.0
57.2	0	62.0
66.1	5.7	56.5
66.1	0	57.5
74.2	2.9	54.0
74.2	0	53.0

Solution:

For the first set of results,

$$\text{Molar ratio } \frac{\text{testosterone propionate}}{\text{chloroform}} = \frac{8.3 \times 119.4}{25.8 \times 344.5} = 0.1$$

Similar calculations give the figures in the first column of the table below.

Percentage intensity = 100 − percentage transmission

Therefore, for the first two lines in the table,

ΔE = intensity of uncomplexed peak − intensity of complexed peak

= $(100 - 87) - (100 - 96) = 9.0$

Similar calculations give the figures in the second column of the table.

Molar ratio of testosterone propionate	ΔE
0.1	9.0
0.2	5.0
0.3	2.0
0.4	−0.5
0.6	−2.5
0.7	−2.0
0.8	−1.0
0.9	1.0

A plot of the first column against the second column gives the graph shown in Fig. 8.8, which gives an inflection at a molecular fraction of 0.5, indicating 1:1 complexation.

In practice, the scatter of the percent transmissions often makes it impossible to construct lines between the points in the plot. In such situations it is useful to prepare plots of percentage transmission against molecular fraction and use the values on the best-fitting plot between the points to calculate values of ΔE. The results given above, for example, give a good binomial correlation.

C. Solubility

The procedure for the preparation of phase solubility diagrams has been described above. An inert solvent is kept saturated with the solute (S) and incremental amounts of complexing agent (L) added. At equilibrium the total amount of S in each mixture is determined by a suitable analytical procedure. The technique has been extended by Higuchi and Connors [6] to the calculation of complexation constants and the procedures will be summarized here.

If S and L combine to form a 1:1 complex and the activities of each species are assumed to be equal to their concentrations, then

$$K_{1,1} = \frac{[SL]}{[S][L]} \qquad (8.23)$$

Concentrations can be expressed in terms of known quantities; that is, $[S] = [S]_o$, where $[S]_o$ is the solubility in the absence of L; $[SL] = [S]_t - [S]_o$, where $[S]_t$ is the total concentration of S in the given mixture; and $[L] = [L]_t - [SL]$, where $[L]_t$ is the concentration of L added. Substitution in Eq. (8.23) gives

$$\frac{1 + K_{1,1}[S]_o}{K_{1,1}[S]_o} = \frac{[L]_t}{[S]_t - [S]_o} \qquad (8.24)$$

or

$$[S]_t = \frac{K_{1,1}[S]_o[L]_t}{1 + K_{1,1}[S]_o} + [S]_o \qquad (8.25)$$

This is an equation of a straight line, so that a plot of $[S]_t$ against the total quantity of complexing solvent added ($[L]_t$) will have a slope of $K_{1,1}[S]_o/(1 + K_{1,1}[S]_o)$ and an intercept of $[S]_o$, from which $K_{1,1}$ can be evaluated.

If 1:1 and 1:2 complexation occur together, as indicated by Eqs. (8.9) and (8.10), $[S]_t$ and $[L]_t$ will be expressed by

$$[S]_t = [S] + [SL] + [SL_2] \qquad (8.26)$$

and

$$[L]_t = [L] + [SL] + 2[SL_2] \qquad (8.27)$$

Rearrangement of the mass action expressions for the complexation processes gives

$$[SL] = K_{1,1}[S][L] \qquad (8.28)$$

and

$$[SL_2] = K_{1,1}K_{1,2}[S][L]^2 \qquad (8.29)$$

and substitution from these, together with $[S] = [S]_o$ in Eq. (8.27), leads to

$$[S]_t = [S]_o + K_{1,1}[S]_o[L] + K_{1,1}K_{1,2}[S]_o[L]^2 \tag{8.30}$$

If the degree of complexation is small, $[L]$ may be approximated to $[L]_t$, giving

$$\frac{[S]_t - [S]_o}{[L]_t} = K_{1,1}[S]_o + K_{1,1}K_{1,2}[S]_o[L]_t \tag{8.31}$$

indicating that a plot of $([S]_t - [S]_o)/[L]_t$ against $[L]_t$ will be rectilinear with slope $K_{1,1}K_{1,2}$ and intercept $K_{1,1}$.

Higuchi et al. [6] suggested that since $[S]_o$ is considered to be constant, the complexation constant could be expressed as an inter-action constant K', defined by

$$K'_{1,1} = \frac{[SL]}{[L]} \tag{8,32}$$

and

$$K'_{1,2} = \frac{[SL_2]}{[L]^2} \tag{8.33}$$

If it is assumed that complexed S is mainly in the form of the 1:1 type, then

$$K_{1,1(\text{apparent})} = \frac{[SL]}{[L]} + \frac{[SL_2]}{[L]} = \frac{[SL] + [SL_2]}{[L]} \tag{8.34}$$

$$= K'_{1,1} + K'_{1,2}[L]$$

where $K_{1,1(\text{apparent})}$ is the apparent 1:1 interaction constant.

Hence a plot of $K_{1,1(\text{apparent})}$ against $[L]$, expressed as $[L]_t - [S]_t + [S]_o$, should give a rectilinear plot, with intercept $K'_{1,1}$ and slope $K'_{1,2}$. This approach also fits if the assumption is that complexation is mainly 1:2, but $[L]$ is then represented by $[L]_t - 2([S]_t - [S]_o)$; hence

$$K'_{1,1(\text{apparent})} = \frac{([S]_t - [S]_o)}{[L]_t - 2([S]_t - [S]_o)} = \frac{[SL] + [SL_2]}{[L]} \tag{8.35}$$

$$= K'_{1,1} + K'_{1,2}[L]$$

This means that a plot of $K'_{1,1(apparent)}$ against $[L]_t - 2([S]_t - [S]_o)$ should give a straight line of slope $K'_{1,2}$ and intercept $K'_{1,1}$.

Example

The solubilities of testosterone in blends of chloroform and cyclo-hexane are shown in the first two columns of the table below. $[L]_t$ and $[S]_t$ represent the concentrations of chloroform and testosterone, respectively, in solution, free plus complexed. Calculate the $K_{1,1}$ and $K_{1,2}$ stability constants, assuming that (a) the degree of complexation is small, (b) complexation is mainly 1,1, and (c) complexation is mainly 1,2.

% v/v CHCl$_3$	$[S]_t$ (m kg^{-1} × 10^2)	$[L]_t$ (m kg^{-1})	$[S]_t - [S]_0$ (m kg^{-1} × 10^2)
0	0.275	0	0
2	0.447	0.313	0.172
4	0.677	0.615	0.402
6	0.955	0.906	0.680
8	1.378	1.191	1.103

% v/v CHCl$_3$	$\dfrac{[S]_t - [S]_o}{[L]_t}$ (× 10^2)	$K_{1,1(app)}$ (× 10^3)	$[L]_t - ([S]_t - [S]_o)$
0	0	0	0
2	0.550	5.53	0.311
4	0.654	6.58	0.611
6	0.751	7.56	0.899
8	0.926	9.35	1.180

Solution:

For 2% v/v CHCl$_3$,

$$[S]_t - [S]_o = (0.447 - 0.275) \times 10^{-2} = 1.72 \times 10^{-3}$$

$$\frac{[S]_t - [S]_o}{[L]_t} = \frac{0.172 \times 10^{-2}}{0.313} = 0.550 \times 10^{-2}$$

$$[L]_t - ([S]_t - [S]_o) = 0.313 - 0.172 \times 10^{-2} = 0.311$$

$$K_{1,1(app)} = \frac{[S]_t - [S]_o}{[L]_t - [S]_t + [S]_o}$$

$$= \frac{0.172 \times 10^{-2}}{0.311} = 5.53 \times 10^{-3}$$

Results for other concentrations of chloroform were calculated in the same way and are shown in the table.

Regression of $([S]_t - [S]_o)/[L]_t$ against $[L]_t$ [Eq. (8.31)]:

	n	r

$$\frac{([S]_t - [S]_o)}{[L]_t} = 6.94 \times 10^{-3}[L]_t + 1.56 \times 10^{-3} \qquad 5 \qquad 0.932$$

$$K_{1,1} = \frac{1.56 \times 10^{-3}}{2.75 \times 10^{-3}} = 0.57 \text{ kg m}^{-1}$$

$$K_{1,2} = \frac{6.94 \times 10^{-3}}{(2.75 \times 10^{-3} \times 0.57)} = 4.43 \text{ kg}^2 \text{ m}^{-2}$$

Regression of $K_{1,1(app)}$ against $([L]_t - [S]_t + [S]_o)$ $(= [L])$ [Eq. (8.34)]:

$$K_{1,1(app)} = 7.08 \times 10^{-3}[L] + 1.56 \times 10^{-3} \qquad 5 \qquad 0.940$$

$$K_{1,1} = \frac{1.56 \times 10^{-3}}{2.75 \times 10^{-3}} = 0.57 \text{ kg m}^{-1}$$

$$K_{1,2} = \frac{7.08 \times 10^{-3}}{2.75 \times 10^{-3}} = 2.57 \text{ kg}^2 \text{ m}^{-2}$$

Regression of $K_{1,1(app)}$* when complexation is mainly 1,2 against $[L]_t - 2([S]_t - [S]_o)$ (= [L]) [Eq. (8.35)] requires construction of an auxiliary table, as follows:

% v/v CHCl$_3$	$K_{1,1(app)}$ × 10^3	$[L]_t - 2([S]_t - [S]_o)$
2	5.55	0.310
4	6.62	0.607
6	7.62	0.892
8	9.44	1.169

which yields,

$$K_{1,1(app)} = 4.42 \times 10^{-3}[L] + 4.02 \times 10^{-3} \qquad \begin{array}{cc} n & r \\ 4 & 0.987 \end{array}$$

$$K_{1,1} = \frac{4.02 \times 10^{-3}}{2.75 \times 10^{-3}} = 1.46 \text{ kg m}^{-1}$$

$$K_{1,2} = \frac{4.42 \times 10^{-3}}{2.75 \times 10^{-3}} = 1.61 \text{ kg}^2 \text{ m}^{-2}$$

Few attempts have been made to quantify solute-solvent complexation in terms of regular solution theory. The ratio experimental solubility/regular solubility has been shown to follow the same rank order as infrared shifts resulting from solute-solvent complexation [18], which have also been shown to be related to l_{12} (Section II.B of Chapter 6) for the solubilities of testosterone in a range of complexing solvents [19]. On a qualitative basis, the observed solubility of a solute in a solvent with which it complexes will be greater than that predicted by regular solution theory, and the greater the stability constant of the complex, or the more negative the free energy of complexation, the greater the solubility.

$$*K_{1,1(app)} = \frac{[S]_t - [S]_o}{[L]_t - 2([S]_t - [S]_o)}.$$

Association between like molecules and association of solute molecules with solvent molecules can be considered as competitive processes. Poor solvents, as exemplified by the paraffins, are random distributions, their molecules do not associate, and when they take a solute into solution, they do little to hinder any interaction of solute molecules with each other. However, because they are poor solvents, and solute-solute association decreases with increasing dilution, it may not be possible to prepare a solution that is sufficiently concentrated for significant solute-solute association to be seen. Solubility can be increased by adding a cosolvent that interacts with the solute, the process usually occurring between a charged site on the solvent molecule and an oppositely charged site on the solute molecule. However, the site on the solute is usually the one that takes part in solute-solute association, so that the increased solubility is achieved at the expense of decreased solute-solute interaction. Complexation with the cosolvent will be predominant in dilute solution, but as the concentration of solute is increased, solute-solute association will become progressively more important.

REFERENCES

1. J. H. Hildebrand and C. A. Jenks Solubility: IV. Solubility relations of naphthalene and iodine in the various solvents, including a method for estimating solubility data, *J. Am. Chem. Soc., 42*, 2180–2189 (1920).
2. J. H. Hildebrand, Solubility: XII. Regular solutions, *J. Am. Chem. Soc., 51*, 66–80 (1929).
3. W. B. Jensen, The Lewis acid-base definitions. A status report, *Chem. Rev. 78*, 1–22 (1978).
4. H. A. Bent, Structural chemistry of donor-acceptor interactions, *Chem. Rev., 68*, 587–648 (1968).
5. A. N. Martin, P. L. Wu, A. Adjei, M. Mehdizadeh, K. C. James, and C. Metzler, Extended Hildebrand solubility approach: testosterone and testosterone propionate in binary solvents, *J. Pharm. Sci., 71*, 1334–1340 (1982).
6. T. Higuchi and K. A. Connors, Phase solubility techniques, in *Advances in Analytical Chemistry and Instrumentation*, Vol. 4 (C. N. Reilley, ed.), Wiley-Interscience, New York, 1965, pp. 117–212.
7. K. C. James and M. Mehdizadeh, Some solute-solvent complexes involving testosterone and testosterone propionate, *J. Pharm. Pharmacol., 33*, 9–13 (1981).
8. K. C. James and M. Ramgoolam, Complexation of some 3-keto-17-hydroxy steroids in polar solvents, *Spectrochim. Acta, 31A*, 1599–1604 (1975).

9. K. C. James and P. R. Noyce, Hydrogen-bonding between testosterone propionate and solvent in chloroform-cyclohexane solutions, *Spectrochim. Acta, 27A,* 691–696 (1971).

10. H. A. Benesi and J. H. Hildebrand, A spectrophotometric investigation of the interaction of iodine with aromatic hydrocarbons, *J. Am. Chem. Soc., 71,* 2703–2707 (1949).

11. T. Higuchi, J. H. Richards, S. S. Davis, A. Kamada, J. P. Hon, M. Nakano, and I. H. Pitman, Solvency and hydrogen-bonding interactions: III. Improvement of the Benesi Hildebrand method for the determination of equilibrium constants, *J. Pharm. Sci., 58,* 661–671 (1969).

12. I. Moriguchi and N. Kaneniwa, Spectroscopic studies on molecular interactions: III. Improvement of the Benesi-Hildebrand method for the determination of equilibrium constants, *Chem. Pharm. Bull., 17,* 2173–2175 (1969).

13. I. D. Kuntz, F. P. Gasparro, M. D. Johnston, and R. P. Taylor, Molecular interactions and the Benesi-Hildebrand equation, *J. Am. Chem. Soc., 90,* 4778–4781 (1968).

14. N. J. Rose and R. S. Drago, Molecular addition compounds of iodine: I. An absolute method for the spectroscopic determination of equilibrium constants, *J. Am. Chem. Soc., 81,* 6138–6141 (1959).

15. K. Kakemi, H. Sezaki, E. Suzuki, and M. Nakano, Studies on molecular interaction of organic molecules in solution: I. Effects of solvent on molecular interaction of salicyclic acid with caffeine, *Chem. Pharm. Bull., 17,* 242–247 (1969).

16. L. J. Bellamy, H. E. Hallam, and R. L. Williams, Infra-red spectra and solvent effects: Part 1. −X−H stretching frequencies, *Trans. Faraday Soc., 54,* 1120–1127 (1958).

17. M. D. Cohen and E. Fischer, Isosbestic points, *J. Chem. Soc.,* 3044–3052 (1962).

18. K. C. James and P. R. Noyce, An infra red study of solute-solvent interactions of testosterone propionate, *J. Pharm. Pharmacol., 22* (Suppl.), 109S–113S (1970).

19. K. C. James, C. T. Ng, and P. R. Noyce, Solubilities of testosterone propionate and related esters in organic solvents, *J. Pharm. Sci., 65,* 656–659 (1976).

9

The Distribution Law

I. FORMAL PARTITION COEFFICIENTS

Liquid-liquid extraction has been used since ancient times, and the
distribution (or partition) law has similar obscure origins. The law
in its simplest sense states that if a solute is distributed between
two immiscible, or partially miscible solvents, the ratio of the concentrations in the two phases will have a constant value, characteristic of the system, and independent of the proportions of the
components.

The concept is a logical consequence of Henry's law and of the
van't Hoff isotherm. Henry's law considers that if a solution (A) of
a volatile solute is enclosed in an isolated system, the partial pressure
of the solute $(\bar{p}_{2(A)})$ in the vapor above the solution will be given by

$$\bar{p}_{2(A)} = p^o_{2(A)} X_{2(A)} f_{2(A)} = H_{2(A)} X_{2(A)} \tag{9.1}$$

$f_{2(A)}$ is the activity coefficient, $H_{2(A)}$ the Henry's law constant,
$X_{2(A)}$ the mole fraction concentration, and $p^o_{2(A)}$ the saturated
vapor pressure, all of the solute in the solvent A. If a second solvent (B), immiscible with A, is introduced and the system allowed
to go to equilibrium, the atmosphere above the solutions will be
common to both, so that

$$\bar{p}_{2(A+B)} = X_{2(A)} H_{2(A)} = X_{2(B)} H_{2(B)} \tag{9.2}$$

Therefore,

$$\frac{X_{2(A)}}{X_{2(B)}} = \frac{H_{2(B)}}{H_{2(A)}} = \text{constant} \tag{9.3}$$

which is the distribution law.

Application of the van't Hoff isotherm to the conjugate solutions
above gives

$$u_{(A)} = u^o_{(A)} + RT \ln a_{(A)} \tag{9.4a}$$

and

$$u_{(B)} = u^o_{(B)} + RT \ln a_{(B)} \tag{9.4b}$$

where a represents activity, u represents chemical potential, and
$u^o_{(A)}$ and $u^o_{(B)}$ are the chemical potentials of the standard states.
When the two systems are in equilibrium, $u_{(A)} = u_{(B)}$, so that

$$\frac{a_{(A)}}{a_{(B)}} = \frac{\exp\ (u^o_{(B)} - u^o_{(A)})}{RT} = \text{constant} \qquad (9.5)$$

This is a more precise form of the distribution law than Eq. (9.3), because it is quoted in terms of activity rather than concentration. Henry's law applies to dilute solutions, for which activity and concentration can be considered equal. The constant in Eqs. (9.3) and (9.5) is the observed, formal distribution or partition coefficient, for which the symbol K_d will be used.

It is essential that it is made clear which solvent is represented by the numerator and which is represented by the denominator. Convention demands that if, for example, the partition coefficient between benzene and water is quoted, it is inferred that the concentration in the first-named solvent, namely benzene, is placed on top of the ratio. To avoid any confusion, it is recommended that the situation be clearly specified, either in the preliminary description of procedures, or as a statement of the form, "The benzene/water partition coefficient is . . . "

The partition coefficient is expressed in terms of formal concentration, which represents total solute concentration, irrespective of the form it takes in the solution. The term formal partition coefficient is therefore used to describe the ratio of the analytically determined concentrations.

A. Extraction

Liquid-liquid extraction is used extensively in all forms of chemical procedures. In analysis, for example, the process can be used to isolate a solute from an aqueous solution. The solution is shaken with a volatile, water-immiscible solvent in a separatary funnel. After standing, the system separates into two phases; the denser layer is removed through the tap and the volatile solution is evaporated to dryness. The method can be scaled up, as in the manufacture of antibiotics and other natural products, or can be modified, as in continuous liquid-liquid extraction. Whatever form the method takes, it is dependent on distribution law.

The quantity of solute that is extracted is dependent mainly on three factors: (1) the partition coefficient between the two solvents, (2) the volumes of the solutions, and (3) the number of extractions. The importance of each of these will be shown through the example given below.

Example

A 1000-liter culture contains 15.42 kg of an antibiotic. Calculate the quantity that would be left in the culture after each of the following treatments: (a) one extraction with 600 liters of amyl acetate; (b) three successive extractions with 200 liters of amyl acetate; and (c) one extraction with 100 liters of amyl acetate which has been used in a previous extraction and contains 1.06% of the antibiotic.   Partition coefficient (amyl acetate/culture) = 103.

Solution:

(a) The example deals with weights, whereas the partition law deals with concentrations.   The volumes of the two phases must therefore be taken into consideration to convert weights to concentrations.

$$\frac{\text{Weight of solute in amyl acetate/volume of amyl acetate}}{\text{Weight of culture/volume of culture}} = \frac{103}{1}$$

Therefore,

$$\frac{\text{Weight of solute in amyl acetate}}{\text{Weight of solute in culture}} = \frac{103 \times 600}{1 \times 1000} = \frac{61.8}{1}$$

$$\text{Amount left in culture} = \frac{15.42 \times 1}{(61.8 + 1)} = 0.246 \text{ kg}$$

The volume of extracting solvent is in the numerator; therefore, the greater the volume, the greater the quantity of antibiotic extracted. By a similar argument, the greater the partition coefficient, the greater the quantity of solute to be found in the solvent, which is represented in the numerator of the coefficient.

(b) By the same mathematical process, after the first extraction,

$$\frac{\text{Weight of solute in amyl acetate}}{\text{Weight of solute in culture}} = \frac{103 \times 200}{1000} = \frac{20.6}{1}$$

Therefore,

$$\text{Amount left in culture} = \frac{15.42}{21.6} = 0.714 \text{ kg}$$

Similarly, after the second extraction,

$$\text{Amount left in culture} = \frac{0.714}{21.6} = 0.033 \text{ kg}$$

and after the third extraction,

$$\text{Amount left in culture} = \frac{0.033}{21.6} = 0.002 \text{ kg}$$

Comparison of the 2 g obtained in process (b) with the 246 g left in the culture after process (a) leads to the conclusion that a series of small extractions is more efficient than one extraction, even when the total volume involved is the same on both occasions.

(c) Total weight of antibiotic = 15.42 + 1.06 = 16.48 kg

$$\frac{\text{Weight of solute in amyl acetate}}{\text{Weight of solute in culture}} = \frac{100 \times 103}{1000} = \frac{10.3}{1}$$

$$\text{Amount left in culture} = \frac{16.48}{11.3} = 1.46 \text{ kg}$$

B. Successive Extractions

The procedure used to calculate the amount of antibiotic remaining in the culture after three extractions was tedious. A simple formula can be obtained in general terms by considering the extraction of V_w milliliters of aqueous phase containing w_o grams of solute, with V_o milliliters of nonaqueous solvent. If the partition coefficient,

$$\frac{\text{Concentration in culture}}{\text{Concentration in amyl acetate}}$$

is called K_d, and the quantity remaining in the culture is w_1,

$$K_d = \frac{w_1/V_w}{(w_o - w_1)/V_o} \qquad (9.6)$$

which on expanding and rearranging yields

$$w_1 = w_o \frac{K_d V_w}{K_d V_w + V_o} \qquad (9.7)$$

If the process is repeated and w_2 grams are left in the culture,

$$w_2 = w_1 \frac{K_d V_w}{K_d V_w + V_o} \qquad (9.8)$$

and substitution in Eq. (9.8) from Eq. (9.7) gives

$$w_2 = w_o \left(\frac{K_d V_w}{K_d V_w + V_o} \right)^2 \qquad (9.9)$$

and for n extractions,

$$w_n = w_o \left(\frac{K_d V_w}{K_d V_w + V_o} \right)^n \tag{9.10}$$

C. Practical and Rational Partition Coefficients

The more commonly used form of the van't Hoff isotherm is

$$\Delta G = \Delta G^o + RT \ln K_d \tag{9.11}$$

ΔG is the free energy of transfer from one solvent to the other, and ΔG^o is the standard free energy, which is the free energy of a hypothetical system in which both phases are at unit concentration and are ideal. The magnitude of the standard free energy depends on the standard state to which the free energy is referred. The commonly used standard states employed are the practical state and the rational state.

In the practical state, concentrations in both phases are expressed in molar units, and the solutions behave as if they were at infinite dilution. Thus, for distribution of a solute between solutions A and B, if the equilibrium concentrations are 0.5 and 1.5 M, respectively, the free energy of transfer will be the free energy required to reduce the concentration in A from 1.0 to 0.5 M, plus the free energy involved in increasing the concentration in B from 1.0 to 1.5 M. Molal concentrations are sometimes used; these are usually considered to be better than molar units because the densities of the solvents are different.

Strictly speaking, since Henry's law is expressed in units of mole fraction, concentrations used to calculate partition coefficients should also be quoted in mole fractions. The resulting coefficient, called the rational or thermodynamic partition coefficient is symbolized as K_d'. On the mole fraction scale, unit concentration represents the pure solute. The standard free energy of transfer will therefore be a constant characteristic of the solute and independent of the solvent system employed.

Practical and rational partition coefficients are directly proportional, provided that the solutions under consideration are dilute. Thus, if we consider a solute distributed between solvents A and B, to give dilute solutions having concentrations c_A and c_B, M, the practical partition coefficient (K_d) will be c_A/c_B. The thermodynamic partition coefficient for dilute solutions is given by $X_{2(A)}/X_{2(B)}$, in which $X_{2(A)}$ and $X_{2(B)}$ are mole fraction concentrations of solute in solvents A and B, respectively. $X_{2(A)}$ is defined by

$$X_{2(A)} = \frac{c_A/(m_2 \times \rho_A)}{[c_A/(m_2 \times \rho_A)] + [(1000 - c_A)/m_A]} \tag{9.12}$$

where m_2 and m_A represent molecular weights of solute and solvent A, respectively, and ρ_A is the density of the solution in solvent A, in $g\ ml^{-1}$. A similar expression and symbols apply to the solution in solvent B. In dilute solutions, ρ_A can be equated to the density of the pure solvent. Additionally, c_A can be ignored in comparison with 1000, and $c_A/m_2\rho_A$ in comparison with $1000/m_A$. The thermodynamic partition coefficient for dilute solutions is therefore defined by

$$K_d' = \frac{c_A m_A}{c_B m_B \rho_A} \tag{9.13}$$

from which follows

$$K_d' = K_d \frac{m_A}{m_B \rho_A} \tag{9.14}$$

providing a factor for conversion of practical partition coefficients to thermodynamic partition coefficients. ρ_A will be a number in the region of $1\ g\ ml^{-1}$ and m_2 will usually be greater than m_A, so mathematically speaking, the effect of concentration will begin to bite when c_A, expressed as a fraction of 1000, approaches the acceptable error in the experimental partition coefficients.

As an example, iodine has a practical partition coefficient of 282 between cyclohexane and water. Thus if the cyclohexane phase contains $28.2\ m\ liter^{-1}$ of iodine and the aqueous phase contains 0.1 mg $liter^{-1}$, the mole fractions will be given by

$$X_{2(cyclohexane)} = \frac{2.82 \times 10^{-2}/(254 \times 0.779)}{(2.82 \times 10^{-2}/254 \times .779) + (1000 - 0.0001)/84}$$

$$= \frac{1.43 \times 10^{-4}}{1.43 \times 10^{-4} + 11.9} = 1.20 \times 10^{-5}$$

$$X_{2(water)} = \frac{1 \times 10^{-4}/254}{1 \times 10^{-4}/254 + (1000 - 0.0001)/18}$$

$$= \frac{3.94 \times 10^{-7}}{3.94 \times 10^{-7} + 55.6} = 7.09 \times 10^{-9}$$

(Molecular weights: water, 18; iodine, 127×2; cyclohexane, 84; density of cyclohexane, 0.779 g ml^{-1}.) The validity of these approximations can be seen from the expressions; 1.37×10^{-4} is negligible in comparison with 11.9, as are 0.0001 and 3.94×10^{-7} in comparison with 1000 and 55.6, respectively. The thermodynamic partition coefficient is therefore given by

$$K'_d = \frac{1.20 \times 10^{-5}}{7.09 \times 10^{-9}} = 1.69 \times 10^3$$

Equation (9.14) gives

$$K'_d = \frac{282 \times 84}{18 \times 0.779} = 1.64 \times 10^3$$

The molecular weight of the solute is required to calculate mole fractions, but since it appears in both numerator and denominator of the partition coefficient, it can be ignored in the calculation. Similar calculations give the results shown in Table 9.1. Deviations appear when the cyclohexane concentration is in excess of 1%, 2.82% iodine in cyclohexane giving a deviation of about 3% from the previous

TABLE 9.1 Calculated Partition Coefficients for Iodine Between Cyclohexane and Water

Iodine concentrations (mg dm^{-3})		Thermodynamic partition coefficient
Cyclohexane	Water	
282	1.0	1.62×10^3
2,820	10.0	1.62×10^3
28,200	100.0	1.66×10^3
282,000	1000.0	1.95×10^3

constant result. Below this limit, partition coefficients are constant and are equal to $84/(18 \times 0.779) = 6.00$ times the practical partition coefficient.

II. INFLUENCE OF ASSOCIATION AND DISSOCIATION ON PARTITIONING

To obey the distribution law, the solute must be in the same state in the two solutions. If, for example, the solute associates in one solvent but not in the other, the ratio of the total concentrations in the solvents will vary with the amount of solute used. The true partition coefficient $(K_{p,1})$ will be the ratio of the concentrations of the monomeric species, as expressed in

$$nS \overset{K_{1,n}}{\rightleftharpoons} S_n \tag{9.15}$$

and

$$K_{p,1} = \frac{\text{monomer concentration in nonaqueous phase}}{\text{monomer concentration in aqueous phase}}$$

$$= \frac{[S]}{c_w} \tag{9.16}$$

where S represents solute and $K_{1,n}$ the association constant for monomers to n-mers. Each associate contains n monomer molecules.

Similar situations occur if the solute is dissociated in one solvent and not in the other, and if the solute is associated in one solvent and dissociated in the other. These three cases will be considered in turn.

A. Association

If association occurs, it is almost always in the nonaqueous phase. Such a situation will be assumed here, although similar arguments can be applied if water is the phase in which association takes place. Application of the law of mass action to Eq. (9.15) gives

$$K_{1,n} = \frac{[S_n]}{[S]^n} = \frac{(c_n)_o}{n(c_1)_o^n} \tag{9.17}$$

where $(c_1)_o$ and $(c_n)_o$ represent monomer and n-mer concentrations in the oil, respectively, expressed in terms of monomer concentration, so that $[S_n] = (c_n)_0/n$. If Eq. (9.15) is predominently to the right, $(c_n)_0$ can be substituted by the total concentration of solute in the nonaqueous phase, $(c_t)_0$, to give

$$\frac{\sqrt{(c_t)_0}}{c_W} = \text{new constant} = K_{p,1}(nK_{1,n})^{1/n} \tag{9.18}$$

Thus if a solute dimerizes in the nonaqueous phase but not in the water, the partition coefficient defined by Eq. (9.3) will vary with the quantity of solute added to the two solvents, but the nth root of the concentration in the oil, divided by the concentration in the water, will give a constant value.

The constant in Eq. (9.3), K_d, is the ratio of two concentrations, so provided that the same units are used for numerator and denominator, K_d is a dimensionless number. In contrast, $K_{p,1}$ $(nK_{1,n})^{1/n}$ is not dimensionless and gives a different value if, for example, concentrations are measured in percentage w/v on one occasion and as grams per liter on another.

The number of molecules involved in the association process can thus be determined by a process of trial and error. Concentrations in the two solutions are determined for a range of quantities of the solute, and ratios calculated, using progressively increasing roots of the concentration in the solvent in which the solute associates. The root that gives a constant ratio corresponds to the number of molecules that associate.

An alternative process involves plotting the log of the concentration in one solvent against the log of the concentration in the other. Taking logs of Eq. (9.18) and rearranging gives

$$\log (c_t)_0 = n \log c_W + \log nK_{1,n} + n \log K_p \tag{9.19}$$

which is an equation of a straight line with slope n.

The foregoing procedures assume that association is virtually complete. However, if the value of $K_{1,n}$ is small, there will be a significant concentration of unassociated solute in the oil, and $\sqrt[n]{(c_t)_0}$ will not be a true measure of $(c_1)_0$. Since association decreases with increasing dilution, the assumption that $K_{1,n}$ is large will be particularly tenuous at concentrations at which the distribution law operates. Despite this limitation, the foregoing methodology is widely quoted, with little reference to its shortcomings.

One of the consequences of this flaw in the theoretical background of the procedure is that curved log-log plots are frequently obtained. Even when the plot is rectilinear, the slope rarely approximates a whole number, and its interpretation is therefore obscure. It is not correct in such circumstances to assume that an experimental value of n between 1 and 2, for example, represents the weighted mean of a population of monomers and dimers. A more valid approach to the calculation of partition coefficients is to assume that at infinite dilution, association is negligible, so that if c_W is plotted against K_d, as expressed in Eq. (9.3), extrapolation to $c_W = 0$ will give the true (monomer-monomer) partition coefficient.

The total concentration of solute in the oil phase, $(c_t)_o$, expressed in units of unassociated molecules, will be equal to $[S]$ + $n[S_n]$. Substitution in Eq. (9.3) gives

$$K_d = \frac{[S] + n[S_n]}{c_W} \tag{9.20}$$

and combination with Eqs. (9.16) and (9.17) gives

$$K_d = K_{p,1} + \frac{nK_{1,n}[S]^n}{c_W} = K_{p,1} + nK_{1,n}K_{p,1}^n c_W^{n-1} \tag{9.21}$$

Davies and Hallam [1] quoted the results shown in Table 9.2 for the distribution of acetic acid between benzene and water. The plot of apparent partition coefficient (K_d) against c_W is shown in Fig. 9.1 and is rectilinear. Regression analysis gave

$$K_d = 0.0228c_W + 0.00800 \tag{9.22}$$

which indicates dimerization, since the power of c_W is unity, and a true partition coefficient ($K_{p,1}$) of 0.00800. The good correlation also suggests that the ionization of acetic acid in the aqueous phase can be ignored. $K_{1,n}$ can be evaluated as $0.0228/(2 \times 0.00800^2) = 178$ dm^3/M^{-1}. Since the units of $K_{1,n}$ are (concentration^{1-n}, its numerical value is dependent on the units of c_W.

TABLE 9.2 Distribution of Acetic Acid Between Benzene and Water at 25°C

Concentration in aqueous phase (M)	0.229	0.433	0.666	0.886	1.090
Apparent partition coefficient	0.0132	0.0179	0.0232	0.0280	0.0329

Source: Abstracted from Ref. 1.

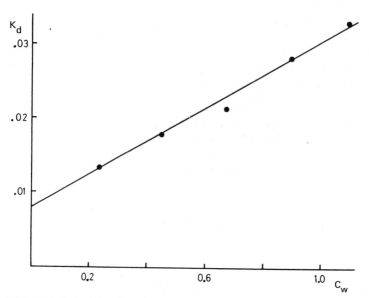

FIGURE 9.1 Distribution of acetic acid between benzene and water at 25°C. (Results from Ref. 1.)

If the degree of association of the solute in the oil is X_o, Eq. (9.15) may be rewritten in the form

$$K_{1,n} = \frac{X_o}{(1 - X_o)^n} \tag{9.23}$$

so that

$$[S] = (1 - X_o)(c_t)_o = \frac{\sqrt[n]{X_o(c_t)_o}}{K_{1,n}} \tag{9.24}$$

Substitution of [S] from Eq. (9.24) into Eq. (9.16) gives

$$\frac{\sqrt[n]{X_o(c_t)_o}}{c_W} = \text{constant} = K_{p,1} \sqrt[n]{K_{1,n}} \tag{9.25}$$

which is a more precise way than Eq. (9.18) of expressing the distribution of associating solutes.

In a similar derivation [2], K_d is substituted by $(c_t)_0/c_W$ in Eq. (9.21), and all the terms divided by c_W^{n-1} to give

$$\frac{(c_t)_0}{c_W} = \frac{K_{p,1}}{c_W^{n-1}} + nK_{p,1}^n K_{1,n} \tag{9.26}$$

This suggests that if $(c_t)_0/c_W^n$ is plotted against $1/c_W^{n-1}$, a straight line of slope $K_{p,1}$ will be obtained. $K_{1,n}$ can be evaluated from the intercept, which is equal to $nK_{p,1}^n K_{1,n}$.

The power series depicted by

$$K_d = K_{p,1} + \frac{2K_{p,1}^2}{K_{2,1}}c_W + \frac{3K_{p,1}^3}{K_{3,1}}c_W^2 + \cdots + \frac{nK_{p,1}^n}{K_{n,1}}c_W^{n-1} \tag{9.27}$$

can be applied to solutes that associate to form a series of progressively increasing complexes. Multiple regression analysis of K_d against c_W can therefore be used to evaluate the intercept and coefficients of c_W, from which the true partition coefficient and the various *dissociation* constants $K_{n,1}$ can be calculated.

Example

Infrared data reveal that acetamide occurs as monomers and trimers in chloroform solution. Total concentrations of acetamide obtained when various quantities were distributed between chloroform and water at 6.2°C [1] are given below. Calculate the true partition coefficient and the association constant of acetamide in chloroform.

Concentration in chloroform (mol dm^{-3} × 10^2)	2.078	3.089	4.321	5.960
Concentration in water (mol dm^{-3})	2.489	3.514	4.573	5.720

Solution:

Calculated values of (concentration in water)^2 (c_W^2), (concentration in water)^3 $(c_W^3)^X$, (concentration in chloroform)$/c_W^3$, and $1/c_W^2$ are as follows:

c_w^2	6.195	12.35	20.88	32.72
c_w^3	15.42	43.40	95.48	187.2
$c_{CHCl_3}/c_w^3 \times 10^4$	13.48	7.118	4.526	3.184
$1/c_w^2 \times 10^2$	16.14	8.097	4.789	3.056

Regression of $1/c_w^2$ against c_{CHCl_3}/c_w^3 gave

$$\frac{c_{CHCl_3}}{c_w^3} = \frac{7.88 \times 10^{-3}}{c_w^2} - 7.602 \times 10^{-5}$$

giving

$$K_p = 7.88 \times 10^{-3}$$

and

$$K_{1,3} = \frac{7.602 \times 10^{-5}}{3 \times (7.88 \times 10^{-3})^3} = 52 \ dm^6 \ M^{-2}$$

B. Dissociation in the Aqueous Phase

1. Strong Electrolytes. If a strong acid, HA, which dissociates in conducting solvents in accord with

$$HA \overset{K_a}{\rightleftharpoons} R^+ + A^- \tag{9.28}$$

is distributed between water and oil, the oil-water partition coefficient, calculated as the ratio of the analytically determined concentrations, will vary with the quantities of solute and solvents used. The true partition coefficient is expressed by

$$K_{p,1} = \frac{[HA]_o}{[HA]_w} \tag{9.29}$$

in which $[HA]_o$ will be the total concentration in the oil and $[HA]_w$ is the concentration of undissociated acid in the water. The concentration of undissociated acid is given by

$$[HA]_w = K_a [H^+][A^-] = K_a [H^+]^2 = K_a [A^-]^2 \qquad (9.30)$$

in which K_a is the acid dissociation constant. Since the acid is strong, K_a will be large and Eq. (9.28) will be almost exclusively to the right. $[H^+]$ can then be approximated to the total concentration in the aqueous phase (c_w), leading to

$$\frac{[HA]_o}{c_w^2} = \text{constant} = K_{p,1} K_a \qquad (9.31)$$

In contrast to a true partition coefficient, this constant is not dimensionless and is dependent on the units of concentration. Thus if the concentrations are $c_w = 1.0\%$ w/v and $[HA]_o = 0.1\%$ w/v, the constant will be $0.1/1^2 = 0.1\%$ v/w, whereas if the units were expressed in grams per liter, it would be $0.01/0.1^2 = 1.0$ dm^3 g^{-1}. Equation (9.31) can be generalized for all strong electrolytes by

$$\text{Undissociated species} \leftrightharpoons \text{n ions} \qquad (9.32)$$

and

$$\frac{\text{Total concentration in oil}}{(\text{Total concentration in water})^n} = \text{constant} \qquad (9.33)$$

2. Weak Electrolytes. If HA is a weak acid, and at the given concentration c_w the concentration of dissociated acid is X,

$$HA \quad \rightleftharpoons \quad H^+ + A^-$$
$$(c_w - X) \quad (X) \quad (X) \qquad (9.34)$$

Therefore,

$$K_a = \frac{X^2}{c_w - X} \qquad (9.35)$$

or

$$K_a c_w - K_a X - X^2 = 0 \qquad (9.36)$$

giving

$$K_{p,1} = \frac{2c_w}{2c_w + K_a \pm \sqrt{K_a^2 + 4K_a c_w}} \qquad (9.37)$$

Equation (9.37) would seem to provide a means of calculating dissociation constants of weak acids, by determining $K_{p,1}$ for two concentration levels and equating the right-hand sides of the two equations. However, the procedure has not enjoyed much success, because the solute does not always behave ideally in the nonaqueous phase. Carboxy acids, which usually dimerize in organic solvents, are particularly notorious in this respect. A further drawback of Eq. (9.37) is that most organic acids have dissociation constants lying between 10^{-5} and 10^{-4}, so that extremely dilute systems would be necessary for K_a to be significant in comparison with c_w. This can be illustrated by calculating partition coefficients from the data given in Table 9.2. The mean formal partition coefficients given by Eq. (9.21) are identical with those obtained with Eq. (9.37).

C. Dissociation in the Aqueous Phase and Association in the Nonaqueous Phase

When a solute that dimerizes in the oil and dissociates into two ions in the water is distributed between the two solvents, the concentration of monomer in the oil will be given by $K_{p,1}(c_w - X)$, and the concentration of dimer in the oil (expressed in units of monomer molecules) by $c_o - K_{p,1}(c_w - X)/2$. X is the concentration of dissociated solute in the aqueous phase, as defined by Eqs. (9.34) and (9.35), and c_o is the analytically determined concentration in the oil. The association constant $(K_{1,2})$ is therefore given by

$$K_{1,2} = \frac{c_o - K_{p,1}(c_w - X)}{2K_{p,1}^2 (c_w - X)^2} \qquad (9.38)$$

This equation can be rationalized by measuring oil- and aqueous-phase concentrations at two different solute concentrations. Total concentrations in the oil phase (monomer plus dimer), represented by $c_{(1)o}$ and $c_{(2)o}$, and in the aqueous phase (dissociated plus undissociated, represented by $c_{(1)w}$ and $c_{(2)w}$, can be determined by analysis. Concentrations of ionized solute, X_1 and X_2, can be calculated from Eq. (9.36). Calling $(c_{(1)w} - X_1)$, M, and $(c_{(2)w} - X_2)$, N, to simplify the algebra, then

$$K_{1,2} = \frac{c_{(1)o} - K_{p,1}M}{2K_{p,1}^2 M^2} = \frac{c_{(2)o} - K_{p,1}N}{2K_{p,1}^2 N^2} \qquad (9.39)$$

and

$$K_{p,1} = \frac{M^2 c_{(2)o} - N^2 c_{(1)o}}{MN(M - N)} \qquad (9.40)$$

from which the true partition coefficient $(K_{p,1})$ can be calculated [3]. Rearrangement of Eq. (9.38) gives

$$\frac{c_o}{(c_w - X)^2} = \frac{K_{p,1}}{c_w - X} + \frac{2K_{p,1}^2}{K_{1,2}} \qquad (9.41)$$

which indicates that a plot of $1/(c_w - X)$ against $c_o/(c_w - X)^2$ should give a straight line of slope $K_{p,1}$ and intercept $2K_{p,1}^2/K_{1,2}$. This provides an alternative means of evaluating $K_{p,1}$ and $K_{1,2}$. The procedure also serves to detect deviation from Eq. (9.38) at extremes of concentration, by inspecting for points that do not follow the rectilinear plot.

Another condition demanded by the distribution law is that the solvents must be mutually insoluble. Even limited solubility can give rise to problems, particularly when the dissolved solvent forms a complex with the solute in the other solvent. Such complexes are different species from molecularly dispersed solute, so that the system does not obey the distribution law.

An example has been reported by Christian et al. [4], who investigated the distribution of acetic acid between benzene and water. They identified four solute species in the benzene layer: H_2O, CH_3COOH, $(CH_3COOH)_2$, and $CH_3COOH \cdot H_2O$. Calling these W, A, A_2, and AW, respectively, the formal concentrations of acetic acid $(c_{A(t)}^b)$ and water $(c_{w(t)}^b)$ in the benzene layer are given by

$$c_{A(t)}^b = c_A^b + c_{A_2}^b + c_{AW}^b \qquad (9.42)$$

and

$$c_{w(t)}^b = c_{AW}^b + c_w^b \qquad (9.43)$$

Equilibrium constants are given by

$$K_{A_2} = \frac{c^b_{A_2}}{c^{b2}_A} \tag{9.44}$$

and

$$K_{AW} = \frac{c^b_{AW}}{c^b_A c^b_W} \tag{9.45}$$

and the partition coefficient for acid monomer by

$$K_{p,1} = \frac{c^b_A}{c^W_A} \tag{9.46}$$

where c^W_A is the concentration of acid monomer in the aqueous phase. Combination of Eqs. (9.42) to (9.46) gives

$$\frac{c^b_{A(t)} - c^b_{w(t)} + c^b_w}{c^W_A} = K_{p,1} + 2K^2_{p,1} K_{A_2} c^W_A = Y \tag{9.47}$$

and

$$\frac{c^b_{A(t)}}{c^W_A} = K_{p,1} + K_{AW} c^b_w K_{p,1} + 2K^2_{p,1} K_{A_2} c^W_A = Z \tag{9.48}$$

which indicate that both Y and Z are rectilinearly related to c^W_A with a slope of $2K^2_{p,1} K_{A2}$. The intercept of the first equation gives $K_{p,1}$. These expressions assume that c^b_w is constant and independent of c^W_A.

Example

Partition and solubility data for the system water-benzene-acetic acid at 15°C [4] are given below. Calculate the monomer partition coefficient of acetic acid between benzene and water, and the dimerization constant of acetic acid in benzene.

Formal concentration of acetic acid in benzene, $c_{A(t)}^b$	Concentration of acetic acid in water, c_A^w (M)	Formal concentration of water in benzene, $c_{W(t)}^b$ (M)
0	0	0.0265
0.0152	0.709	0.0287
0.0206	0.851	0.0280
0.0294	1.047	0.0291
0.0474	1.366	0.0307
0.0691	1.680	0.0310

Solution:

For the second line of the table,

$$\frac{c_{A(t)}^b}{c_A^w} = \frac{0.0152}{0.709} = 2.144 \times 10^{-2}$$

Similar calculations give the figures in the second column of the table below.

It is assumed that c_W^b is constant and equal to the solubility of water in benzene. This is given as $c_{W(t)}^b$ at zero acetic acid concentration (i.e., 0.0265). Hence for the second line of the table above,

$$\frac{c_{A(t)}^b - c_{W(t)}^b + c_W^b}{c_A^w} = \frac{0.0152 - 0.0287 + 0.0265}{0.709} = 1.834 \times 10^{-2}$$

Similar calculations give the figures in the third column of the table below.

Linear regression of the first column against the second column gives

$$\frac{c_{A(t)}^b}{c_A^w} = 2.03 \times 10^{-2} c_A^w + 6.91 \times 10^{-3} \qquad \begin{array}{c} r \\ 1.000 \end{array} \qquad (a)$$

c_A^w	$\dfrac{c_{A(t)}^b}{c_A^w} \times 10^2$	$\dfrac{c_{A(t)}^b - c_{W(t)}^b + c_W^b}{c_A^w} \times 10^2$
0.709	2.14	1.83
0.851	2.42	2.24
1.047	2.81	2.56
1.366	3.47	3.16
1.680	4.11	3.85

$$\frac{c_{A(t)}^b - c_{W(t)}^b + c_W^b}{c_A^w} = 2.00 \times 10^{-2} c_A^w + 4.64 \times 10^{-3} \qquad 0.998 \qquad \text{(b)}$$

The monomer partition coefficient $(K_{d,1})$ is given by the intercept of Eq. (b), that is,

$$K_{p,1} = 4.64 \times 10^{-3}$$

The dimerization constant of acetic acid in benzene is the slope of either Eq. (a) or (b) divided by $2K_{p,1}^2$, that is

$$K_{A_2} = \frac{2.03 \times 10^{-2}}{2(4.64 \times 10^{-3})^2} = 471 \text{ dm}^3 \text{ mol}^{-1}$$

or

$$= \frac{2.00 \times 10^{-2}}{2(4.64 \times 10^{-3})^2} = 464 \text{ dm}^3 \text{ mol}^{-1}$$

If both monomer and dimer form hydrates, symbolized AW_j and A_2W_k, respectively, the hydration constants will be given by

$$K_{h,1} = \frac{AW_j}{c_A^b (c_W^b)^j} \qquad (9.49)$$

TABLE 9.3 Tests for Hydration Using Eqs. (9.51) and (9.52)

Slope, Y − Z	Intercept, Y − Z	Hydration	
		Monomer	Dimer
O	O	No	No
O	-ve	Yes	No
-ve	O	No	Yes
-ve	-ve	Yes	Yes

and

$$K_{h,2} = \frac{A_2 W_k}{(c_A^b)^2 (c_W^b)^k}$$ (9.50)

Substitution of these expressions into Eqs (9.47) and (9.48) yields

$$Y = K_{p,1}[1 + (1 - j)K_{h,1}(c_w^b)^j] + K_{p,1}^2 2K_{A_2}$$

$$+ (2 - k)K_{n,2}(c_w^b)^k c_A^w$$ (9.51)

and

$$Z = K_{p,1}[1 + K_{h,1}(c_w^b)^j] + K_{p,1}^2 [2K_{A_2} + 2K_{h,2}(c_w^b)^k]c_A^w$$ (9.52)

Comparison of the intercepts and slopes of Eqs. (9.51) and (9.52) provides a test for determining which species is hydrated. Thus, if neither monomer nor dimer is hydrated, j - k = O, and the right-hand sides of Eqs. (9.51) and (9.52) become identical. Similarly, if monomer is hydrated and dimer is not, j > 1 and k = O, so that the intercept of Eq. (9.52) will be greater than that of Eq. (9.51). The four possible situations and their effects on Eqs. (9.51) and (9.52) are given in Table 9.3.

III. THE COLLANDER EQUATION

The standard state for partition coefficients is that in which the concentration in each solvent is unity. Unit concentration in mole fraction units is the pure solute, so that the thermodynamic standard free energy of transfer is constant for a given solute and independent of the solvent system which is used. Thus if the distribution of a given solute between a pair of immiscible solvents, described as system A, is compared with the distribution between a pair of solvents, called system B, the standard free energy of transfer of the two systems will be zero; hence

$$G_A - RT \ln K'_{d(A)} = G_B - RT \ln K'_{d(B)} \tag{9.53}$$

or

$$\ln K'_{d(A)} = \ln K'_{d(B)} + \frac{G_A - G_B}{RT} \tag{9.54}$$

Since the solute is the same in both systems, $G_A - G_B$ must be dependent solely on the nature of systems A and B, and in no way influenced by the nature of the solute. Therefore

$$\ln K'_{d(A)} = \ln K'_{d(B)} + constant \tag{9.55}$$

Equation (9.55) provides a theoretical basis for using partition coefficients obtained with one solvent system to estimate partition coefficients for another solvent system. Collander [5,6] made the first quantitative attempt to follow this approach by deriving the following equation empirically from experimental data:

$$\log K_{d(A)} = a \log K_{d(B)} + b \tag{9.56}$$

where a and b are constants. Equation (9.56) is universally known as the Collander equation and is invariably quoted as justification for using partition coefficients measured with one solvent system as an estimate of the partition coefficients in another solvent system. Most of the quantitative structure-activity relationships (QSAR) in the medical literature, for example, depend on the use of 1-octanol/water partition coefficients as a model for the biological solvent systems in vivo. Collander used molar concentrations to calculate his partition coefficients and made no allowance for association or dissociation, assuming that complications of this sort would be insignificant. He described his partition coefficients as "of no great accuracy" and hinted that his equation was based on rather shaky foundations. The constants in the equation varied from one solvent system to another and also with the type of solute used.

Leo and Hansch [3,7] tried to rationalize the problems encountered by Collander by considering the electron-donor and electron-acceptor properties of the solutes and solvents. They used

1-octanol/water as a reference system [i.e., as system B in Eq. (9.56)] and found that if the nonaqueous solvent in system A was similar in properties to 1-octanol, one equation could be derived to fit all solutes. Oleyl alcohol was an example. The equation is shown in Table 9.4; it has a slope close to unity and a good correlation coefficient. In contrast, nonaqueous solvents that were not similar to 1-octanol gave poor correlations. Cyclohexane is an example; its equation is shown in Table 9.4. Such relationships were improved if the solutes were grouped into electron acceptors and electron donors, and separate equations allocated to each group. Solutes were allocated to the groups by observing whether they fell above or below the regression lines obtained when all solutes were considered together. The classification into groups is given in Table 9.5.

When chloroform and carbon tetrachloride were considered as solvents, two equations had to be allocated to the electron acceptors. All the electron acceptors in subgroup I of Table 9.5 follow equations I for carbon tetrachloride and chloroform in Table 9.4. Some of the electron acceptors in subgroup II comply with equation II of the solvent under investigation, and the remainder follow equation I.

Example

Use the mean log octanol-water partition coefficients given below to estimate the corresponding partition coefficients between diethyl ether and water and between chloroform and water.

Solute	1-Octanol/water partition coefficient
(a) Ethanol	0.490
(b) Propionic acid	1.95
(c) Aniline	9.94

Solution:

(a) Ethanol is listed in Table 9.5 as an electron acceptor. The diethyl ether-water partition coefficient is therefore given by

$$\log K_d = 1.130 \times \log 0.490 - 0.170$$
$$= 1.130 \times -0.31 - 0.170 = -0.52 \quad (\text{or } K_d = 0.302)$$

(Mean experimental $\log K_d = -0.55$.) It appears in subgroup II of the electron acceptors; the chloroform-water partition is given by either

TABLE 9.4 Statistical Parameters for Correlation Equations[a]

$\log K_{d(A)} = a \log K_{d(octanol)} + b$

Solvent		a	b	n	r	s
Cyclohexane	All solutes	0.872	−1.241	56	0.649	1.015
	Electron acceptors	0.675	−1.842	26	0.761	0.503
	Electron donors	1.063	−0.734	30	0.957	0.360
Heptane	All solutes	1.566	−2.661	21	0.731	1.354
	Electron acceptors	1.056	−2.851	10	0.764	0.916
	Electron donors	1.848	−2.223	11	0.954	0.534
Carbon tetra-chloride	All solutes	1.307	−1.592	41	0.797	0.937
	Electron acceptors					
	(I)	1.168	−2.163	24	0.974	0.282
	(II)	0.862	−0.626	6	0.809	0.462
	Electron donors	1.207	−0.219	11	0.959	0.347
Xylene	All solutes	1.033	−1.180	40	0.862	0.661
	Electron acceptors	0.942	−1.694	19	0.963	0.225
	Electron donors	1.027	−0.595	21	0.986	0.230
Toluene	All solutes	1.328	−1.560	36	0.852	0.664
	Electron acceptors	1.135	−1.770	22	0.980	0.194

Benzene	Electron donors	1.398	−0.922	14	0.971	0.274
	All solutes	0.979	−1.005	52	0.815	0.555
	Electron acceptors	1.015	−1.402	33	0.962	0.234
Chloroform	Electron donors	1.223	−0.573	19	0.958	0.291
	All solutes	1.012	−0.512	72	0.811	0.734
	Electron acceptors (I)	1.126	−1.343	28	0.967	0.308
	(II)	1.100	−0.649	23	0.971	0.292
	Electron donors	1.276	0.171	21	0.976	0.251
Oils	All solutes	1.096	−1.147	79	0.945	0.470
	Electron acceptors	1.099	−1.310	65	0.981	0.271
	Electron donors	1.119	−0.325	14	0.988	0.233
Nitrobenzene	Electron acceptors	1.176	−1.072	9	0.977	0.217
Isopentyl acetate	Electron acceptors	1.027	0.072	22	0.986	0.209
Diethyl ether	All solutes	1.184	−0.474	103	0.929	0.477
	Electron acceptors	1.130	−0.170	71	0.988	0.186
	Electron donors	1.142	−1.070	32	0.957	0.326
Oleyl alcohol	All solutes	0.999	−0.575	37	0.985	0.225

TABLE 9.4 (Continued)

Solvent		a	b	n	r	s
Methyl isobutyl ketone	All solutes	1.094	0.050	17	0.993	0.184
Ethyl acetate	All solutes	0.932	0.052	9	0.969	0.202
Cyclohexanone	All solutes	1.035	0.896	10	0.972	0.340
Primary pentanols	All solutes	0.808	0.0271	19	0.987	0.161
Secondary and tertiary pentanols	All solutes	0.892	0.288	11	0.996	0.091
2-Butanone	All solutes	0.493	0.315	9	0.987	0.093
Cyclohexanol	All solutes	0.745	0.866	12	0.985	0.100
Primary butanols	All solutes	0.697	0.381	57	0.993	0.123

[a]n, Number of solutes used for correlation; r, correlation coefficient; s, standard deviation.
Source: Abstracted from Ref. 7.

TABLE 9.5 Solute Classes for Collander-Type Equations

Electron acceptors	
Subgroup I	Acids, phenols.
Subgroup II	Barbiturates, alcohols, amides (negatively substituted but not disubstituted), sulfonamides, nitriles, imides, amides, aromatic amines (not di-N-substituted)
Electron donors	Aliphatic amines and imines, tertiary amines, including ring N compounds, ketones, ethers, esters, compounds with intramolecular hydrogen bonds, aromatic hydrocarbons, miscellaneous electron donors

Source: Abstracted from Ref. 7.

$$\log K_d = 1.126 \times -0.31 - 1.343 = -1.69$$

or

$$\log K_d = 1.100 \times -0.31 - 0.649 = -0.99$$

The first equation is the general equation for electron acceptors, and in this case, for interaction between the hydrogen of ethanolic hydroxyl and an electron-rich site on the solvent. Chloroform would be expected to function as an electron acceptor, through its hydrogen atom, and the tendency would therefore be for ethanol to interact as an electron donor through the oxygen of the hydroxyl group. One would not therefore anticipate that the first equation would apply to this situation, and would choose the second equation. Comparison with the mean experimental value of -0.85 for $\log K_d$ confirms this assumption. The calculated partition coefficient is therefore antilog $-0.99 = 0.102$.

(b) Propionic acid is found in subgroup I of the electron acceptors. The estimated partition coefficients are therefore given by:
Diethyl ether-water:

$$\log K_d = 1.130 \times 0.29 - 0.170 = 0.158$$

$$K_d = \text{antilog } 0.158 = 1.44$$

Chloroform-water:

$$\log K_d = 1.126 \times 0.29 - 1.343 = -1.02$$

$$K_d = \text{antilog } -1.02 = 0.095$$

(Mean experimental $\log K_d$ values: diethyl ether-water, 0.207; chloroform-water, −0.83.)

Aniline is also in subgroup II of the electron acceptors. The estimated partition coefficients are therefore given by:

Diethyl ether-water:

$$\log K_d = 1.130 \times 0.9 - 0.170 = 0.85$$

$$K_d = \text{antilog } 0.85 = 0.71$$

(Mean experimental $\log K_d = 0.85$.)

Chloroform-water:

$$\log K_d = 1.126 \times 0.9 - 1.343 = -0.330$$

$$K_d = 0.47$$

or

$$\log K_d = 1.10 \times 0.9 - 0.649 = 0.341$$

$$K_d = 2.19$$

(Mean experimental $\log K_d = 1.32$.) This does not agree with either of the calculated results. The amino group is known to strongly potentiate the electron density of an aromatic ring to which it is attached, so in view of the electron-attracting properties of the chloroform hydrogen, it seems more likely that aniline would behave as an electron donor in this solvent. Application of the electron donor equation gives

$$\log K_d = 1.276 \times 0.9 + 0.171 = 1.32$$

in perfect agreement with the experimental result.

Leo and Hansch [7] pointed out that the slopes of all the equations in Table 9.4 should be unity (see Eq. (9.55)], and that the deviations from this value were due to hydrogen-bonding interactions. They used association constants (K_{HB}) between sarin (isopropoxy-methylphosphoryl fluoride) and a series of substituted phenols [8] as a measure of the hydrogen-bonding ability of the phenols, and introduced constants into Collander-type equations as a correction for this effect. These are represented by

$$\log K_{d(octanol)} = 0.50 \log K_{d(cyclohexane)} \qquad \begin{array}{ccc} n & r & s \\ 9 & 0.791 & 0.391 \end{array}$$

$$+ 2.43 \qquad\qquad (9.57)$$

and

$$\log K_{d(octanol)} = 1.00 \log K_{d(cyclohexane)} \qquad 9 \quad 0.979 \quad 0.140$$

$$+ 1.20 \log K_{HB} + 2.35 \qquad (9.58)$$

where n represents the number of terms, r the correlation coefficient, and s the standard deviation. Equations (9.57) and (9.58) indicate that such an assumption is reasonable. Although Eq. (9.58) serves to support the proposals of Leo and Hansch [7], it has little predictive value without the support of a wide selection of K_{HB} values. Only 21 were quoted by Higuchi et al. [8], and all these refered to phenols. A parameter that can be calculated or easily determined experimentally, analogous to K_{HB}, would rectify this problem.

A saturated solution is defined as a solution that is in equilibrium with undissolved solute. If the solute is a liquid, the system can be considered as the distribution of the solute between itself and the solvent, so that solubilities and partition coefficients should be related by equations of the form of Eq. (9.56). Hansch et al. [9] examined the aqueous solubilities and 1-octanol/water partition coefficients of 156 organic liquids, and fitted them into equations of the form

$$\log \frac{1}{S_w} = a \log K_d + b \qquad\qquad (9.59)$$

where S_w represents molal aqueous solubility and a and b are constants. An equation spanning all 156 solutes gave a reasonable correlation, but better relationships followed when solutes were grouped into chemical classes. The equations, reproduced in Table 9.6, were recommended [9] as a means of estimating aqueous solubilities from Hansch substituent constants (see Section IV.A). They also provide a procedure for estimating 1-octanol/water partition coefficients from aqueous solubilities. Valvani et al. [10] related the aqueous solubilities and 1-octanol/water partition coefficients of 111 liquid nonelectrolytes, and obtained

TABLE 9.6 Statistical Parameters for Eq. (9.59)

Compound class	a	b	Number of compounds	Correlation coefficient	Standard deviation
Alcohols	1.113	−0.926	41	0.967	0.136
Ketones	1.229	−0.720	13	0.980	0.164
Esters	1.013	−0.520	18	0.990	0.201
Ethers	1.182	−0.935	12	0.938	0.160
Alkyl halides	1.221	−0.832	20	0.928	0.235
Alkynes	1.294	−1.043	7	0.953	0.319
Alkenes	1.294	−0.248	12	0.985	0.131
Aromatics	0.996	−0.339	16	0.975	0.179
Alkanes	1.237	0.248	16	0.953	0.199
All compounds less alkanes	1.214	−0.850	140	0.955	0.344
All compounds	1.339	−0.978	156	0.935	0.472

Source: Abstracted from Ref. 9.

$$\text{Log } c'_w = -1.016 \text{ log } K_d \qquad \begin{array}{ccc} n & r & s \\ 111 & 0.931 & 0.421 \end{array}$$

$$+ 0.515 \tag{9.60}$$

and

$$\text{log } X_{2(w)} = -1.026 \text{ log } K_d \qquad \begin{array}{ccc} 111 & 0.931 & 0.427 \end{array}$$

$$- 0.23 \tag{9.61}$$

where c'_w represents molar and $X_{2(w)}$ mole fraction solubilities in water. The authors pointed out that the slopes are closer to the theoretical value of -1.0 than were those obtained by Leo and Hansch [7] and attributed the improvement to better raw data. Procedures of this nature are better suited for the estimation of aqueous solubilities and are therefore discussed in more detail in Chapter 10.

IV. LINEAR FREE-ENERGY RELATIONSHIPS

If the standard free energy ($\Delta G°$) in Eq. (9.11) is set as that of two infinitely dilute solutions in equilibrium, the standard state will approximate a mixture of the two pure solvents. The standard free energy of transfer then becomes a constant for a given solvent system and independent of the nature of the solute under scrutiny. Equation (9.55) therefore applies to such situations, but this time the partition coefficients are for two different solutes, A and B, distributed between identical solvent mixtures. The equation in this form is the basis for applying linear free-energy relationships to distribution coefficients.

The concept of linear free-energy relationships is based on the assumption that the total free energy of a given transition for a particular molecule is the sum of the free-energy contributions of the individual chemical groups comprising the molecule. A standard transition is used to allocate to the various chemical groups characteristic free-energy increments, or substituent constants, which may be used to sum estimated free energies of transition of molecules for which experimental data are not available. Suppose that Eq. (9.54) is converted to logs to the base 10 and applied to the 1-octanol/water partition coefficients of compounds A-H and A-X, to give

$$\text{log } K_{d(A-X)} = \text{Log } K_{d(A-H)} + \frac{\Delta G_{(A-X)} - \Delta G_{(A-H)}}{2.303RT} \tag{9.62}$$

where H represents hydrogen, X a substituent group, and A-X the derivative of A-H in which hydrogen has been replaced by X. Then

$$\log K_{d(A-X)} = \log K_{d(A-H)} + \frac{\Delta \Delta G_X}{2.303RT} \qquad (9.63)$$

where the second term on the right-hand side represents the substituent constant for the group X.

A. Hansch Substituent Constants

The application of linear free-energy relationships to distribution was first proposed by Iwasa et al. [11], and the concept has been used extensively in Hansch's subsequent publications. The subject has mushroomed, and since it is concerned more with (biological) quantitative structure-activity relationships than with physicochemical problems, it will not be considered here in great detail. There are many treatises on the subject (e.g., [3,12,13]) for readers who require further information. A substituent constant π, defined by

$$\pi_X = \frac{K_{d(X)}}{K_{d(H)}} \qquad (9.64)$$

was introduced [11]. $K_{d(H)}$ represents the 1-octanol/water partition coefficient for a standard compound, and $K_{d(X)}$ the corresponding coefficient for a derivative in which a hydrogen atom in the standard compound has been replaced by the group X. Iwasa et al. [11] derived aliphatic π values for a range of chemical groups (X), by measuring the 1-octanol/water partition coefficients of the compounds $C_6H_5(CH_2)_nX$, in which n was varied from 0 to 3. The aromatic group provided a chromophore for spectrophotometric analysis. Some of their results are reproduced in Table 9.7, which suggests that π values are not always reliable when the group is attached directly to the benzene ring or separated by only one methylene group. However, good agreement was obtained between the compounds in which n was 2 or 3. Currently accepted π values are based on more extensive data. A selection is reproduced in Table 9.8; more comprehensive lists are available elsewhere [3,13]. Aliphatic π values can be used to estimate 1-octanol/water partition coefficients when the group X does not interact with the parent molecule. For example, given that the log of the 1-octanol/water partition coefficient of propionic acid is 0.33, the log value for 1-hexanoic acid can be estimated as $0.33 + 3 \times 0.50 = 1.83$. Literature values for $\log K_{d(1-hexanoic\ acid)}$ are 1.88 and 1.92, which are in good

TABLE 9.7 1-Octanol/Water Partition Coefficients for Side-Chain-Substituted Benzene Derivatives, and Derived Aliphatic π Values

$$C_6H_5(CH_2)_n X$$

Group	n = 3		n = 2		n = 1		n = 0	
	log K_d	π	log K_d	π	log K_d	π	log K_d	π
H	3.68	—	3.15	—	2.69	—	2.13	—
OH	1.88	−1.80	1.36	−1.79	1.10	−1.59	1.46	−0.67
NH_2	1.83	−1.85	1.41	−1.74	1.09	−1.60	0.90	−1.23
$COOCH_3$	2.77	−0.91	2.32	−0.83	1.83	−0.86	2.12	−0.01
COOH	2.42	−1.26	1.84	−1.31	1.41	−1.28	1.85	−0.28
$CONH_2$	1.41	−2.27	0.91	−2.24	0.45	−2.24	0.64	−1.49

Source: Abstracted from Ref. 11.

TABLE 9.8 π Values for Aliphatic Substitutions

Group	π	Group	π	Group	π
OH	−1.12	F	−0.17	CH_3	0.50
NH_2	−1.19	Cl	0.39	CH_2	0.50
$N(CH_3)_2$	−0.30	Br	0.60	$CONH_2$	−1.71
NO_2	−0.85	I	1.00	$C\equiv CH$	0.48
CN	−0.84	C_6H_5	2.15	$COCH_3$	−0.62

Source: Abstracted from Ref. 11.

agreement. However, they are not so encouraging when the actual partition coefficients are compared (i.e., calculated = 67.6, observed = 75.9 or 83.2). This illustrates a pitfall in using estimates of this nature, in that the log form of the estimate inspires undue confidence in its accuracy.

Similar calculations can be carried out using the data given in Table 9.7. Thus the 1-octanol/water partition for methanol is given by

$$\log K_{d(C_6H_5(CH_2)_3OH)} - \log K_{d(C_6H_5(CH_2)_2H)} = 1.88 - 3.15$$
$$= -1.27$$

or

$$\log K_{d(C_6H_5(CH_2)_2OH)} - \log K_{d(C_6H_5CH_2H)} = 1.36 - 2.69$$
$$= -1.33$$

The mean value is −1.30.

In another paper [14], π was evaluated for a variety of systems in which the substituent groups were linked directly to a benzene ring. Some of the results are reproduced in Table 9.9. All refer to partition coefficients between 1-octanol and water. The substituent constant for 3- and 4-methyl remained reasonably constant for all the substrates examined, and the mean value of 0.51 agreed well with the accepted aliphatic π value of 0.50. Other n-alkyl groups gave results that approximated the requisite multiples of 0.50. However, as the degree of interaction with the aromatic ring increased, increasingly more variation from one type of substrate to another was observed. Thus the halogens gave reasonably constant results, across the board, but with, for example, 3-hydroxyl, the π values obtained when the group was attached to either phenoxyacetic or

TABLE 9.9 Hansch Substituent Constants, Derived Using Aromatic Substrates

Substituent group	Group already attached to the benzene ring								Mean π
	OCH_2COOH	CH_2COOH	COOH	CH_2OH	OH	NH_2	NO_2	H	
3-CH_3	0.51	0.49	0.52	0.50	0.56	0.50	0.57	0.57	0.51 ± 0.06
4-CH_3	0.52	0.45	0.42	0.48	0.48	0.49	0.52	0.56	
3-F	0.13	0.19	0.28	–	0.47	0.40	–	0.14	0.23 ± 0.10
4-F	0.15	0.14	0.19	–	0.31	0.25	–	0.14	
3-Cl	0.76	0.68	0.83	0.84	1.04	0.98	0.61	0.71	0.78 ± 0.11
4-Cl	0.78	0.70	0.87	0.86	0.93	–	0.54	0.71	
3-Br	0.94	0.91	0.99	–	1.17	–	0.79	0.86	0.96 ± 0.11
4-Br	1.02	0.90	0.98	–	1.13	–	–	0.86	
3-I	1.15	1.22	1.28	–	1.47	–	–	–	1.28 ± 0.15
4-I	1.26	1.23	1.14	–	1.45	–	–	–	
3-NO_2	0.11	-0.10	-0.05	0.11	0.54	0.47	-0.36	-0.28	0.08 ± 0.23
4-NO_2	0.24	-0.04	0.02	0.16	0.50	0.49	-0.39	-0.28	
3-OH	-0.49	-0.52	-0.38	-0.61	-0.66	-0.73	0.15	-0.67	–
4-OCH_3	-0.04	0.01	0.08	0.00	-0.12	–	0.18	-0.02	–

Source: Abstracted from Ref. 17.

phenylacetic acid were significantly different from those obtained when
the substituted molecule was benzyl alcohol, phenol, aniline, or benzene. Fujita et al. [14] recognized these problems and suggested
that although π varies for a given substituent from system to system, the variance within similar systems is not great. They therefore proposed that phenoxyacetic acid be used when strongly interacting groups are not involved, and that phenol be used when phenols or amines form the parent compound.

Nys and Rekker [15] have suggested that the principles involved
in the Hansch substituent constant concept are sometimes misinter-
preted, with the result that some of the calculations found in the
literature are not correct. Hansch substituent constants are
obtained from

$$\pi_X = \log K_{d(AX)} - \log K_{d(AH)} \tag{9.65}$$

AH represents a "marker compound" and AX is a derivative of the
marker compound in which one of the hydrogen atoms has been replaced by group X. Ethylbenzene, $C_6H_5CH_2CH_3$, was one of the
marker compounds used by Hansch to calculate π values and was
chosen because the phenyl group provided a convenient chromophore
for the experimental determination of the partition coefficient. The
logarithm of the 1-octanol/water partition coefficient of ethylbenzene
is 3.15, and the mean experimental value for n-propylbenzene is
3.63. If these two figures are introduced into Eq. (9.65), a π value
of 0.48 is obtained *for the methyl group*. However, one would logically assume that the π value is that for CH_2, since this is the
group that is actually added to the molecule. This is not so, because Eq. (9.65) clearly states that the π value applies to the group
that replaces the hydrogen atom, not to the group that is inserted
into the molecule. Put in another way, the process is given by

$$C_6H_5CH_2CH_3 + CH_3 = C_6H_5CH_2CH_2CH_3 + H \tag{9.66}$$

and not by

$$C_6H_5CH_2CH_3 + CH_2 = C_6H_5CH_2CH_2CH_3 \tag{9.67}$$

Practically speaking, the difference between the two interpretations
is not important in this example, because CH_3 and CH_2 have been
allocated the same π value of 0.50, but it is a convenient way of
showing a misconception that sometimes arises in the interpretation
of linear free-energy relationships. These misconceptions usually
occur in the calculation of partition coefficients rather than the calculation of π values. The following is sometimes quoted as a means
of calculating partition coefficients:

$$\log K_d = \sum_1^n \pi_n \qquad (9.68)$$

If this equation is used to calculate the partition coefficient of n-propylbenzene, assuming that the marker compound for expressing the π value of the phenyl group is H-H, and progressively building up the molecule by adding π values, the following equations are obtained:

$$\pi_{C_6H_5} = \log K_{d(C_6H_6)} - \log K_{d(H-H)} \qquad (9.69)$$

$$\pi_{CH_3} = \log K_{d(C_6H_5CH_3)} - \log K_{d(C_6H_6)} \qquad (9.70)$$

$$\pi_{CH_3} = \log K_{d(C_6H_5CH_2CH_3)} - \log K_{d(C_6H_5CH_3)} \qquad (9.71)$$

$$\pi_{CH_3} = \log K_{d(C_6H_5CH_2CH_2CH_3)} - \log K_{d(C_6H_5CH_2CH_3)} \qquad (9.72)$$

Summation leads to

$$\sum \pi = \log K_{d(C_6H_5CH_2CH_2CH_3)} - \log K_{d(H-H)} \qquad (9.73)$$

which indicates that Eq. (9.68) gives the logarithm of the octanol/water partition coefficient of n-propylbenzene less an increment representative of an imaginary partition coefficient for a hydrogen molecule.

This error can be eliminated by beginning the calculation with $\log K_{d(C_6H_6)}$ rather than $\pi_{C_6H_5}$. Equation (9.68) gives

$$\log K_{d(C_6H_5CH_2CH_2CH_3)} = \pi_{C_6H_5} + 3 \times \pi_{CH_3}$$

$$= 1.96 + 3 \times 0.50 = 2.94$$

and the alternative calculation gives

$$\log K_{d(C_6H_5CH_2CH_2CH_3)} = \log K_{d(C_6H_6)} + 3\pi_{CH_3}$$

$$= 2.3 + 3 \times 0.50 = 3.63$$

The mean experimental value is 3.63.

A similar error can occur in summing $\log K_d$ values. $\log K_d$ for toluene has been reported as 2.69, 2.73, and 2.80, giving a mean value of 2.74. It is incorrect to say that the $\log K_d$ for bibenzyl ($C_6H_5CH_2CH_2C_6H_5$) is $2 \times 2.74 = 5.58$. The mean experimental log K_d is 4.81, compared with 5.10 given by log $K_{d(C_6H_6)}$ + $2\pi C_6H_5$.

The situation can therefore be summarized by saying that partition coefficients must be calculated by the summation of one, and not more than one, partition coefficient plus the π values of the remaining chemical groups in the molecule.

B. Fragmental Constants

The procedure in which Hansch substituent constants (π) are used to estimate partition coefficients is described as a substitution process, because it involves substitution of a hydrogen atom in a compound for which the partition coefficient is known, with the relevant chemical group, and adding the π value of the group to the log of the partition coefficient of the original compound. The method depends on the assignation of an arbitrary value of zero to the hydrogen atom, which implies that every hydrogen atom behaves in the same way, irrespective of its environment. The fragmental method is an alternative procedure. In this, the contributions of the individual elements or groups are summed to give the partition coefficient of the parent compound. The procedure is described mathematically by

$$\log K_d = \Sigma \; af \tag{9.74}$$

where f represents the fragmental constant of each "fragment" that makes up the compound, and a the number of times it occurs.

1. Rekker Fragmental Constants. The first fragmental constants [15] were derived by multiple regression analysis of 128 compounds for which reliable partition coefficients had been reported. These were designated as primary fragmental constants and are listed in Table 9.10. A small intercept to Eq. (9.74) was obtained and was ignored. 1-Octanol/water partition coefficients could be obtained from these constants by simple addition; for example:
Ethyl acetate, $CH_3COOCH_2CH_3$

$$\log K_d = 2 \times f_{CH_3} + f_{CH_2} + f_{COO}$$

$$= 2 \times 0.702 + 0.527 - 1.281 = 0.650$$

(Mean experimental log $K_d = 0.68$.) A supplementary set of secondary constants was obtained by substituting primary constants into experimental log K_d values. These are also given in Table 9.10.

An additional factor was introduced to correct for proximity effects. This effect occurs when two hydrophilic groups are

TABLE 9.10 Nys and Rekker Fragmental Constants[a]

Fragment	Constant	Fragment	Constant
H	0.21	COO	−1.281
CH	0.236	Br	0.24
N	−2.133	CN	−1.13
COOH	−1.003	$CH=CH_2$	0.93
Cl	0.06	CH_2	0.527
$CONH_2$	−1.99	NH	−1.864
C=O	−1.69	O	−1.536
CH_3	0.702	F	−0.51
NH_2	−1.380	I	0.59
C_6H_5	1.896	NO_2	−1.06
OH	−1.440	C(quat)	0.14

[a]Proximity effects:

pe 1 (two hydrophilic groups separated by one CH_2): add 0.80.

pe 2 (two hydrophilic groups separated by two CH_2 groups): add 0.46.

The constants quoted to three decimal places are primary constants, obtained from the multiple regression analysis calculations. Those quoted to only two decimal places are secondary constants, obtained by substituting primary constants into $\log K_d$ values.

Source: Abstracted from Ref. 15.

positioned close together and as a result, bind fewer water molecules than they would if they were independent. The result is an increase in lipophilicity and positive corrections are necessary: 0.80 for groups separated by one methylene group, and 0.46 for groups separated by two methylene groups. An example of the proximity effect is:

2-Aminoethanol, $NH_2CH_2CH_2OH$

$$\log K_d = f_{NH_2} + 2 \times f_{CH_2} + f_{OH} + 0.46$$

$$= -1.380 + 2 \times 0.527 - 1.440 + 0.46 = -1.31$$

(Experimental $\log K_d = -1.31$.)

The fragmental constants for carbon and hydrogen do not normally change when moved from an aliphatic to an aromatic environment; for example:

1,2-Cyclopentanobenzene,

$$\log K_d = f_{C_6H_4} + 3 \times f_{CH_2} = 1.719 + 3 \times 0.527 = 3.303$$

(Experimental $\log K_d = 3.30$.)

In contrast, a new set of constants had to be allocated to other groups conjugated to aromatic systems. These are listed in Table 9.11. Thus for,

4-Chlorophenol,

$$\log K_d = f_{C_6H_4} + f_{Cl} + f_{OH} = 1.719 + 0.943 - 0.359 = 2.303$$

(Experimental $\log K_d = 2.42$.)

Condensation of aromatic rings leads to higher $\log K_d$ values than those predicted by simple fragmental constants. The carbon atoms forming the fusion of the rings are designated $C^\bullet$ and have a fragmental constant of 0.314. Thus for

Quinoline,

$$\log K_d = \log K_{d(pyridine)} + 4 \times f_{CH_{ar}} + 2f_{C^\bullet} - 2f_{CH_{ar}}$$

$$= 0.65 + 4 \times 0.356 + 2 \times 0.314 - 2 \times 0.356 = 1.99$$

(Experimental $\log K_d = 2.04$.)   0.65 is the experimentally determined $\log K_d$.

$f_{C^\bullet}$ is also used in cross-conjugated systems such as diphenyl ether and styrene; for example:

Cinnamic acid, $C_6H_5\overset{\bullet}{C}H = \overset{\bullet}{C}H-\overset{\bullet}{C}OOH$

$$\log K_d = f_{C_6H_5} + f_{CH_2=CH} - f_H + 4(f_{C^\bullet} - f_{C_{ar}}) + f_{COOH}$$

$$= 1.896 + 0.93 - 0.21 + 4(0.314 - 0.15) - 1.003 = 2.27$$

(Mean experimental $\log K_d = 2.11$.)

TABLE 9.11 Nys and Rekker Aromatic Fragmental Constants

Fragment	Constant	Fragment	Constant	Fragment	Constant
H	0.21	OCH_2COOH	-0.588	COO	-0.43
F	0.412	(ar)OCONH(al)	-1.370	NH	-0.93
Cl	0.943	(ar)CO(al)	-0.869	N	-1.06
Br	1.168	SO_2NH	-1.506	CF_2	1.25
I	1.460	$CONH_2$	-1.120	CN	-0.23
OH	-0.359	COOH	0.00	SH	0.62
O	-0.454	NH_2	-0.897	SO	-2.05
NO_2	-0.077	S	0.11	SO_2	-1.87
C_6H_5	1.90	C_6H_4	1.719	C_6H_3	1.440

Source: Abstracted from Ref. 16.

Another variation occurs with hydrogen atoms joined to electron-withdrawing groups, such as carbonyl and carboxyl. These are assigned a higher fragmental constant (0.47) than usual; for example:

Benzaldehyde, C_6H_5CHO

$$\log K_d = f_{C_6H_5} + f_{alCO_{ar}} + 0.47 = 1.896 - 0.869 + 0.47 = 1.50$$

(Mean Experimental $\log K_d = 1.50$.)

2. Hansch-Leo Fragmental Constants

a. General. The fragmental constant for hydrogen is the fundamental unit of the Hansch-Leo approach [13]. It was calculated from the octanol/water partition coefficient of the hydrogen dimer (H_2), which is 0.45, giving a value of $0.45/2 = 0.225$ for f_H. All other fragmental constants were obtained by substituting this value into reliable octanol-water partition coefficients. Thus f_C was derived from the partition coefficient of methane, which is 12.3 ($\log 12.3 = 1.09$), as follows:

$$f_C = \log K_{d(CH_4)} - 4f_H = 1.09 - 4 \times 0.225 = 0.19$$

The number was rounded off to 0.20, so that for propane, $CH_3CH_2CH_3$,

$$\log K_d = 3f_C + 8f_H = 3 \times 0.20 + 8 \times 0.225 = 2.40$$

(Experimental $\log K_d = 2.36$.)

Deviations from additive behavior were adjusted by means of correction factors, which were given the blanket symbol F, so that Eq. (9.74) is modified to

$$\log K_d = \Sigma \, af + \Sigma \, bF \tag{9.75}$$

in which b represents the number of times each correction is used. The flexibility correction (F_b) is an example and is applied to paraffin chains containing more than two carbon-carbon bonds. The flexibility factor corrects for a loss of degree of order and is therefore negative. It has been evaluated as -0.12 for every bond after the first C-C bond, but it applies only when the carbon number is 3 or more. Thus for

n-Hexane, $CH_3(CH_2)_4CH_3$

$$\log K_d = 6 \times 0.20 + 14 \times 0.225 - 4 \times 0.12 = 3.87$$

(Experimental $\log K_d = 3.85.$)

For cyclic compounds the correction factor is -0.09 and applies to all carbon-carbon bonds; for example:

Cyclohexane

$$\log K_d = 6 \times 0.20 + 12 \times 0.225 - 5 \times 0.09 = 3.45$$

(Experimental $\log K_d = 3.44.$) Constants for cyclic factors are underlined.

A double bond counts as $--0\ 55$; thus for

Cyclohexene,

$$\log K_d = 3.45 - 0.55 = 2.90$$

(Experimental $\log K_d = 2.86.$)

Branching favors aqueous solubility, with a resulting decrease in 1-octanol/water partition coefficient. A negative correction ($F_{C_{Br}}$) is therefore applied and is equal to -0.13. The butanes serve to illustrate the importance of this factor.

n-Butane, $CH_3CH_2CH_2CH_3$

$$\log K_d = 4 \times 0.20 + 10 \times 0.225 - 2 \times 0.12 = 2.81$$

(Experimental $\log K_d = 2.89.$)

i-Butane, $CH_3CH\ CH_3$
$\qquad\qquad |$
$\qquad\quad CH_3$

$$\log K_d = 4 \times 0.20 + 10 \times 0.225 - 2 \times 0.12 - 0.13 = 2.76$$

(Experimental $\log K_d = 2.76.$)

TABLE 9.12 Fragmental and Factor Constants for Hydrocarbons

Aliphatic fragmental constants (f)

  -C-   0.20   H   0.225

Aromatic fragmental constants (f^ϕ)

  $\underline{C}$ 0.13   (carbon atom forming part of an aromatic
                                       ring)

  $\underline{\overset{.}{C}}$ 0.225   (carbon atom forming part of more than one
                                       aromatic ring)

  H   0.225   (hydrogen atom bound to an aromatic system)

Aliphatic factor constants (F)

  F_b −0.12   (chain flexibility constant, for chains consist-
                                       ing of three or more carbon atoms; multi-
                                       plied by n − 1, where n is the number of
                                       carbon atoms)

  $\underline{F}_b$ −0.09   (ring flexibility constant; multiplied by the
                                       number of bonds in the ring; the constant
                                       does not apply to aromatics, which have
                                       their own built-in corrections)

  $F_=$ −0.55   (unsaturation, double bond)

  $F_\equiv$ −1.42   (unsaturation, triple bond)

  $F_{C_{Br}}$ −0.13   (chain branching)

Aromatic factor constants (F^ϕ)

  $F^\phi_{(=)}$ −0.42   (double bond conjugated to one aromatic
                                       system)

  $F^{\phi\phi}_{(=)}$ 0.00   (double bond conjugated to two aromatic
                                       systems)

  $F^{\phi\phi}_{(\equiv)}$ 0.00   (triple bond conjugated to two aromatic
                                       systems)

Source: Abstracted from Ref. 13.

Fragmental and factor constants applicable to hydrocarbons are given in Table 9.12.

When compounds containing heteroatoms are considered, fragments are divided into two groups, single-atom fundamental fragments and multiple-atom fundamental fragments. A single-atom fundamental fragment is an isolating carbon, hydrogen, or heteroatom bound solely to hydrogen or other isolated carbon atoms. Isolating carbon atoms are, in turn, defined as carbon atoms with at least two valencies satisfied by bonding to carbon or hydrogen, and the remainder satisfied by single bonding to one or two heteroatoms. All other carbon atoms are nonisolating. Examples of both classes are given in Table 9.13.

Fragmental constants for compounds containing only isolated carbon atoms and not more than one heteroatom are additive; for example, using the values given in Table 9.14.

TABLE 9.13 Isolating and Nonisolating Carbon Atoms

Isolating	Nonisolating
$\begin{array}{c} H \\ \| \\ H- \underset{\sim}{C} -H \\ \| \\ H \end{array}$	
$\begin{array}{c} CH_3 \\ \| \\ H- \underset{\sim}{C} =CH_2 \\ \| \\ H \end{array}$	$\begin{array}{c} OH \\ \| \\ CH_3- \underset{\sim}{C} =O \end{array}$
$\begin{array}{c} CH_3- \underset{\sim}{C} -OH \\ \| \\ H \end{array}$	$\begin{array}{c} H \\ \| \\ CH_3- \underset{\sim}{C} =O \end{array}$
$CH_3- \underset{\sim}{C} \equiv C-H$	

TABLE 9.14 Single-Atom Fragmental Constants

Fragment	f	Fragment	f
H	0.225	C	0.20
Br	0.20	N	−2.18
Cl	0.06	O	−1.82
F	−0.38	S	−0.79
I	0.59		

Source: Abstracted from Ref. 13.

Diethyl ether, $CH_3CH_2-O-CH_2CH_3$

$$\text{Log } K_d = 4 \times f_C + 10 \times f_H + f_C + (4 - 1)F_b$$
$$= 4 \times 0.20 + 10 \times 0.225 + (-1.82) + 3 \times (-0.12) = 0.87$$

(Experimental log K_d = 0.83.)

Piperidine, ⬡NH

$$\log K_d = 5 \times f_C + 11 \times f_H + f_N + (6 - 1)F_b$$
$$= 5 \times 0.20 + 11 \times 0.225 + (-2.18) + 5 \times (-0.09) = 0.85$$

(Experimental log K_d = 0.85.)
The procedure should apply equally well to compounds containing more than one heteroatom, provided that they are well separated.

b. Halogenated alkanes. These compounds appear to behave in the same simple fashion as those given above when no carbon is substituted with more than one halogen atom. However, when carbons are substituted with more than one halogen each, or adjacent atoms are substituted, corrections must be made for shielding of the dipole created by the halogen by that of the adjacent halogen. There are four factors, as follows:

Number of halogens involved	Factor
Two on the same carbon	$F_{mhG_2} = 0.30 \times n$
Three on the same carbon	$F_{mhG_3} = 0.53 \times n$

Number of halogens involved	Factor
Four on the same carbon	$F_{mhG_4} = 0.72 \times n$
Adjacent monosubstituted carbons	$F_{mhV_n} = (n - 1) \times 0.28$

where n represents the number of halogen atoms involved. Some examples are:

Chloroform, $CHCl_3$

$$Log\ K_d = f_C + f_H + 3 \times f_{Cl} + 3 \times F_{mhG_3} + (3 - 1)F_b$$
$$= 0.20 + 0.225 + 3 \times 0.06 + 3 \times 0.53 + 2 \times (-0.12)$$
$$= 1.96$$

(Experimental log K_d = 1.96.)
   Methyl chloride, CH_3Cl

$$log\ K_d = f_C + 3 \times f_H + f_{Cl} = 0.20 + 3 \times 0.225 + 0.06 = 0.94$$

(Experimental log K_d = 0.91.)

1,1-Dichloroethane, CH_3CHCl_2

$$log\ K_d = 2 \times f_C + 4 \times f_H + 2 \times f_{Cl} + 2 \times F_b + 2 \times F_{mhG_2}$$
$$= 2 \times 0.20 + 4 \times 0.225 + 2 \times 0.06 + 2 \times (-0.12) + 2 \times 0.30$$
$$= 1.78$$

(Experimental log K_d = 1.79.)

c. Multiple-atom fragmental constants. Fragmental constants for nonisolated carbon atoms cannot be calculated by adding together single-atom fragmental constants. Overall multiple-atom fragmentation constants have therefore been obtained from experimental results, and allocated to chemical groups rather than individual atoms. Some multiple-atom fragmentation constants are given in Table 9.15. Examples of their usage follow.

TABLE 9.15   Multiple-Atom Fragmental Constants

Fragment	f	f^ϕ	Fragment	f	f^ϕ	$f^{1/\phi}$
NO_2	−1.16	−0.03	CN	−1.27	−0.34	
NH	−2.15	−1.03	−CON	−3.04	−2.80	−2.20
OH	−1.64	−0.44	−SCN	−0.48	0.64	
SH	−0.23	0.62	C)	−1.90	−1.09	
NH_2	−1.54	−1.00	COO	−1.49	−0.56	
CONH	−2.71	−1.81	OCONH	−1.79	−1.46	−0.91
COOH	−1.11	−0.03	CH=NOH	−1.02	−0.15	
$OCONH_2$	−1.58	−0.82	NHCONH	−2.18	−1.07	
$NHCONH_2$	−2.18	−1.07				

Butylamine, $CH_3CH_2CH_2CH_2NH_2$

$$\log K_d = 4 \times f_c + 9 \times f_H + f_{NH_2} + (4 - 1)F_b$$

$$= 4 \times 0.20 + 9 \times 0.225 + (-1.54) + 3 \times (-0.12) = 0.93$$

(Experimental $\log K_d = 0.88$.)
Butane-1-thiol, $CH_3CH_2CH_2CH_2SH$

$$\log K_d = 4 \times f_C + 9 \times f_H + f_{SH} + (4 - 1)F_b$$

$$= 4 \times 0.20 + 9 \times 0.225 + (-0.23) + 3 \times (-0.12) = 2.24$$

(Experimental $\log K_d = 2.28$.)
N-methylacetamide, $CH_3NHCOCH_3$

$$\log K_d = 2 \times f_C + 6 \times f_H + f_{CONH}$$

$$= 2 \times 0.20 + 6 \times 0.225 + (-2.71) = -0.96$$

(Experimental $\log K_d = -1.05$.)

d. Aromatics. Aromatic fragmental constants are based on the 1-octanol/water partition coefficient of benzene, which is 135, giving $\log K_d = 2.13$. Thus the fragmental constant of the phenyl group is given by

$$f_{C_6H_5} = \log K_{d(C_6H_6)} - f_H = 2.13 - 0.225 = 1.905$$

which is normally rounded down to 1.90. Similarly, the fragmental constant for aromatic $-C=$ is obtained from

$$f_{-CH} = \frac{\log K_{d(C_6H_6)}}{6} = \frac{2.13}{6} = 0.355$$

and for aromatic carbon,

$$f_{-C} = 0.355 - 0.255 = 0.13$$

Fragmental constants for groups forming part of an aromatic ring are given in Table 9.16.

TABLE 9.16 Fragmental Constants for Groups Fused in Aromatic Rings

Group	f^{ϕ}	Group	f^{ϕ}	Group	f^{ϕ}
—N=	−1.12	—O—	−0.08	$\underset{|}{C}$	0.13
—N$\diagdown$	−1.60	—S—	0.36	$\underset{|}{\overset{\cdot}{C}}$	0.22$_5$
—N$\overset{\phi}{\diagup}$	−0.56	—Se—	0.45	(for atoms involved in two rings)	
—N=N—	−2.14	—OC— ‖ O	−1.40	$\overset{*}{C}$	0.44
—NH—	−0.65	—CH=N—NH—	−0.47	(for atoms involved in two hetero rings)	
—C— ‖ O	−0.59	—N=CH—S—	−0.29	—N=CH—NH—	0.79
—N=CH—O—	−0.71			—NH—C— ‖ O	−2.00

Source: Abstracted from Ref. 13.

Groups linked to aromatic systems usually have fragmental constants different from the aliphatic values. They are distinguished by designating the aromatic constants f^{ϕ}. The symbol $f^{\phi\phi}$ represents an atom that forms part of more than one aromatic ring. If the substituent group has an unsatisfied bond at both ends, the symbol f^{ϕ} represents the contribution when the aromatic system is linked to the left of the group, and $f^{1/\phi}$ when it is conjugated to the right. Thus for the group $-CONH-$,

$$f^{\phi} \equiv -CONH- \quad \text{and} \quad f^{1/\phi} \equiv -CONH-$$

The following examples illustrate the use of aromatic fragmental con- constants.

Naphthalene

$$\log K_d = 8 \times f_{-C} + 2 \times f_{-C}^{\phi} + 8 \times f_H^{\phi}$$

$$= 8 \times 0.13 + 2 \times 0.225 + 8 \times 0.225 = 3.29$$

(Experimental $\log K_d = 3.20$.)

Styrene, $CH=CH_2$

$$\log K_d = 6 \times f_{-C}^{\phi} + 2 \times f_C + 5 \times f_H^{\phi} + 3 \times f_H + F_{(=)}^{\phi}$$

$$= 6 \times 0.13 + 2 \times 0.20 + 5 \times 0.225 + 3 \times 0.225 + (-0.42)$$

$$= 2.56$$

(Experimental $\log K_d = 2.95$.)

Thiophene,

$$\log K_d = 4 \times f_{-C}^{\phi} + 4 \times f_H^{\phi} + f_{-S}^{\phi}$$

$$= 4 0.13 + 4 \times 0.225 + 0.36 = 1.78$$

(Experimental $\log K_d = 1.81$.)

Pyridine,

$$\log K_d = 5 \times f_{-C}^{\phi} + 5 \times f_H + f_N^{\phi}$$

$$= 5 \times 0.13 + 5 \times 0.225 - 1.12 = 0.66$$

(Mean experimental $\log K_d = 0.64$.)

Nitrobenzene,

$$\log K_d = 6 \times f_{-C}^{\phi} + 5 \times f_H + f_{-NO_2}^{\phi}$$

$$= 6 \times 0.13 + 5 \times 0.225 - 0.03 = 1.88$$

(Mean experimental $\log K_d = 1.84$.)

e. Interactions. The methods and examples quoted so far involve comparatively simple compounds in which there is little or no interaction between one part of the molecule and another. The methodology breaks down when interactions occur, and there is no comprehensive procedure for dealing with the problem. Methods have been developed for specific situations. Some of these are given below.

(1) Disubstituted aromatics. Introduction on a benzene ring of a second substituent can influence the properties of a hydrogen-bonding group already present on the ring. The effect of the second group on the electron distribution of the molecule can be assessed from its Hammett substituent constant (σ). The Hammett constant, or sigma value, is a number assigned to chemical groups to indicate their electron-attracting or withdrawing properties. Positive σ values are given to electron-withdrawing groups; for example, the values for 4-chloro and 4-nitro are +0.23 and +0.78, respectively, the higher numerical value for nitro signifying that it is a stronger electron-withdrawing group than is chloro. Negative values signify electron donation; for example, $\sigma_{4-OCH_3} = -0.27$ and $\sigma_{3-CH_3} = -0.07$. Hansch and Leo [13] have allocated f^X values for some hydrogen-bonding groups that are influenced in this way. f^{X1} represents the fragmental constant which is applied when there is a second group having a σ value of 0.30 to 0.60, and f^{X2} applied to σ values greater than 0.6. The ether group $-O-$ has an f^{X1} of -0.22, and 4-carboxyl has a σ value of 0.45, so that the 1-octanol/water partition coefficient of 4-methoxybenzoic acid is calculated as

$$\log K_d = 6 \times f^{\phi}_{-C} + f_C + 7 \times f_H + f^{X1}_{-O-} + f^{\phi}_{-COOH}$$

$$= 6 \times 0.13 + 0.20 + 7 \times 0.225 - 0.22 - 0.03 = 2.31$$

(Experimental $\log K_d$ = 2.33.) Further information on Hammett constants can be obtained elsewhere [12,17,18].

(2) Benzyl fragmental constants. Chemical groups separated from an aromatic system by only one methylene group are not conjugated to the system, but frequently have properties intermediate between aromatic and aliphatic. The constant f^{1R} is sometimes assigned for such groups. Given that f^{1R}_{COOH} = -1.03, the 1-octanol/water partition for phenylacetic acid is calculated as

$$\log K_d = 6 \times f^{\phi}_{-C} + f_C + 7 \times f_H + f^{1R}_{COOH}$$

$$= 6 \times 0.13 + 0.20 + 7 \times 0.225 - 1.03 = 1.53$$

(Mean experimental $\log K_d$ = 1.46.) In contrast, 3-methylbenzoic acid gives

$$\log K_d = 6 \times f^{\phi}_{-C} + f_C + 7 \times f_H + f^{\phi}_{COOH}$$

$$= 6 \times 0.13 + 0.20 + 7 \times 0.225 - 0.03 = 2.53$$

(Experimental $\log K_d$ = 2.37.)

V. OTHER METHODS OF PREDICTING PARTITION COEFFICIENTS

A. Molecular Connectivities

This is a procedure by which numbers can be allocated to molecular structures to give a quantitative assessment of skeletal complexity. Methods of calculating connectivities will be given here, but the text will be confined to the minimum necessary to demonstrate that there are correlations with partition coefficients. For the rationale behind the concept and further detail on methodology, the reader is referred to the original references [19–21].

The zero-order connectivity ($^0\chi$) is the simplest parameter. It is calculated from

$$^0\chi = \Sigma \; (\delta_i)^{-1/2} \tag{9.76}$$

where δ_i is a number assigned to each non-hydrogen atom, reflecting the number of nonhydrogen atoms bonded to it. Thus for n-pentane,

```
    H   H   H   H   H
    |   |   |   |   |
H − C  − C  − C  − C  − C  − H
    |a  |b  |c  |d  |e
    H   H   H   H   H
```

$\delta_{C_a} = 1$ (C_a is bonded to C_b), $\delta_{C_b} = 2$ (C_b is bonded to C_a and C_c), and so on. Therefore,

$$^0\chi = \frac{1}{\sqrt{\delta_{C_a}}} + \frac{1}{\sqrt{\delta_{C_b}}} + \frac{1}{\sqrt{\delta_{C_c}}} + \frac{1}{\sqrt{\delta_{C_d}}} + \frac{1}{\sqrt{\delta_{C_e}}}$$

$$= \frac{1}{\sqrt{1}} + \frac{1}{\sqrt{2}} + \frac{1}{\sqrt{2}} + \frac{1}{\sqrt{2}} + \frac{1}{\sqrt{1}} = 4.121$$

The first-order connectivity ($^1\chi$) is derived for each bond by calculating the product of the numbers associated with the two atoms of the bond. The reciprocal of the square root of this number is then computed and becomes the bond value. The sum of the bond values gives the first-order connectivity of the molecule. Again, hydrogen atoms are not counted. Thus for n-pentane:

Bonding value for $C_a - C_b = (\delta_{C_a}\delta_{C_b}) = 1$ (because C_a is bonded to C_b) $\times$ 2 (because C_a is bonded to C_a and C_c) = 2. Similarly,

$$(\delta_{C_d}\delta_{C_e}) = 2 \text{ and } (\delta_{C_b}\delta_{C_c}) = (\delta_{C_c}\delta_{C_d}) = 2 \times 2 = 4$$

giving

$$^1\chi = \Sigma(\delta_i\delta_j)^{-1/2} = 2\chi\frac{1}{\sqrt{2}} + 2\chi\frac{1}{\sqrt{4}} = 2.414$$

Murray et al. [20] correlated the first-order connectivities of 183 compounds with their octanol-water partition coefficients and obtained the results given in Table 9.17. The hydrocarbons gave a slope entirely different from those obtained with the other solutes and were therefore placed in a class of their own. The remaining compounds could be grouped together to give a reasonable correlation, shown on the bottom line of Table 9.17. Better correlations were obtained when the compound types were considered independently.

TABLE 9.17 Regression Equations for Correlation of Log Partition Coefficients with First-Order Connectivity Index

Compound class	Number of compounds	Slope	Intercept	Correlation coefficient	Standard deviation
Carboxylic acids	9	0.927	−1.41	0.996	0.122
Esters	24	0.996	−1.71	0.999	0.060
Ethers	12	0.964	−1.30	0.976	0.080
Alcohols	49	0.966	−1.53	0.997	0.151
Amines	28	0.977	−1.51	0.979	0.179
Ketones	16	0.982	−1.61	0.993	0.094
Hydrocarbons	45	0.884	0.406	0.975	0.160
All compounds except hydrocarbons	138	0.950	−1.48	0.986	0.152

Source: Abstracted from Ref. 20.

Hetero atoms were treated on the basis that OH and NH_2 were assigned the value 1, analogous to CH_3, and ether oxygen was given the value 2. Nitrogen in the groups RNH and R_2N were assigned connectivities of 2 and 3, respectively, carboxy oxygen in carboxylic acids and ketones 1, and $=CH_2$ assigned connectivity 2, RHC= and HC= connectivity 3, and $R_2C=$ connectivity 4. Examples of calculations using these values are:

Benzene,

Each carbon atom contributes 3 units, 2 for C= and 1 for C−; therefore each bond is worth $3 \times 3 = 9$, so that

$$1\chi = 6 \times \frac{1}{\sqrt{9}} = 2.00$$

Substitution in the equation for hydrocarbons in Table 9.17 gives $\log K_d = 2.17$; observed $\log K_d = 2.13$.

$$
\text{4-Methylpentan-3-one, } CH_3CH-\overset{\overset{\displaystyle O}{\|}}{C}\text{--}CH_2CH_3
$$
$$
\underset{\displaystyle CH_3}{|}
$$

Taking the bonds from left to right, we have

$$
{}^1\chi = \frac{1}{\sqrt{1 \times 3}} + \frac{1}{\sqrt{1 \times 3}} + \frac{1}{\sqrt{3 \times (2 + 2)}} + \frac{1}{\sqrt{2 \times (2 + 2)}}
$$
$$
+ \frac{1}{\sqrt{2 \times (2 + 2)}} + \frac{1}{\sqrt{1 \times 2}}
$$
$$
= \frac{1}{\sqrt{3}} + \frac{1}{\sqrt{3}} + \frac{1}{\sqrt{12}} + \frac{1}{\sqrt{8}} + \frac{1}{\sqrt{8}} + \frac{1}{\sqrt{2}} = 2.858
$$

Substitution in the equation for ketones in Table 9.17 gives $\log K_d = 1.19$; observed $\log K_d = 1.09$

n-Butyric Acid, $CH_3CH_2CH_2COOH$

$$
{}^1\chi = \frac{1}{\sqrt{2}} + \frac{1}{\sqrt{4}} + \frac{1}{\sqrt{8}} + \frac{1}{\sqrt{8}} + \frac{1}{\sqrt{4}} = 2.414
$$

giving $\log K_d = 0.83$; observed $\log K_d = 0.79$.

Some of the partition coefficients used to obtain the results given in Table 9.17 were calculated using Hansch π values. Boyd et al. [22] reinvestigated these relationships, using experimentally obtained partition coefficients, and obtained the equations shown in Table 9.18. Better correlations were obtained with phenols, anilines, and carboxylic acids when higher-order connectivities were considered.

B. Parachor and Molar Volume

Most theories of solution are based on the simple concept of the creation of a cavity in the solvent, followed by its occupation by a molecule of the solute. The quasi-crystalline model of regular solutions is a typical example. The total cavity volume for 1 mol of solute will be equal to the molar volume of the solute (V_2), and the free-energy change per mole (ΔG) will be equal to $V_2 P_i$, where P_i is the internal pressure of the solvent. In a distribution situation, where solutions in a solvent A and a solvent B are in equilibrium, the free energy of transfer ($\Delta \Delta G$) will be given by

$$\Delta \Delta G = \Delta G_A - \Delta G_B = -RT \ln X_{2(A)} + RT \ln X_{2(B)}$$

$$= V_2 P_{i(A)} - V_2 P_{i(B)} \tag{9.77}$$

which arrangement gives

$$-\log \frac{X_{2(A)}}{X_{2(B)}} = \frac{P_{i(A)} - P_{i(B)}}{2.303\ RT} \times V_2 = -\log K_d \tag{9.78}$$

and provides a means of evaluating the partition coefficient (K_d).

McGowan [23] pointed out that whereas the internal pressures of most organic liquids lie between 1500 and 2000 atm, that of water is about 15,000 atm, so that for distributions between organic solvents and water, $(P_{i(A)} - P_{i(B)}) \cong 13{,}000$ atm. Substitution for this and $R = 82.06\ cm^3\ atm\ K^{-1}\ mol^{-1}$ in Eq. (9.78) gives, at 298 K,

$$-\log K_d = 0.2 V_2$$

McGowan [24] used the parachor [P] as a measure of molar volume, and evaluated a constant of 0.012 for hydrocarbons and halogenated hydrocarbons from experimental results. An additional constant (E_A) had to be introduced to account for solute-solvent interactions, as shown in

$$\log K_d = 0.012[P] + E_A \tag{9.79}$$

TABLE 9.18 Regression Equations for Correlation of Log Partition Coefficients with First-order Connectivity Index

Compound class	Number of compounds	Slope	Intercept	Correlation coefficient	Standard deviation
Alcohols	14	1.090	−1.353	0.995	0.157
Amines	12	0.887	−1.104	0.987	0.175
Phenols	16	0.640	0.467	0.883	0.219
Anilines	16	1.148	−1.285	0.958	0.220
Acids	8	1.070	−1.148	0.993	0.197

Source: Abstracted from Ref. 22.

TABLE 9.19 E_A Values

	Diethyl ether-water	Isobutanol-water
Amine	−2.8	−1.6
Ester	−1.9	−1.6
Hydroxyl	−1.9	−1.1

Source: Abstracted from Ref. 23.

E_A values, evaluated experimentally [23], are given in Table 9.19. Parachors were chosen for these relationships because they were easy to calculate compared with molar volumes. Substituent constants for parachor [25] are reproduced in Table 9.20. Parachors are calculated by simple addition, followed by subtraction of 18.6 cm^3 for every bond, regardless of whether single, double, or treble. Two specimen calculations are given below.

$$\begin{array}{ccc}
& H \quad O & H \quad H \\
& | \quad\ \| & | \quad | \\
\text{Ethyl Acetate,} & H-C-C-O-C-C-H & \\
& | & | \quad | \\
& H & H \quad H
\end{array}$$

$$4C = 4 \times 46.35 = 185.4$$
$$8H = 8 \times 24.7\ = 197.6$$
$$\underline{2O = 2 \times 35.25 = \ \ 70.5}$$
$$453.5$$
$$\underline{13 \text{ bonds} \qquad\quad 241.8}$$

$$[P] = 211.7; \text{ literature } [P] = 217.1 \ [25].$$

TABLE 9.20 Atomic Parachors

H	B	C	N	O	F
24.7	51.9	46.35	40.8	35.25	29.7
Si	P	S	Cl	Br	I
76.05	70.5	64.95	59.4	74.3	97.9

Source: Abstracted from J. C. McGowan, *Recp. Trav. Chim. Pays-Bas Belg.*, 75, 193−208 (1956).

log K_d = 0.012 × 211.7 − 1.9 = 0.64; literature log K_d = 0.93.

Benzene

6C = 6 × 46.35 = 278.1
6H = 6 × 24.7 = 148.2
                 426.3
12 bonds   223.2
[P] = 203.1; literature [P] = 206.8 [25].

log K_d = 0.012 × 203.1 = 2.44; the mean log K_d between 1-octanol, chloroform, "oils," heptane, and hexane, and water [13] = 2.23 ± 0.21 (P' = 0.01).

The procedure described above has been compared with alternative methods for calculating parachors [18].

An extension of this approach [26], specifically for partition coefficients of steroids between diethyl ether and water, uses

$$log\ K_d = 36,000V_x - E \qquad\qquad (9.80)$$

V_x is the characteristic volume of the solute in $m^3\ mol^{-1}$, and E is an interaction factor, which is equal to --0.15 for each fluorine atom and 1.9 for each ester, carbonyl, or hydroxyl group, except when two such groups are close together. Characteristic volumes are calculated by summation of the atomic constants given in Table 9.21, less 6.56 × 10^{-6} for every bond, irrespective of its type. Thus cortisone-21-acetate (XXVIII), which contains 62 chemical bonds, has a characteristic volume of (23 × 1.635 + 30 × 0.871 + 6 × 1.243) × 10^{-5} − (62 × 6.56 × 10^{-6}) = 3.052 × $10^{-4}\ m^3\ mol^{-1}$. There are four carbonyl groups and one hydroxyl, so that E = 5 × 1.9 = 9.5.

TABLE 9.21 Atomic Constants ($m^3\ mol^{-1}$ × 10^5) for Characteristic Volumes[a]

H	C	N	O	F	Si
0.871	1.635	1.439	1.243	1.048	2.683

P	S	Cl	Br	I
2.487	2.291	2.095	2.621	3.453

[a]For a bond between two atoms, subtract 6.56 × 10^{-6}.
Source: Abstracted from Ref. 26.

TABLE 9.22 Substituent Constants (π_e) for Diethyl Ether-Water Partition Coefficients of Steroids[a]

	n	π_e
6α-CH_3	3	0.458
9α-F	4	0.155
16α-CH_3	1	0.403
16α-OH	1	−0.305
16α-Cl	1	0.696
17 ··· OH / 16 ··· OH $\longrightarrow$ ··· O / ··· O $\rangle C(CH_3)_2$	1	1.286
HO 11 $\longrightarrow$ H	1	1.061
21 C−OH $\longrightarrow$ 21 C−H	1	0.895
O 11 $\longrightarrow$ HO	2	0.043
16 CH_3 $\longrightarrow$ CH_3	1	0.899
[b] $-CH_2CH_2CH_2-$ $\longrightarrow$ $-CH$ $\langle CH_2- / CH_2-$	1	−0.038
6α-F	4	0.248
16α−CH_3	1	0.403
16β-CH_3	1	0.493
16α-F	2	0.176
17−$OCOCH_3$	1	0.456
21−$OCOCH_3$	10	1.265
17 C−OH $\longrightarrow$ CH	2	0.609

TABLE 9.22   (Continued)

	n·	π_e
$21-OCOCH_3 \longrightarrow C-H$	1	-0.401
	3	0.182

[a]n, Number of pairs of compounds used for the
calculation.
[b]21-*n*-butyl ester; 21-isobutyl ester.
Source: Abstracted from Ref. 27.

$$\log K_d = 36,000 \times 3.052 \times 10^{-4} - 9.5 = 1.49$$

and literature $\log K_d = 1.4$.

The scheme works well for the 27 compounds quoted in the paper
but appears to be confined to corticosteroids, since testosterone,
estradiol, and progesterone, for example, give $\log K_d$ values of 4.96,
4.12, and 5.64, respectively, compared with literature results of
1.94, 1.81, and 2.78.

Flynn [27] examined the ether-water partition coefficients of 46
steroids and assigned π_e substituent constants, analogous to Hansch
π values.   As an example, cortisol has a mean ether-water partition
coefficient of 1.60, compared with 26.0 for cortisol-21-acetate.   This
yields a π_e for 21-acetate of $\log(26.0/1.60) = 1.211$.   Comparison of
a further nine pairs of compounds gave a range of estimates of π_e
for 21-acetate, from which a mean value of 1.265 was obtained.   The
full set of substituent constants is reproduced in Table 9.22.   Flynn's
substituent constants are useful for predicting the ether-water partition coefficients of a derivative when the partition coefficient for the
parent compound is known.   For example, the mean ether-water partition coefficient of cortisone reported by Flynn was 1.40; the calculated

ether-water partition coefficient for cortisone-21-acetate is therefore 1.40 × antilog 1.265 = 25.8, in comparison with an observed value of 25.1. The scheme applies mainly to corticosteroids, although testosterone and progesterone were included. Estrogens were not considered, however.

VI. MEASUREMENT OF PARTITION COEFFICIENTS

A. Classical Methods

In simple situations in which the solute has reasonable solubilities in both solvents and the partition coefficient lies roughly in the region of 0.1 to 10, the only apparatus required are a beaker or flask to hold the mixture, a constant-temperature bath to maintain the mixture at the required temperature, and a pair of pipets for withdrawing samples from the two phases. The two solvents and the solute are placed in the vessel, and stirred for a suitable period of time, after which the phases are allowed to separate, and samples taken. A refinement is that a bored cork or rubber bung can be slid onto the stem of a pipet and adjusted to a position whereby the tip of the pipet is located in the required liquid layer when the cork or bung comes in contact with the lip of the vessel.

This basic technique is described as an undergraduate exercise in many physical chemistry textbooks. Two popular systems are iodine between carbon tetrachloride and water, which may be analyzed by titration against standard thiosulfate, and ammonia between chloroform and water, involving acid-base titration.

Most so-called immiscible binary liquid systems have finite mutual solubilities and should be saturated with each other before introducing the solute. If a series of experiments are to be carried out with the same pair of solvents, the usual technique is to shake together large quantities of the two solvents in a separatory funnel and use them as a reservoir. When required, the denser liquid is withdrawn through the tap, and the other, by pipet, from the top. The solute should not be added to the mixed liquids, but instead, dissolved in one of the solvents before mixing with the other solvent.

Removal of a sample of the lower layer by passing a pipet through the upper layer is feasible when the solubilities in the two solvents are not greatly different. Even then, picking up some of the upper-layer as the pipet is passed through into the lower layer must be avoided by blocking the open end of the pipet. Additionally, the stem must be wiped with a tissue before discharging the sample. If the solute is considerably more soluble in the upper layer than in the lower layer, even a minute quantity of the upper layer picked up in the pipet used for sampling the lower layer will give rise to a large error in the determination. The problem can be avoided by

setting up the equilibrium in a separatory funnel and withdrawing
the lower layer through the tap. However, it must be ensured that
none of the lighter solution is trapped in the tap or on the lower
sides of the funnel, from which it can be sucked out when the tap
is opened.

The temperature of the mixture in a separatory funnel should
not be controlled by immersing the funnel in a constant-temperature
water bath, because of the difficulties of removing bath water from
the stem of the tap. The problem is best avoided by using a jacketed separatory funnel, through which water at the necessary temperature can be circulated. This has the advantage that it can be agitated in a mechanical shaker.

It was recommended in Chapter 1 that saturated solutions can be
prepared more rapidly by heating to an elevated temperature, then
dropping the temperature to the required level. This procedure will
give no benefit in preparing partitioned systems; equilibrium must
be reached by agitating for a sufficient time at the required temperature. The period of agitation must be established by trial and error,
as also must the resting period following agitation, when the phases
are allowed to separate. Leo and Hansch [3] consider that repeated
inversion of the containing vessel for 1 or 2 min is sufficient for
most systems. However, personal experience with solutes having
partition coefficients highly in favor of one phase indicates that hours
rather than minutes are necessary to yield reproducible partition coefficients. Separating the two phases is sometimes difficult, particularly when the solute is surface active. In these circumstances centrifugation may help, but it is not always successful. Probably the
only effective way to deal with surface-active solutes is to agitate
the mixture very gently, but this will require a protracted time to
reach equilibrium.

When the concentrations in the two phases are not too different,
only one phase need be assayed, and the concentration of the other
calculated by difference. However, when the concentrations in the
two phases are very different, the procedure is possible only if the
weaker solution is assayed. Unfortunately, it is usually this solution
that presents the analytical problems. Analysis of the stronger phase
under these circumstances *could* give, by difference, a concentration
in the weaker phase, within the analytical error of the result for the
stronger phase. A further problem associated with analysis is that
concentrations involved in partitioning processes are less than the
solubilities in the isolated solvents, with the result that analytical
procedures that are adequate for determining solubilities may not be
sufficiently sensitive for determining partition coefficients. Radio-
active labeling, followed by scintillation or Geiger counting, is a very
sensitive technique and is often successful when other techniques
have failed.

An alternative method for systems with partition coefficients widely removed from unity is to arrange the system so that there is a greater volume of the less favored solvent than for the other solvent. Thus, if a solute has a partition coefficient of 100 in favor of the oil in an oil-water mixture, if the system contains 50 mg of solute, distributed between 100 ml each of oil and water, the water will contain 0.5 mg. However, if 100 ml of water and 5 ml of oil were used, the water would contain 8.3 mg, representing a 16-fold increase in concentration in the aqueous phase. Another way of overcoming the problem is to concentrate the weaker phase by extraction or evaporation.

Any technique applied to partitions in which the solubility in one solvent is considerably greater than in the other suffers the disadvantage that even the smallest contamination of the weaker phase by the stronger phase will give rise to large errors in the partition coefficient.

B. Automated Methods

Several devices for rapid, semiautomatic determination of partition coefficients have been developed over recent years. The AKUFVE system [28] uses a conventional mixing chamber equipped with thermostatically controlled heating coil and paddle stirrer. While the mixture is agitated, the mixed phases are continuously drawn off into a specially designed centrifuge, which separates the phases and passes them along separate paths, either to waste or back to the mixing chamber. Measuring cells are placed in the flow paths leaving the centrifuge and are monitored spectrophotometrically or radiometrically. The apparatus has been evaluated by Davis and coworkers [29,30], who found that equilibrium is normally attained in a matter of minutes but that it is unsuitable for single determinations, because the stripping and cleaning after use is too involved. However, the apparatus was recommended for situations where one system was examined under a range of conditions, such as pH or temperature. Two other disadvantages were the quantities involved, 500 ml of each solvent, which are too large for most situations, and the possibility that volatile solvents could escape.

An apparatus in which the solutions are equilibrated as they flow through a helical tube has been described [31]. The phases were mixed in a T piece, designed to disperse the aqueous phase as segments, in the nonaqueous phase, as shown in Fig. 9.2a. As they left the helical tube, the solutions were separated by a phase splitter (Fig. 9.2b), in which the mixture passed through a chamber lined on one side with (PTFE) and on the other with glass. The nonaqueous phase followed the hydrophobic PTFE surface through one exit, and the aqueous phase followed the glass surface through the

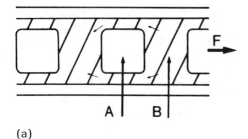

(a)

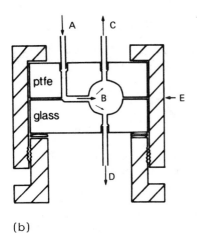

(b)

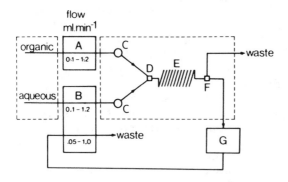

(c)

FIGURE 9.2 (a) Segmentation of (A) aqueous and (B) organic phases;
(b) phase splitter; (c) construction of segmented flow and phase
splitter apparatus for determination of partition coefficients. (From
Ref. 31.)

other. Both phases were run to waste, one through a flow cell that monitored the solute concentration. The complete apparatus is shown diagramatically in Fig. 9.2c. Kinkel and Tomlinson [31] evaluated the apparatus and recommended it for single as well as repetative determinations with systems having log partition coefficients between ±2.5. Not all systems were well separated by the phase splitter, but emulsions were broken by contact with the PTFE surface.

The principles involved in the phase splitter, described above, have been used to construct filter probes for sampling aqueous and nonaqueous phases in partitioning systems [32,33]. In an evaluation of the technique [32], two probes were immersed in the equilibrating mixture. One probe used a cellulose filter, which allowed only the aqueous phase to pass through, and the second probe, containing a PTFE filter, selectively withdrew the nonaqueous phase. Both solutions were passed through flow cells and returned to the bulk mixture. Results obtained with 4-chloraniline between pH 7.0 buffer and 2,2,4-trimethylpentane at 35°C were indistinguishable from those obtained by the conventional shake flask procedure.

C. Chromatographic Techniques

When chromatography is applied to the determination of partition coefficients, it is frequently used solely as an analytical tool for measuring solute concentrations in equilibrium mixtures set up by standard methods. The remaining applications are based on the knowledge that most chromatographic procedures involve partitions between conjugate solutions, with consequent relationships between partition coefficients and chromatographic parameters. The best known of these relationships [34] is represented by

$$\log K_d = R_m + \text{constant} \tag{9.81}$$

and

$$R_m = \log\left(\frac{1}{R_f} - 1\right) \tag{9.82}$$

which define the parameter R_m and relates R_f value to partition coefficient (K_d).

If chromatography is used specifically for determining partition coefficients, the decision to employ the technique is usually motivated by difficulties encountered in applying traditional methods for the system under test. The difficulties are, in turn, usually due to the solute being considerably more soluble in one solvent than in the other. Although chromatography is not as sensitive to this problem as are traditional techniques, it is often difficult to adapt, particularly when very high or very low partition coefficients are involved. The relationship expressed in Eq. (9.81) does not apply when either the solute migrates too near the solvent front, or when it travels only a small way from the point or time of application. R_f values between about 0.15 and 0.75 are desirable, and procedures working within these restrictions have to be employed. A thin-layer chromatography (TLC) procedure described by Boyce and Milborrow [35] for measuring R_m values of a series of *N-n*-alkyltritylamines between paraffin and water is typical of the ingenuity and adaptability that are sometimes required. A silica gel layer was impregnated with liquid paraffin by allowing a 5% solution in hexane to run to the top of the plate, and then volatilizing off the hexane at 40°C. Solutions of solute in acetone-water mixtures were run and found to give satisfactory R_f values with solvent mixtures containing up to 50% v/v of water. Plots of R_m against proportion of acetone in the solvent were rectilinear and were extrapolated to zero acetone content to give estimated paraffin-water R_m values. The results were not compared with conventional partition coefficients, but they showed the anticipated rectilinear relationship to the numbers of carbon atoms in the alkyl chains and the binomial relationship with biological activities.

Reverse-phase paper chromatography, described by Bush [36], is another technique that can be adapted to the estimation of partition coefficients. In this, the paper is soaked in one of the solvents and the other is used as developing solvent. The method was examined by Bowen et al. [37] as a means of predicting the ethyl oleate-water partition coefficients of some androgen esters. Partition coefficients, estimated as the ratios of the solubilities in the two solvents, were found to be rectilinearly related to R_m values obtained with the solvent mixture, formic acid-methanol-light petroleum (10-100-90), in which the methanol rich phase was used to impregnate the paper and the petroleum-rich phase used as developing solvent. When R_f values less than 0.15 are obtained, more realistic migrations may be achieved by overrunning; the solvent is allowed to drip off the end of the paper, using the descending technique, until adequate movement is obtained, and the R_f value calculated by comparison with the distance traveled by a marker compound of known R_f. This refinement was used to estimate the R_m value of testosterone decanoate and give excellent correlation with biological observations [38].

The partition coefficient expressed in Eq. (9.81) obviously relates specifically to the solvent system operating in the chromatographic apparatus, and Boyce and Milborrow [35] adapted their process so that the solvent system they were interested in was used. Chromatographic methods of predicting partition coefficients usually invoke the Collander equation [Eq. (9.56)]. Thus if $K_{d(B)}$ in Eq. (9.56) represents the partition efficient operating in the chromatographic system and $K_{d(A)}$ is the partition coefficient in another solvent system, substitution for log K_d in Eq. (9.81) by log $K_{d(B)}$ from Eq. (9.56) yields

$$\log K_{d(A)} = aR_m + \text{constant} \tag{9.83}$$

The retention time (t_R) of a component passing through a GLC column is given by [39,40]

$$t_R = t_A(1 + qK_d) \tag{9.84}$$

where t_A is the elution time for the unabsorbed gas and q is the volume ratio of stationary and mobile phases. Rearrangement of Eq. (9.84) gives

$$\log K_d = \log \left(\frac{t_R}{t_A} - 1 \right) + \log \frac{1}{q} \tag{9.85}$$

which indicates that the first term on the right-hand side is analogous to the R_m value and can be substituted in Eq. (9.83) to give

$$\log K_{d(A)} = a \log \left(\frac{t_R}{t_A} - 1 \right) + \text{constant} \tag{9.86}$$

The intercept in Eq. (9.85) and t_A are difficult to evaluate directly but can be obtained indirectly by measuring the retention time of two compounds (1 and 2) having known partition coefficients, $K_{d(1)}$ and $K_{d(2)}$, and inserting the results in

$$q = \frac{t_{R(2)} - t_{R(1)}}{t_{R(1)}K_{d(2)} - t_{R(2)}K_{d(1)}} \tag{9.87}$$

and

$$t_A = \frac{t_{R(1)}K_{d(2)} - t_{R(2)}K_{d(1)}}{K_{d(2)} - K_{d(1)}} \tag{9.88}$$

The method is practicable for volatile solutes, which can be processed at reasonably low temperatures, but application to solutes that must be developed at high temperatures requires the assumption that the enthalpy of transfer is constant over the temperature range separating the operating temperature from the temperature for which the estimated partition coefficient is required. One must be particularly wary when the process is used to estimate a partition coefficient at a temperature at which the solute exists as a solid [41].

High-pressure liquid chromatography (HPLC) is a natural extension of these techniques. With HPLC, partition coefficient can be expressed in terms of the retention volume (V_R), and the term corresponding to R_m is log k', defined by

$$k' = \frac{V_R - V_0}{V_0} \qquad (9.89)$$

V_0 is the retention volume with no solute on the column. The method has the advantage that the same solutes can be used in the column as those to which the partition coefficient applies. Mirrless et al. [42] estimated 1-octanol-water partition coefficients by covering trimethylchlorosilane treated silica with a thin layer of octanol and developing with water saturated with octanol. Others [43,44] have used similar techniques.

Even HPLC sometimes lacks the flexibility to deal with a selection of solutes that cover a wide range of partition coefficients. Solutes that favor the stationary phase will have inconveniently long retention times, coupled with detection difficulties, and those with a low affinity for the stationary phase will pass through the column too quickly. Chromatographic methods are frequently looked to in quantitative structure-activity relationship (QSAR) investigations, which usually involve such wide-ranging collections of partition coefficients, and can be found not to provide too many advantages over traditional methods of measuring them. Mirrlees et al. [42] did, in fact, find that their method was limited to solutes having octanol-water partition coefficients between 0.5 and 5000.

Extra flexibility can be achieved by changing the solvent system. Konemann et al. [45] were able to adapt HPLC to the determination of high octanol-water partition coefficients by using 70% methanol in water as eluent instead of water alone. This gave measurable retention volumes for compounds having octanol-water partition coefficients in excess of 5000. Partition coefficients were calculated from retention volumes by using the empirically derived link equation,

$$\log K_d = (2.50 \pm 0.07) \log k' + (2.12 \pm 0.05) \qquad (9.90)$$

It is feasible that the technique could be extended to wider ranges of partition coefficients by using a less lipophilic stationary phase and two different solvent combinations as eluents. A low concentration of methanol in water would be used for the more hydrophilic substrates, and a high concentration of methanol in water for the more lipophilic substrates. The two sets of conditions could be

linked by submitting standard intermediate partition coefficient substrates to both regimes. However, care must be taken in the interpretation of the results, with respect to potential hydrogen bonding
and to ionizing solvents [44].

An interesting procedure was used by Huber et al. [40] to determine partition coefficients of steroids between two solvent systems
A and B. Sufficient solute was dissolved in solvent A to give a
suitable spectrophotometer reading (E_A^o), and a volume V_A of this
solution equilibrated with V_B of solvent B. A sample of phase A
was then removed and a spectrophotometer reading (E_A) taken. If
w_t is the weight of solute present in solvent A at zero time, and
w_A and w_B the weights in the respective phases at equilibrium, then

$$w_t = \frac{E_A^o V_A}{E^{1\%}} \qquad (9.91)$$

$$w_A = \frac{E_A V_A}{E^{1\%}} \qquad (9.92)$$

$$w_B = \frac{(E_A^o - E_A)V_A}{E^{1\%}} \qquad (9.93)$$

$E^{1\%}$ is the extinction coefficient. Since concentration (c) = weight
of solute/volume of solution,

$$K_d = \frac{c_A}{c_B} = \frac{(E_A^o - E_A)V_A}{E_A V_B} \qquad (9.94)$$

from which the partition coefficient can be calculated. Alternatively,
$(E_A^o - E_A)/E_A$ for a range of volume V_A and V_B can be plotted
against V_B/V_A. If the graph is rectilinear, the indication is that
the partition coefficient is not dependent on concentration, and is
given directly by the slope of the line.

Huber et al. [40] expressed partition coefficients in the form of

$$\log K_d = \sum_p^1 a_{i,p} x_{i,p} \qquad (9.95)$$

in which $a_{i,p}$ represents a range of constants characteristic of the
solute and $x_{i,p}$ represents similar values characteristic of the solvent

system. Constants were evaluated by computer, from experimental data, for two-term (p = 2) and three-term (p = 3) calculations. Thus for progesterone:

For p = 2: $a_{i,1} = 8.91$ $a_{i,2} = 9.01$

For p = 3: $a_{i,1} = 7.11$ $a_{i,2} = 5.22$ $a_{i,3} = 7.07$

while for the solvent system water:ethanol:2,2,4-trimethylpentane (2.5:31.7:65.8),

For p = 2: $x_{i,1} = 1.15$ $x_{i,2} = -0.98$

For p = 3: $x_{i,1} = 1.65$ $x_{i,2} = -0.424$ $x_{i,3} = -1.14$

Using these figures, we obtain

$$\log K_d = 8.91 \times 1.15 - 9.01 \times 0.98 = 1.42$$

and

$$\log K_d = 7.11 \times 1.65 - 5.22 \times 0.424 - 7.07 \times 1.14 = 1.46$$

REFERENCES

1. M. Davies and H. E. Hallam, The determination of molecular association equilibria from distribution and related measurements, *J. Chem. Educ.*, *33*, 322—327 (1956).
2. T. Higuchi and K. A. Connors, Phase solubility techniques, in *Advances in Analytical Chemistry and Instrumentation*, Vol. 4 (C. N. Reilley, ed.), Wiley-Interscience, New York, 1965, pp. 117—212.
3. A. Leo, C. Hansch, and D. Elkins, Partition coefficients and their uses, *Chem. Rev.*, *71*, 525—612 (1971).
4. S. D. Christian, H. E. Affsprung, and S. A. Taylor, The role of dissolved water in partition equilibria of carboxylic acids, *J. Phys. Chem.*, *67*, 187—189 (1963).
5. R. Collander, On lipid solubility, *Acta Physiol. Scand.*, *13*, 363—381 (1947).
6. R. Collander, The distribution of organic compounds between iso-butanol and water, *Acta Chem. Scand.*, *4*, 1085—1098 (1950).
7. A. Leo and C. Hansch, Linear free energy relationships between partitioning solvent systems, *J. Org. Chem.*, *36*, 1539—1544 (1971).

8. T. Higuchi, J. H. Richards, S. S. Davis, A. Kamada, J. P. Hou, M. Nakano, N. I. Nakano, and I. H. Pitman, Solvency and hydrogen bonding interactions in non-aqueous systems, *J. Pharm. Sci.*, *58*, 661—671 (1969).

9. C. Hansch, J. E. Quinlan, and G. L. Lawrence, The linear free energy relationship between partition coefficients and the aqueous solubility of organic liquids, *J. Org. Chem.*, *33*, 347—350 (1968).

10. S. C. Valvani, S. H Yalkowsky, and T. J. Roseman, Solubility and partitioning: IV. Aqueous solubility and octanol-water partition coefficients of non-electrolytes, *J. Pharm. Sci.*, *70*, 502—507 (1981).

11. J. Iwasa, T. Fujita, and C. Hansch, Substituent constants for aliphatic functions obtained from partition coefficients, *J. Med. Chem.*, *8*, 150—153 (1965).

12. K. C. James, Linear free energy relationships and biological action, in *Progress in Medicinal Chemistry*, Vol. 10 (G. P. Ellis and G. B. West, eds.), Elsevier, Amsterdam, 1973, pp. 205—243.

13. C. Hansch and A. Leo, *Substituent Constants for Correlation Analysis in Chemistry and Biology*, Wiley, New York, 1979.

14. T. Fujita, J. Iwasa, and C. Hansch, A new substituent constant π, derived from partition coefficients, *J. Am. Chem. Soc.*, *86*, 5175—5180 (1964).

15. G. G. Nys and R. F. Rekker, Statistical analysis of a series of partition coefficients with special reference to the predictability of folding of drug molecules. The introduction of hydrophobic fragmental constants (f values), *Chem. Ther.*, *5*, 521—535 (1973).

16. R. F. Rekker, *The Hydrophobic Fragmental Constant*, Elsevier, New York, 1977.

17. P. R. Wells, *Linear Free Energy Relationships*, Academic Press, London, 1968.

18. L. P. Hammett, *Physical Organic Chemistry*, McGraw-Hill, New York, 1940.

19. L. B. Kier, L. H. Hall, N. J. Murray, and M. Randic, Molecular connectivity: II. Relationship to non specific anesthesia, *J. Pharm. Sci.*, *64*, 1971—1974 (1975).

20. W. J. Murray, L. H. Hall, and L. B. Kier, Molecular connectivity: III. Relationship to partition coefficients, *J. Pharm. Sci.*, *64*, 1978—1981 (1975).

21. L. B. Kier and L. H. Hall, *Molecular Connectivity in Chemistry and Drug Research*, Academic Press, New York, 1976.

22. J. C. Boyd, J. S. Millership, and A. D. Woolfson, The relationship between molecular connectivity and partition coefficients, *J. Pharm. Pharmacol.*, *34*, 364—366 (1982).

23. J. C. McGowan, The physical toxicity of chemicals: IV. Solubilities, partition coefficients and physical toxicities, *J. Appl. Chem.*, *4*, 41–47 (1954).

24. J. C. McGowan, The physical toxicity of chemicals: II. Factors affecting physical toxicity in aqueous solutions, *J. Appl. Chem.*, *2*, 323–328 (1952).

25. J. C. McGowan, Molecular volumes and the periodic table, *Chem. Ind.*, 495–496 (1952).

26. J. C. McGowan, P. Ahmad, and A. Mellors, The estimation of partition coefficients of steroids between water and ether, *Can. J. Pharm. Sci.*, *14*, 72–74 (1979).

27. G. L. Flynn, Structural approach to partitioning: estimation of steroid partition coefficients based on molecular constitution, *J. Pharm. Sci.*, *60*, 345–353 (1971).

28. H. Reinhardt and J. Rydberg, A rapid and continuous system for measuring the distribution ratios in solvent extraction, *Chem. Ind.*, 488–491 (1970).

29. S. S. Davis and G. Elson, The determination of partition coefficients data using the AKUFVE method, *J. Pharm. Pharmacol.*, *26* (Suppl.), 90P (1974).

30. S. S. Davis, G. Elson, E. Tomlinson, G. Harrison, and J. C. Deardon, The rapid determination of partition coefficient data using a continuous solvent extraction system (AKUFVE), *Chem. Ind.*, 677–683 (1976).

31. J. F. M. Kinkel and E. Tomlinson, Drug liquid-liquid distribution based on the fundamentals of segmented flow, *Int. J. Pharm.*, *6*, 261–275 (1980).

32. J. F. M. Kinkel, E. Tomlinson, and P. Smit, Thermodynamics and extrathermodynamics of organic solute liquid-liquid distribution between water and 2,2,4-trimethylpentane, *Int. J. Pharm.*, *9*, 121–136 (1981).

33. E. Tomlinson, Filter-probe extractor: a tool for the rapid determination of oil-water partition coefficients, *J. Pharm. Sci.*, *71*, 602–604 (1982).

34. E. C. Bate-Smith and R. G. Westall, Chromatographic behaviour and chemical structure: I. Some naturally occurring phenolic substances, *Biochim. Biophys. Acta*, *4*, 427–440 (1950).

35. C. B. C. Boyce and B. V. Milborrow, A simple assessment of partition data for correlating structure and biological activity using thin layer chromatography, *Nature*, *208*, 537–539 (1965).

36. I. E. Bush, *The Chromatography of Steroids*, Pergamon, London, 1961.

37. D. B. Bowen, K. C. James, and M. Roberts, An investigation of the distribution coefficients of some androgen esters using paper chromatography, *J. Pharm. Pharmacol.*, *22*, 518–522 (1970).

38. K. C. James, R_m values and biological action of testosterone esters, *Experientia*, *28*, 479–480 (1972).
39. B. L. Karger and W. D. Cooke, Lightly loaded columns, in *Advances in Chromatography*, Vol. 1 (J. C. Giddings, and R. A. Keller, eds.), Marcel Dekker, New York, 1965, pp. 309–334.
40. J. F. K. Huber, C. A. M. Meijers, and J. A. R. J. Hulsman, New method for prediction of partition coefficients in liquid-liquid systems and its experimental verification for steroids by static and chromatographic methods, *Anal. Chem.*, *44*, 111–116 (1972).
41. K. C. James, G. T. Richards, and T. D. Turner, A comparison of chromatographic methods for the assessment of the distribution coefficients of androgen esters, *J. Chromatogr.*, *69*, 141–149 (1972).
42. M. S. Mirlees, S. J. Moulton, C. T. Murphy, and P. J. Taylor, Direct measurement of octanol-water partition coefficients by high pressure liquid chromatography, *J. Med. Chem.*, *19*, 615–619 (1976).
43. D. Henry, J. H. Block, J. L. Anderson, and G. R. Carlson, Use of high pressure liquid chromatography for quantitative structure-activity relationship studies of sulfonamides and barbiturates, *J. Med. Chem.*, *19*, 619–626 (1976).
44. S. H. Unger, J. R. Cook, and J. S. Hollenberg, Simple procedure for determining octanol-aqueous partition distribution and ionization coefficients by reverse-phase, high pressure liquid chromatography, *J. Pharm. Sci.*, *67*, 1364–1367 (1978).
45. H. Konemann, R. Zelle, F. Busser, and W. E. Hammers, Determination of log P_{oct} values of chloro-substituted benzenes, toulene and anilines by high performance liquid chromatography, *J. Chromatogr.*, *178*, 559–565 (1979).

10

Aqueous Solubilities

I. AQUEOUS SOLUBILITIES OF NONELECTROLYTES

A. Predictions Involving Carbon Number

It is generally recognized that water is a highly irregular solvent, so that the behavior of aqueous solutions does not comply with

regular solution theory. If, however, the solute is sufficiently inert, similarities to regular solution behavior can be observed. Paraffins are an example. The lower paraffins beginning with n-pentane,
are liquids at ambient temperatures, and so have ideal mole fraction
solubilities of unity. Regular solubilities are therefore dependent
solely on the activity coefficient (f), defined by

$$RT \ln f = V_2 \phi_1^2 \left[\frac{c_1}{V_1} - \left(\frac{2c_1 c_2}{V_1 V_2} \right)^{1/2} + \frac{c_2}{V_2} \right] \qquad (10.1)$$

The aqueous solubilities of paraffins are low, so ϕ_1, the volume
fraction of solvent, can be approximated to 1. V represents molar
volume and c the cohesive energy density (see Section II.D in Chapter 5), so that since the solvent is always the same (water), c_1 and
V_1 will be independent of the nature of the solute. Homologous
series are ascended by progressively adding methylene groups, and
with the normal paraffins, the process does not markedly change
the molecular geometry. It is therefore reasonable to assume that
with this series, c_2 and V_2 change in a similar manner as the series
is ascended, and that c_2/V_2 remains constant, as will the geometric
mean term in Eq. (10.1). It follows that at constant temperature,
ln f should be a rectilinear function of the molar volume of the solute,
and therefore also of carbon number.

There is support for this suggestion in the literature. McAuliffe
[1] determined the aqueous solubilities of a range of hydrocarbons.
His results for the n-paraffins gave a perfect rectilinear plot of ln
molar solubility against carbon number, and similar plots can be obtained with his results for normal olefins and acetylenes. The three
series yield a family of parallel straight lines, as shown in Fig. 10.1.
The regression equations are:

Paraffins

$$-\ln \text{ molar solubility} = -\ln M_s = 1.49n + 0.09 \qquad (10.2)$$

Olefins

$$-\ln M_s = 1.51n - 1.50 \qquad (10.3)$$

Acetylenes

$$-\ln M_s = 1.50n - 3.62 \qquad (10.4)$$

indicating that the contribution of the methylene group is constant
and independent of the basic structure of the series, adding an increment of $1.5 \times 8.315 \times 298 = 3.7$ kJ per methylene group to the

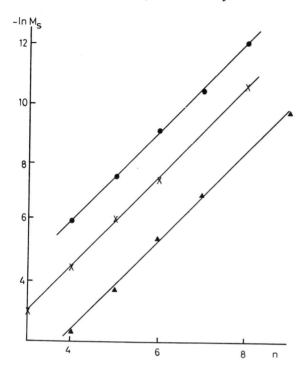

FIGURE 10.1 Solubilities of normal aliphatic hydrocarbons in water.
--•--, Paraffins; --×--, olefins; --▲--, acetylenes.

molar free energy of solution at 25°C. Davis et al. [2] calculated excess molar free energies of solution in water for 34 homologous series,
most of which involved atoms additional to carbon and hydrogen, and
found remarkably good agreement, with a mean free energy of solution of 3.55 ± 0.17 kJ mol^{-1}. An increment of 3.8 kJ has since been
suggested for substituted benzoic and phenoxyacetic acids [3], but
lower values, 1.80 and 2.18 kJ, have been proposed for steroid esters and long-chain fatty acids, respectively [4]. Yalkowsky et al.
[5] obtained solubilities for alkyl-p-aminobenzoates which yielded a
molar free-energy increment of 5.40 kJ mol^{-1} [4]. It thus appears
that while a free energy of 3.55 kJ can be used to calculate aqueous
solubilities of fairly simple molecules, it must be used with caution,
particularly with more complex systems.

The intercepts of Eqs. (10.2) to (10.4) indicate the contributions
of the skeleton structures of the series and suggest that a double
bond reduces molar free energy by 3.49 kJ, and a triple bond by
9.19 kJ, in line with the known fact that unsaturation contributes

to aqueous solubility. Consideration of all the paraffins examined
by McAuliffe [1], involving straight and branched-chain compounds,
gives a less satisfactory relationship, suggesting that molecular configuration plays an important role in determining the aqueous solubilities of these compounds. McAuliffe obtained a reasonable rectilinear plot of log solubility in grams per 10^6 g of water. The choice
of units of concentration was unfortunate, since the units do not take
molecular weight into consideration, so that some of the variation in
solubility must be due to changes in molecular weight, which in turn
are related to molar volume. Part of the proposed relationship between solubility and molar volume is therefore inevitable. Regression
using molar solubilities, gives a poor correlation with molar volume,
as shown in Fig. 10.2. This is because there is a general decrease

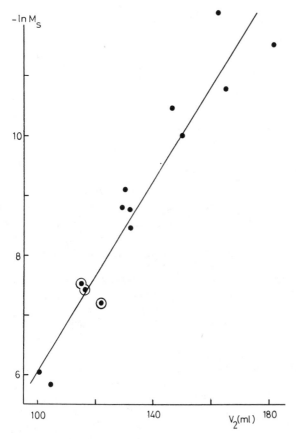

FIGURE 10.2 Solubilities of normal and branched paraffins in water.

in solubility with increasing carbon number, and hence with increasing molar volume, while for a given carbon number, increased molar volume due to increased branching results in an increase in solubility. Molar volume therefore affects solubility in two opposing ways, and the relationship must be considered as an artifact brought about by a loose association between carbon number and molar volume. The criticism can be appreciated if the solubilities of the three pentanes, indicated by the circled points in Fig. 10.2, are considered. The solubilities increase with increased branching, in the order n-pentane, isopentane, and 2,2-dimethylpropane, and the molar volumes increase in the same rank order. However, the overall plot exhibits a decrease in solubility with increasing molecular weight, and hence increasing molar volume.

The situation can be improved by separating the effects of branching and carbon number. Thus the equation

$$-\ln M_s = 1.49n - 0.321m + 0.787 \qquad \begin{array}{ccc} n & r & s \\ 14 & 0.998 & 0.128 \end{array} \quad (10.5)$$

where n represents the total number of carbon atoms and m the number of methyl groups, predicts the results more accurately than the equation

$$-\ln M_s = 7.85 \times 10^{-2} V_2 - 1.74 \qquad \begin{array}{ccc} n & r & s \\ 14 & 0.957 & 0.562 \end{array} \quad (10.6)$$

which expresses the relationship shown in Fig. 10.2. The goodness of fit of Eq. (10.5) is shown in Fig. 10.3.

B. Predictions Involving Molar Volume and Parachor

McGowan [6] considered the solubilities of gases and vapors in terms of the creation of a hole in the solvent and the accommodation of the solute therein. He proposed that only two energy changes need be considered: U_C for formation of cavities to accommodate gas molecules, and U_A for the transfer of gas molecules into these cavities. He suggested that since both these terms are proportional to molar volume, they could be represented by the parachor [P], molar volume which has been corrected for forces of intermolecular attraction by multiplying by the fourth root of surface tension. Parachors can be predicted from the contributions of the atoms forming the molecule. McGowan's procedure [7,8] has been described in Chapter 9. Sugden [9] allocated parachor equivalents for this purpose; they were additive, and unlike McGowan's method, some allowance was made

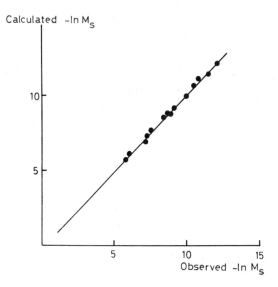

FIGURE 10.3 Observed and predicted solubilities of normal and branched paraffins in water. Predicted results calculated from Eq. (10.5).

for the ways in which the atoms were combined. Vogel et al. [10] assigned parachor equivalents to bonds rather than to atoms. The measured and calculated parachors of a selection of compounds are compared in Table 10.1. It is recommended that McGowan's constants be used with his solubility calculations, which will be described later.

McGowan [11] correlated parachor with the toxic concentrations (C_t) of a range of hydrocarbons and halogenated hydrocarbons in living organisms, and found that the results followed

$$-\log\ C_t = 0.012[P] + \text{constant} \tag{10.7}$$

The constant varied with the biological indicator and was considered to be dependent on the concentration of the solute in the biophase (C_{bio}), corresponding to the concentration (C_t) in the external phase in equilibrium with the biophase. The equation was therefore rewritten in the form

$$-\log\ C_t = -\log\ C_{bio} + 0.012[P] \tag{10.8}$$

which applies generally to all systems in which two immiscible solutions are in equilibrium, and in the limiting case of a saturated solution in equilibrium with the pure liquid solute, Eq. (10.8) can be extended to [12].

$$-\log C_s = -\log C_L + k[P] \qquad (10.9)$$

where C_s is the aqueous solubility and C_L the concentration of solute in the pure liquid.

Equation (10.9) was tested [12] by correlating the aqueous solubilities of 15 liquids with parachor, and yielded a proportionality constant of 0.0134 when C_s and C_L were expressed in moles per kilogram. Solubilities predicted by antilog(0.0134[P] − log C_L) were in good agreement with observed values. This relationship was based on parachors calculated by subtracting 19 cm^3 for each bond; the amended correction of 18.6 cm^3, together with modified atomic values, were introduced in a later paper [8]. Results obtained using the amended procedure are reproduced in Table 10.2, which shows that McGowan's treatment can be extended to solutes other than

TABLE 10.1 Measured and Calculated Parachors

Compound	Measured parachor	Calculated parachor		
		Sugden	McGowan	Vogel
Acetamide	148	151	143	144
Acetone	162	160	155	158
Acetonitrile	122	120	115	120
Benzene	206	207	203	206
Chloroform	183	185	175	190
Diethyl ether	211	210	192	212
Ethyl acetate	217	216	212	216
n-Hexane	272	268	271	271
Nitrobenzene	264	265	253	264
n-Propylamine	179	188	185	191
n-Propyl chloride	190	188	185	191

TABLE 10.2 Estimation of the Aqueous Solubilities of a
Selection of Liquids from Their Parachors

Liquid	$-\log_{10}$ solubility (mol dm^{-3})	
	Measured	Calculated
Benzene	1.64	1.62
Bromobenzene	2.58	2.60
Chlorobenzene	2.36	2.24
Ethylbenzene	2.71	2.82
Fluorobenzene	1.80	1.77
Iodobenzene	3.06	3.01
Bromoform	1.92	2.35
Carbon tetrachloride	2.30	2.00
Chloroform	1.21	1.34
Ethyl bromide	1.08	1.05
n-Pentane	2.30	2.15
Toluene	2.17	2.32
m-Xylene	2.73	2.92
p-Xylene	2.73	2.92

Source: McGowan's parachors Refs. 11 and 12, were
used for these calculations.

hydrocarbons. The geometry of the molecules is such that one
would not anticipate the chain-branching problems associated with
McAuliffe's work [1]. Furthermore, the substituent groups are not
normally involved in significant solute-solute or solute-water interactions. McGowan recognized this and extended his technique to
oxygenated solutes by examining 40 alcohols, aldehydes, esters, and
ketones. A rectilinear relationship with slope 0.0134 between log
solubility and parachor was again obtained, but with an intercept
of -1.75.

Example

Estimate the solubility of benzene in water at ambient temperature,
using the parachor. The molecular weight of benzene is 78.

Solution:

Using McGowan's constants from Table 9.20, we obtain

$$[P] = (6 \times 46.35) + (6 \times 24.7) - (12 \times 18.6) = 203.1$$

$$1 \text{ kg of benzene} = \frac{1000}{78} = 12.8 \text{ mol of benzene}$$

Therefore,

$$-\log \text{ solubility} = -\log 12.8 + 0.0134 \times 203.1$$
$$= -1.615$$
$$\text{solubility} = \text{antilog} - 1.615 = 0.024 \text{ mol kg}^{-1}$$

Since the solution is dilute, this is equivalent to 0.024 mol dm^{-3}, which compares favorably with the experimental value of 0.018 mol dm^{-3}.

C. Predictions Involving Cavity Surface Area

It has been shown in Chapter 5 that the enthalpy of mixing expression of the regular solubility equation can be modified by replacing cohesive energy density with surface energy and volume fraction with surface area. The process of solution is then considered in terms of the changes in interfacial tension in creating a cavity in the solvent, withdrawing a molecule from the bulk solute and inserting that solute molecule into the cavity in the solvent.
Butler et al. [13,14] considered the free energy of hydration (ΔG_{hyd}) in terms of the work done in carrying out these three operations, as expressed by

$$\Delta G_{hyd} = \gamma_{w-w} - \gamma_{A-w} \tag{10.10}$$

where γ_{w-w} represents the work done in separating the water molecules to form a cavity, and γ_{A-w} the work required to separate a solute molecule (A) from a water molecule (W). Since the treatment involved only liquid solutes, γ_{A-A}, the work required to separate a solute molecule from the bulk solute was considered to be small and was ignored. They calculated the free energies of hydration of various liquids from

$$\Delta G_{hyd} = -RT \ln \frac{\bar{p}_2}{X_2} \tag{10.11}$$

and evaluated the interaction constants shown in Table 10.3. $\bar{p}_2$ represents the partial pressure of the solute and X_2 its mole fraction concentration in the solution.

A simple arrangement of solute and solvent molecules was assumed, namely that in an aqueous solution a methyl group and a hydroxyl group were each surrounded by three water molecules and a methylene group by two. Thus for 1-butanol (XXIX), in which the circles represent the positions of water molecules

$$OCH_3CH_2CH_2CH_2OH \qquad XXIX$$

$$\text{Total interaction} = \frac{12}{2}\gamma_{W-W} - 9\gamma_{C-W} - 3\gamma_{OH-W} \qquad (10.12)$$

The experimental values of ΔG_{hyd} had been obtained using units, such as millimeters of mercury for $\bar{p}_2$, which necessitated a correction to Eq. (10.12), giving

$$\text{Total interaction} = \frac{12}{2}\gamma_{W-W} - 9\gamma_{C-W} - 3\gamma_{OH-W} + 36,000 \qquad (10.13)$$

The result can be equated to $RT \ln(\bar{p}_2/X_2)$, from which by substitution of the partial pressure of the solute, mole fraction concentration can be calculated. When the solubility is low, the saturated vapor pressure of the solute can be substituted for $\bar{p}_2$, to give the mole fraction solubility. Thus for 1-butanol,

$$\text{Total interaction} = 6 \times 25,100 - 9 \times 12,100 - 3 \times 20,900 \qquad (10.14)$$
$$+ 36,000 = 15,000 \text{ J mol}^{-1}$$

Therefore, $\qquad \dfrac{\bar{p}_2}{X_2} = \exp\left(\dfrac{15,000}{8.315 \times 298}\right) = 426$

TABLE 10.3 Interaction Constants (kJ mol^{-1})

Interaction	γ	Interaction	γ	Interaction	γ
W-W	25.1	C-W	12.1	OH-W	20.9
O(ether)-W	19.7	O(ketone)-W	18.8	NH$_2$-W	20.5

Source: Abstracted from Ref. 14, and converted to S. I. units.

The experimental saturated vapor pressure of 1-butanol at 298 K is 6.78 mmHg [12].

$$X_2 = \frac{6.78}{426} = 0.0159$$

This is approximately equal to a molarity of

$$\frac{0.0159 \times 1000}{18} = 0.88 \text{ mol dm}^{-3}$$

The experimental value is 1.01 mol dm^{-3} [15].

The procedure therefore appears to give reliable results, but it is limited to sparingly soluble, volatile liquids. It is presumably also applicable to solids with finite vapor pressures, such as menthol and camphor, but would require a knowledge of enthalpy of fusion in order to calculate and correct for the ideal solubility.

Herman [16] used a more precise assessment of the number of interacting water molecules. His parameter was the cavity surface area, a surface running parallel to the profile of the solute molecule and lying a distance r_W outside. The water molecules were assumed to be spheres of radius r_W, so that the cavity surface area was proportional to the number of water molecules that could be packed around each solute molecule. The three-dimensional profile of the solute molecule was mapped out by locating the center of each atom at fixed coordinates, x, y, and z, and constructing a spherical surface corresponding to the radius of that atom. The procedure is shown in two dimensions in Fig. 10.4. It was considered that the free energy per solute molecule of a saturated solution of hydrocarbon would be logarithmically related to solubility (C_S), in accordance with the van't Hoff isotherm, so that a plot of cavity surface area against log C_S should be rectilinear. Two good rectilinear plots were in fact obtained, one for aromatics and the other for alkanes and cycloalkanes. The difference was attributed to the aromatic ring being more soluble in water than an aliphatic system of similar size.

Amidon et al. [15] used Herman's procedure [16] to calculate the cavity surface areas (CSA) of 73 aliphatic and alicyclic alcohols and saturated hydrocarbons and attempted to relate them to the logarithms of their aqueous solubilities. The correlations were poor, even when the cavity surface areas were split up into hydroxyl surface area (OHSA) and hydrocarbon surface area (HYSA). However, introduction of the term IOH, equal to unity for alcohols and zero for hydrocarbons, yielded

$$\begin{array}{cccc} & \text{n} & \text{r} & \text{s} \\ \ln C_S = -0.043 OHYSA + 8.003 IOH & 73 & 0.992 & 0.452 \\ \quad\; -\; 0.0586 OHSA + 4.420 & & & (10.15) \end{array}$$

which explained 98.4% of the variation in solubility. The theoretical
intercept is dependent on the units of concentration. Molal concentrations were used in deriving Eq. (10.15) which gives an intercept of 4.0, in good agreement with the observed value of 4.420.
The 73 compounds included three solid alkanols, whose observed
solubilities, as expected, deviated significantly from Eq. (10.15).
On correcting for the enthalpy required for liquefaction, surprisingly,
the solubilities of the supercooled liquids deviated even more from the
equation. The method has been extended to other aliphatic monofunctional compounds [17] using the general form of Eq. (10.15),
expressed by

$$\ln C_S = HYSA \theta_1 + FGSA \theta_2 + IFG \theta_3 + \theta_4 \qquad (10.16)$$

FGSA is the functional group surface area and is equal to CSA –
HYSA. IFG, the functional group index, is analogous to IOH and
is equal to zero for hydrocarbons and unity for compounds contain-
ing a functional group. θ_1, θ_2, θ_3, and θ_4 are the coefficients of
the equation. Alcohols, ethers, aldehydes, and ketones, esters,

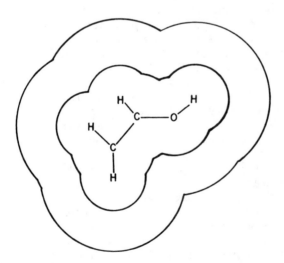

FIGURE 10.4 Cavity surface of ethanol. The inner line represents
the surface of ethanol, and the outer line represents the surface
formed by a 1.5-Å-thick layer of solvent molecules. (From Ref. 15.)

TABLE 10.4 Calculation of Methylene Group Contribution to Cavity Surface Area

$$CH_2SA = CSA_1 - CSA_2$$

Compounds		Cavity surface area ($nm^2 \times 10^2$)		
1	2	1	2	CH_2SA
n-Propane	Ethane	223.4	191.5	31.9
n-Butane	n-Propane	255.2	223.4	31.8
n-Pentane	n-Butane	287.0	255.2	31.8
n-Hexane	n-Pentane	318.0	287.0	32.0
n-Heptane	n-Hexane	351.0	319.0	32.0
n-Octane	n-Heptane	383.0	351.0	32.0
1-Pentanol	1-Butanol	303.9	272.1	31.8
1-Hexanol	1-Pentanol	335.7	303.9	31.8
1-Heptanol	1-Hexanol	367.5	335.7	31.8
1-Octanol	1-Heptanol	399.4	367.5	31.9
1-Nonanol	1-Octanol	431.2	399.4	31.8
1-Decanol	1-Nonanol	463.0	431.2	31.8
(P' = 0.01)				Mean = 31.9 ± 0.1

Source: Raw data abstracted from Refs. 15 and 16.

and carboxylic acids each gave good correlations within their particular groups, but olefins alone and hydrocarbons in general were not so good.

In an attempt to improve the technique, Valvani and Yalkowsky [18] have investigated other methods for calculating cavity surface areas, but all appear to be just as complicated as determining the solubility experimentally. An alternative possibility for calculating cavity surface areas is to sum contributions for substituent groups, in a similar approach to fragmental analysis (see Section IV.B in Chapter 9). Thus the contribution of a methylene group (CH_2SA) in an alkyl chain can be calculated as the difference between the cavity surface areas of n-propane and n-ethane. This and similar calculations are listed in Table 10.4 and show that in n-alkanes and 1-alkanols, the contribution per methylene group to surface area is constant and equal to 0.319 ± 0.001 nm^2 (or 31.9 A^2). The contribution of the methyl group can be calculated from this figure, using expressions of the form

$$CH_3SA = \frac{n\text{-butane CSA} - 2 \times 0.319)}{2} \qquad (10.17)$$

Similar calculations, using the C_3 to C_8 n-alkanes, gave a mean value of 0.957 ± 0.001 nm^2. The two results are in the ratio CH_3/CH_2 = 3:1, in contrast to Butler's ratio of 3:2 [14]. A selection of cavity surface group contributions, calculated in this way, is given in Table 10.5

Example

Using the contributions cited in Table 10.5, calculate the cavity surface area of 5-nonanol.

Solution:

Cavity surface area contributions for 1-nonanol are as follows:

$$CH_3 - (CH_2)_8 - OH$$

$$0.957 + 8 \times 0.319 + 0.802 = 4.311 \text{ nm}^2$$

TABLE 10.5 Substituent Constants for Cavity Surface Areas

	Contribution (nm$^2 \times 10^2$)
CH_3 in alkyl chain	95.7 ± 0.1
CH_2 in alkyl chain	31.9 ± 0.1
Primary OH attached to alkyl chain	80.2 ± 0.2
Primary OH to secondary OH	
1-OH in alkyl chain	
To 2-OH	-81.0 ± 6.0
To other positions	-104.0 ± 0.0
n-Alkyl to methyl branching	12.6 ± 0.2

$(P' = 0.01)$

Source: Raw data abstracted from Refs. 15 and 16.

The factor for conversion from 1-primary alcohol to 5-secondary alcohol is -0.104 nm^2.

$$\text{CSA for 5-nonanol} = 4.311 - 0.104 = 4.207 \text{ nm}^2$$

Previously calculated value [15] $= 4.208$ nm^2.

D. Predictions Involving Partitioning

Relationships between aqueous solubilities of liquids and their octanol-water partition coefficients were discussed briefly in Chapter 9. The rationale for relating aqueous solubility with octanol-water partition coefficient [19] has been based on the cavity concept, described above. Thus the activity coefficient ($f_{x(o)}$) of a solute dissolved in octanol can be described by

$$RT \ln f_{x(o)} = DD + OO - 2DO \qquad (10.18)$$

in which DD, OO, and DO represent solute-solute, solvent-solvent, and solute-solvent interactions, respectively. Partition coefficients (K_d) of liquid solutes can be expressed in the form

$$K_d = \frac{f_{x(w)}}{f_{x(o)}} \qquad (10.19)$$

in which $f_{x(w)}$ and $f_{x(o)}$ are the rational activity coefficients of the solute in water and octanol, respectively, Substitution for $f_{x(o)}$ from Eq. (10.19) in Eq. (10.18) gives

$$RT \ln f_{x(w)} = \ln K_d + DD + OO - 2DO \qquad (10.20)$$

Yalkowsky and Valvani [19] considered that octanol is a desirable solvent for such studies, because it is in the solubility parameter range of most organic compounds, so that its polarity will not be very different from those of most organic liquids. They therefore suggested that for such solutes, a cohesive energy similar to that of octanol would apply. The adhesive interaction between solute and solvent were considered to be equal to the average of the interactions between solute and solute and between solvent and solvent:

$$DD + OO \cong 2DO \qquad (10.21)$$

so that all the terms on the right-hand side of Eq. (10.20), except $\ln K_d$, disappear, to give

$$\ln f_{x(w)} \cong \ln K_d \qquad\qquad (10.22)$$

This concept is reminiscent of regular solution theory, in which co-hesive energy density between solute and solvent is equated to the geometric mean of the cohesive energy densities between like mole-cules. The theory was tested by correlating the octanol-water par-tition coefficients of 417 organic liquids with aqueous solubilities $(X_{s(w)})$ to obtain

$$
\begin{array}{cccc}
 & & n & r & s \\
-\log f_{x(w)} = \log X_{s(w)} & & 417 & 0.946 & 0.356 \\
 = -1.08 \log K_d - 1.04 & & & & (10.23)
\end{array}
$$

Logarithms to the base 10 are used to come into line with the original publication. The intercept of -1.04 arises because Eq. (10.22) uses mole fraction concentrations, whereas the partition coefficients used to develop Eq. (10.23) used molar concentrations. It is equiv-alent to the logarithm of the ratio of the molarities of pure octanol and pure water and has a theoretical value of -0.94.

The relationship was tested more rigorously [20] by examining 111 liquids for which reliable experimental partition coefficients were available. Much of the data used to compile Eq. (10.23) was obtained by calculation. The equation

$$
\begin{array}{cccc}
 & n & r & s \\
-\log M_{s(w)} = -1.016 \log K_d & 111 & 0.931 & 0.421 \\
 + 0.515 & & & (10.24)
\end{array}
$$

was obtained, whose slope is similar to that of Eq. (10.23), but whose intercept is different, because the units of the aqueous solu-bilities were molar, in contrast to mole fraction in Eq. (10.23). Such was the enthusiasm of the authors for this equation that they recommended it as a means of verifying the accuracy of experimental aqueous solubilities.

Equation (4.16) was developed in Chapter 4 as a method for predicting the ideal solubilities of rigid, nonspherical solids. The precise value of the slope in Eq. (4.16) is 1.84×10^{-2}, so that conversion to logarithms to the base 10 leads to

$$\log X_2^i = 0.01(mp - 25) \qquad\qquad (10.25)$$

where X_2^i is the ideal mole fraction solubility of the solute and mp the melting point in degrees Celsius. The theoretical form of Eq. (10.23) is

$$\log X_{s(w)} = -\log K_d - 0.94 \tag{10.26}$$

and can be combined with Eq. (10.25) to give

$$\log X_{s(w)} = -\log K_d - 0.01(mp - 25) - 0.94$$

$$= -\log K_d - 0.01\ mp - 0.69 \tag{10.27}$$

The intercept 0.94 has been explained above. Alternative versions are

$$\log X_{s(w)} = -\log K_d - \frac{\Delta H^f(mp - 25)}{1364\ T_m} - 0.94 \tag{10.28}$$

$$\log X_{s(w)} = -\log K_d - \frac{\Delta S^f(mp - 25)}{1364} - 0.94 \tag{10.29}$$

Equations (10.27) and (10.29) applied to molar concentrations are

$$\log M_{s(w)} = -\log K_d - 0.01\ mp + 1.05 \tag{10.30}$$

$$\log M_{s(w)} = -\log K_d - \frac{\Delta S^f(mp - 25)}{1364} + 0.80 \tag{10.31}$$

Equations (10.30) and (10.31) are based on the fact that for dilute solutions, molar concentration is equal to mole fraction concentration multiplied by the molarity of pure water (55.5), so that

$$\log M = \log X + 1.74 \tag{10.32}$$

ΔH^f and ΔS^f are enthalpy and entropy of fusion of the solute, respectively, expressed in calories, and T_m the melting point in kelvin. Yalkowsky and Valvani [19] have tested these equations, using a universal melting point of 25°C for the liquids, and claimed good predictions with alkanols, halobenzenes, aromatic hydrocarbons, and steroids [19]. The following is a modification of Eq. (10.31), derived experimentally and found to fit the observed results more closely than Eq. (10.31).

$$\log M_{s(w)} = -\log K_d - 1.11 \frac{\Delta S^f(mp - 25)}{1364} + 0.54 \qquad (10.33)$$

Example

Use the information provided below to predict the molar aqueous solubilities of (a) 1-butanol, (b) naphthalene, and (c) 1-hexadecanol.

	m.p. (C)	ΔS^f (eu)	$\log K_d$
1-Butanol	Liquid	Liquid	0.84
Naphthalene	80	12.7	3.35
1-Hexadecanol	49	43.5	7.17

Solution:

(a) 1-Butanol

[Eq. (10.30)] $\log M_{s(w)} = -0.84 + 1.05 = 0.21$

[Eq. (10.31)] $\log M_{s(w)} = -0.84 + 0 + 0.80 = -0.04$

[Eq. (10.33)] $\log M_{s(w)} = -0.84 + 0.54 = -0.30$

Observed $\log M_{s(w)} = -0.01$.

(b) Naphthalene

[Eq. (10.30)] $\log M_{s(w)} = -3.35 - 0.01 \times 80 + 1.05 = -3.10$

[Eq. (10.31)] $\log M_{s(w)} = -3.35 - 12.7(80 - 25)/1364 + 0.80$

$$= -3.06$$

or since $\Delta S^f = 13.5$ eu (56.5 J deg^{-1}) for rigid, nonspherical molecules (page 138),

[Eq. (10.31)] $\log M_{s(w)} = -3.35 - \dfrac{13.5(80 - 25)}{1364} + 0.80 = -3.09$

[Eq. (10.33)] $\log M_{s(w)} = -3.35 - 1.11 \times \dfrac{13.5(80 - 25)}{1364} + 0.54$

$$= -3.41$$

Observed $\log M_{s(w)} = -3.61$.

(c) 1-Hexadecanol

[Eq. (10.30)] $\log M_{s(w)} = -7,17 - 0.01 \times 49 + 1.05 = -6.61$

[Eq. (10.31)] $\log M_{s(w)} = -7.17 - \dfrac{43.5(49 - 25)}{1364} + 0.80 = -7.14$

or since hexadecanol is a chain of more than five atoms (i.e., n = 17), entropy of fusion can be estimated from 2.5(n − 5) (page 138); hence

[Eq. (10.31)] $\log M_{s(w)} = -7.17 - \dfrac{2.5(17 - 5)(49 - 25)}{1364} + 0.82$

$$= -7.68$$

[Eq. (10.33)] $\log M_{s(w)} = -7.17 - 1.11 \times 12 \times \dfrac{24}{1364} + 0.54$

$$= -6.86$$

Observed $\log M_{s(w)} = -7.00$.

E. Predictions Involving Solubility Parameters

Equation (5.45) is used to calculate regular solubilities of solids in liquids. As pointed out in Chapter 5, the equation is successful only with low-polarity solutes and solvents, and fails badly with aqueous solubilities. Amidon and Williams [21] assumed that 1-octanol behaved as a regular solvent. Substitution of the known solubility parameter of 10.3 H for octanol, and approximating ϕ_1^2 to unity, gives

$$\log X = \frac{-\Delta S^f}{2.303 \times 1.987 \times 298}(T_m - 298) - \frac{V_2(10.3 - \delta_2)^2}{2.303 \times 1.987 \times 298}$$

$$= -7.3 \times 10^{-4}(T_m - 298)\,\Delta S^f - V_2(10.3 - \delta_2)^2 \qquad (10.34)$$

for solubilities at 25°C. R and ΔS^f are expressed in calories, because the units of the solubility parameter are $cal^{1/2}\ cm^{-3/2}$.

Practical partition coefficients (K_d) and rational partition coefficients (K_d') are related by

$$\log K_d' = \log K_d + 0.94 \qquad (10.35)$$

in which the factor 0.94 represents the logarithm to the base 10 of the molarity of pure octanol divided by the molarity of pure water. Then

$$\log X_{s(w)} = \log X_{s(o)} - \log K_d'$$

$$= \log X_{s(o)} - \log K_d - 0.94 \qquad (10.36)$$

and substitution of $\log X_{s(o)}$ from Eq. (10.34) gives

$$\log X_{s(w)} = -0.94 - 7.3 \times 10^{-4} [T_m - 298) \Delta S^f +$$

$$(10.3 - \delta_2)^2 V_2] - \log K_d \qquad (10.37)$$

providing a method for calculating aqueous solubilities. The equivalent equation for molar solubility is

$$\log M_{s(w)} = 0.80 - 7.3 \times 10^{-4} [(T_m - 298) \Delta S^f +$$

$$(10.3 - \delta_2)^2 V_2] - \log K_d \qquad (10.38)$$

Example

Using the data given below, calculate the molar solubilities of (a) carbon tetrachloride and (b) naphthalene in water at 25°C.

	$\log K_d$	V_2 (cm^3)	δ_2 (H)	ΔS^f (eu)	m.p. (°C)
Carbon tetra-chloride	2.83	97.1	8.6	Liquid	Liquid
Naphthalene	3.30	126	10.2	12.7	80

Solution:

(a) Carbon tetrachloride

$$\log M_{s(w)} = 0.80 - 7.3 \times 10^{-4}(10.3 - 8.6)^2 \times 97.1 - 2.83$$

$$= -2.23$$

$$M_{s(w)} = \text{antilog} - 2.23 = 5.8 \times 10^{-3} \text{ mol dm}^{-3}$$

Observed solubility $= 6.0 \times 10^{-3}$ mol dm^{-3}.

(b) Naphthalene

$$\log M_{s(w)} = 0.80 - 7.3 \times 10^{-4}[(353 - 298) \times 12.7 +$$

$$(10.3 - 10.2)^2 \times 126] - 3.30 = -3.01$$

$$M_{s(w)} = \text{antilog} - 3.01 = 9.8 \times 10^{-4} \text{ mol dm}^{-3}$$

Observed solubility $= 2.5 \times 10^{-4}$ mol dm^{-3}.

In the absence of experimental data, the entropy term can be substituted by the ideal solubility, estimated from Eq. (10.25), and δ_2 and V_2 can be predicted using the methods described in Chapter 5.

II. EFFECT OF ADDITIVES ON AQUEOUS SOLUBILITIES OF NONELECTROLYTES

A. Electrolytes

In most situations, addition of electrolyte to water decreases the quantity of nonelectrolyte that can be dissolved. Put in another way, if an electrolyte is dissolved in a saturated solution of a non-electrolyte, the usual consequence is that some of the nonelectrolyte will be precipitated. The process, termed *salting-out*, is not universal sometimes salting-in occurs, and solubility increases with increasing electrolyte concentration. Both effects are described mathematically by the empirically derived Setschenow equation,

$$\log \frac{M_s^o}{M_s} = K_s M_{salt} \tag{10.39}$$

where M_s^o is the solubility of the nonelectrolyte in pure water and M_s the solubility in the electrolyte solution of electrolyte concentration M_{salt}. Molar concentrations are shown here, but the equation applies equally well to other units of concentration. K_s is the Setschenow or salting-out constant.

The equation can be justified theoretically for dilute solutions. Since M_s^o and M_s represent saturated solutions, they are, by definition, in equilibrium with the pure nonelectrolyte, and therefore in equilibrium with each other. They therefore have the same activity, so

$$f_m^o M_s^o = f_m M_s \tag{10.40}$$

where f_m^o and f_m are the activity coefficients of the nonelectrolyte in water and in nonelectrolyte solution, respectively. Rearrangement and conversion to logs gives

$$\log f_m = \log f_m^o + \log \frac{M_s^o}{M_s} \tag{10.41}$$

where $f_m^o M_s^o$ is a constant, independent of electrolyte concentration, so that Eq. (10.41) indicates that a rise in the activity coefficient of the electrolyte solution results in a fall in the solubility of the nonelectrolyte. Activity coefficients are dependent on the total concentrations of the various species in solution and can be represented by a power series involving all the solutes. For example,

$$\log f_m = \sum_{m,n=0}^{\infty} (k_m M_s^m + k_n M_{salt}^n) \tag{10.42}$$

applies to a system containing one nonelectrolyte and one electrolyte. The first term of the series is the most important, so that higher terms can be ignored to give

$$\log f_m = k_{s_1} M_s + k_{salt_1} M_{salt} \tag{10.43}$$

where k_m and k_n represent the power series coefficients for nonelectrolyte and electrolyte, respectively, and k_{s_1} and k_{salt_1} the specific coefficients for the linear term of the series. Combining Eqs. (10.41) and (10.43) yields

$$\log f_m = \log f_m^o + \log \frac{M_s^o}{M_s} = k_{s_1} M_s + k_{salt_1} M_{salt} \tag{10.44}$$

which since $\log f_m^o = k_{s_1} M_s$, leads to

$$\log \frac{f_m}{f_m^o} = \log \frac{M_s^o}{M_s} = k_{salt_1} M_{salt} + k_{s_1} (M_s - M_s^o) \tag{10.45}$$

If M_s and M_s^o are small in comparison with M_{salt}, the last term can be neglected, to give Eq. (10.39), in which $K_s = k_{salt_1}$.

Example

The table below gives the number of moles (w) of water required to dissolve 1 mol of ethyl acetate in the presence of m moles of ammonium chloride [22].   Calculate the salting-out constant.

m	0	0.525	1.568	4.280	8.410	14.95
w	66.15	76.54	89.14	112.4	139.7	174.5

Molecular weights: ethyl acetate, 88; water, 18; ammonium chloride, 53.5.

Solution:

When m = 0,

$$\text{Molality of ethyl acetate} = \frac{1 \times 1000}{88 + 66.15 \times 18} = 0.782$$

When m = 0.525,

$$\text{Molality of ethyl acetate} = \frac{1000}{88 + 76.54 \times 18 + 0.525 \times 53.5} = 0.669$$

and

$$\text{Molality of ammonium chloride} = \frac{0.525 \times 1000}{88 + 76.54 \times 18 + 0.525 \times 53.5}$$

$$= 0.351$$

Therefore,

$$K_s = \frac{\log (0.782/0.669)}{0.351} = 0.193$$

Similarly,

m	1.568	4.280	8.410	14.95
Molality of ethyl acetate, M	0.563	0.427	0.328	0.248
$\log M_s^o/M_s$	0.143	0.262	0.378	0.498

Molality of ammonium chloride	0.883	1.829	2.755	3.711
K_S	0.161	0.143	0.137	0.134

giving a mean K_S of 0.154 kg mol^{-1}, with a standard deviation of 0.024. This is too large, and the progressive decrease in K_S with increasing ammonium chloride concentration is not satisfactory. An improvement would be anticipated if activities were used instead of concentrations. Activity coefficients for ammonium chloride at 25°C are as follows [23]:

Molality	0.3	0.5	0.7	1.0	1.4	2.0	3.0	4.0
f_m	0.687	0.649	0.625	0.603	0.584	0.570	0.561	0.560

Activity coefficients corresponding to the relevant concentrations can be obtained by interpolation and salting-out constants calculated as follows:

Molality of NH_4Cl	0.351	0.883	1.829	2.755	3.711
Activity of coefficient, f_m	0.677	0.631	0.574	0.563	0.560
Activity, a	0.238	0.557	1.050	1.552	2.079
$\log (M_S^0/M_S)/a = K_S$	0.285	0.257	0.250	0.244	0.240

giving a mean K_S of 0.255 kg mol^{-1}, with a standard deviation of 0.002, which is a more acceptable variation.

Example

The solubility of benzoic acid at ambient temperature is 1 in 350. Given that the thermodynamic salting-out parameter for benzoic acid/NaCl is 0.152 dm^3 mol^{-1} at 25°C, estimate the solubility of benzoic acid in molar NaCl. The activity coefficient of molar NaCl is 0.657. The molecular weight of benzoic acid is 122.

Solution:

$$1 \text{ in } 350 = \frac{1000 \times 1}{350 \times 122} = 0.0234 \text{ M}$$

Activity of NaCl = 1×0.657

$$\log \frac{M_s^o}{M_s} = 0.152 \times 0.657 = 0.0999$$

$$\frac{0.0234}{M_s} = \text{antilog } 0.0999 = 1.259$$

$$M_s = \frac{0.0234}{1.259} = 0.019 \text{ M}$$

$$= 0.019 \times 122 = 2.27 \text{ g dm}^{-3}$$

or

$$\frac{1 \text{ in } 1000}{2.27} = 441$$

Several theories have been advanced in attempts to explain the influence of electrolytes on the aqueous solubilities of nonelectrolytes. The hydration theory suggests that the electrolyte competes with the nonelectrolyte for water, each making less solvent available for the other. This approach suggests that the effectiveness of a given electrolyte is specific to that electrolyte and independent of the nature of the nonelectrolyte. Some Setschenow constants are given in Table 10.6. The constants follow the same electrolyte rank order, and the relative values, in which the constants for sodium chloride are allocated the value of unity, are similar. There are discrepancies, however, suggesting that other factors are operating. The biggest objection to the hydration theory is that it does not explain salting-in.

The electrostatic theory is based on the fact that electrolytes bring about an increase in the dielectric constant of water. The concept has been approached in a similar manner to that used to develop the Debye-Hückel limiting law (Section III.A of Chapter 1). The work necessary to remove the electrostatic charge on an ion in water, and replace it with the charge associated with the ion in the solution containing the nonelectrolyte, was calculated [26] and related to $-(RT/N) \ln f_m$, where N is Avogadro's number, to yield

TABLE 10.6 Setschenow Coefficients[a] ($dm^3 mol^{-1}$ at 25°C)

	NaCl	LiCl	KCl	NaBr	KBr
Benzene	0.198	0.141	0.166	0.155	0.119
	(1.0)	(0.7)	(0.8)	(0.8)	(0.6)
Naphthalene	0.260	0.180	0.204	0.169	—
	(1.0)	(0.7)	(0.8)	(0.7)	—
Biphenyl	0.276	0.218	0.295	0.209	—
	(1.0)	(0.8)	(1.1)	(0.8)	—
Ethyl acetate	0.166	0.088	0.105	0.119	0.105
	(1.0)	(0.5)	(0.6)	(0.7)	(0.6)
Phenol	0.220	0.181	0.245	—	—
	(1.0)	(0.8)	(1.1)	—	—

[a]The figures in parentheses represent the coefficient relative to that for NaCl.
Source: Abstracted from Refs. 22, 24, and 25.

$$\ln f_m = \frac{(\varepsilon_0 - \varepsilon)e^2}{2kT\varepsilon_0^2 M_s} \sum_i \frac{0 \; M_i z_i^2}{r_i} \tag{10.46}$$

where ε_0 and ε represent dielectric constants of water and solution containing the nonelectrolyte respectively, M_s is molar concentration of the nonelectrolyte, and i represents the various ionic species. M_i is molarity of each ion, z_i its valency, and r its ionic radius. k is the Boltzmann constant and e is the electronic charge. Substitution of the known constants gives

$$\ln f_m = 1.82 \times 10^{-6} \frac{\varepsilon - \varepsilon_0}{M_s} \sum_i \frac{0 \; M_i z_i^2}{r_i} \tag{10.47}$$

in which ionic radius is expressed in meters. Similar approaches and equations have followed, but none have been entirely successful, and all have failed to explain the process of salting-in.

An extension of the electrostatic theory suggests that dispersion forces play a part in the process and are responsible for salting-in

by large ions. Activity coefficient, according to this theory, is
equal to the electrostatic effect, taking a form similar to that expressed in Eq. (10.46), divided by a polarizability term. When
the influence of the dispersion forces is greater than the electrostatic effect, f_m becomes less than 1 and salting-in results.

Another theory is based on internal pressures and their influence on the volume of the solvent. Thus if the internal pressure
causes a contraction of the solvent, there will be less room available for the nonelectrolyte, which is salted out. Further information on the processes of salting-in and salting-out may be obtained
elsewhere (e.g., [23,25]).

Polar and nonpolar nonelectrolytes, as expressed by their dipole moments, fall into two groups with respect to the influence of
electrolytes on their solubilities in water. With nonpolar nonelectrolytes, the degree of salting-out appears to be solely dependent
on the nature of the electrolyte, the Setschetow coefficients falling
in approximately the same order for all the nonelectrolytes. The
degree of salting-out decreases with ionic size, and the effect of a
given ion appears to be independent of the nature of the counterion; for example, the difference between NaCl and KCl would be
roughly the same as that between NaBr and KBr. Nonpolar nonelectrolytes therefore seem to fit the hydration and internal pressure
theories, both of which are governed by the amount of water available to the nonelectrolyte. Contraction of the water will result from
the attraction of the solvent dipoles by the electrostatic field of the
ion, but this is opposed by the volume taken up by the ion. The
electrostatic field strength also falls with increasing ionic size. The
overall result is that the degree of salting-out tends to decrease with
ionic size. There are exceptions, however, particularly with respect
to lithium, which is less effective than its size suggests.

The influence of electrolytes on the solubilities of polar nonelectrolytes follows roughly the same order as with nonpolar molecules, but the extent of the differences between electrolytes varies
with the nature of the nonelectrolyte. These differences are undoubtedly due to interactions involving dipoles on the nonelectrolytes.

The activity coefficients of weak electrolytes have also been found
to follow the Setschenow equation; Harned and Owen [23], for example, quote salting-out constants for a selection of organic acids.
Miyazaki et al. [27] published salting-out constants for hydrochlorides of weak bases in aqueous sodium chloride solutions and obtained
good rectilinear plots of log (S_0/S) against sodium chloride concentration. S_0 and S represent solubilities in mg ml^{-1} in water and sodium chloride solution, respectively. They used their observations
to suggest that the solubilities of salts of weak bases are lower in
the gastric environment than in pure water. Their systems were
more specific than those embraced by the Setschenow equation,

because they involve a common (chloride) ion. The approach is interesting, however, because it appears to provide a method of quantitating the common-ion effect at concentrations in excess of those at which the solubility product operates (page 396).

The process of salting-in has been known for many years and has acquired the description *hydrotropism*. It occurs with large ions, such as phenate, alkyl sulfate, and quaternary ammonium ions, and is probabably due to a large extent to the expansion of water on the introduction of these ions. Ion-dipole interaction with polar nonelectrolytes is also a contributory factor.

The degree of salting-in by homologous series of ions increases with increasing size of the ion. This effect has been observed with sodium salts of normal fatty acids, and it has been suggested [25] that salting-in progresses continously to the associated phenomenon of solubilization as the series is ascended. A similar concept can be applied to the formation of specific complexes between large ions and nonelectrolytes, such as sodium benzoate and caffeine. This type of behavior has been discussed in Chapter 8, when 1:1 association between a substrate S and complexing agent L, to give a soluble complex SL, has been shown to follow the law of mass action according to

$$K_{1,1} = \frac{[SL]}{[S][L]} \tag{10.48}$$

[S] was equated to the solubility of the substrate in the pure solvent, and [SL] to the apparent increase in solubility in the presence of L. With sparingly soluble substrates, $[SL] \gg [S]$, and Eq. (10.48) can be simplified and rearranged to give

$$\frac{[SL]}{[S]} = \frac{M_s}{M_s^o} = K_{1,1}[L] \tag{10.49}$$

which has a form that is similar (although nonlogarithmic) to that of the Setschenow equation. It is possible therefore, that salting-in and complexation are extremes of what is basically the same process.

B. Nonelectrolytes

Regular solution theory has, understandably, proved to be of little value in predicting solubilities of nonelectrolytes in aqueous systems. It does, however, provide a useful basis for explaining why mixtures of water and water-miscible organic liquids are usually better sol-

vents for organic nonelectrolytes than water alone. The following
is a form of the regular solubility equation [Eq. (5.45)] and predicts
solubilities in solutions in which molecular interactions are small.

$$-\ln X_2 = -\ln X_2^i + \frac{V_2 \phi_1^2 (\delta_1 - \delta_2)^2}{RT} \tag{10.50}$$

δ_1 represents the solubility parameter of the solvent and δ_2 that
of the solute. The closer the values of δ_1 and δ_2, the smaller will
be the term within the parentheses, and when $\delta_1 = \delta_2$, the second
term on the right-hand side disappears. At this point regular solubility is maximal and equal to ideal solubility (X_2^i). Water has a solubility parameter of 23.4 H, which is greater than those of organic
nonelectrolytes, so that addition of an organic cosolvent will decrease
the net solubility parameter of the solvent mixture, with a resulting
increase in the quantity of nonelectrolyte it is capable of dissolving.

The effects of increasing concentrations of cosolvent will depend
on the solubility parameters of solute and cosolvent. If the solubility parameter of the cosolvent is greater than that of the solute,
solubility will increase progressively with increasing cosolvent concentration, but if the solubility parameter of the solute is greater than
that of the cosolvent, solubility will increase to a maximum, corresponding to the solubility parameter of the solute, and then decline.
By the same argument, if the solute has a solubility parameter greater than or equal to that of water, addition of an organic cosolvent
will result in a reduction in solubility.

Experimental results normally follow this pattern; for example,
the behavior of sulfamethoxazole in ethanol-water mixtures [28] is
typical of the relative solubility parameters of the components.
These are: sulfamethoxazole = 16.4 H, ethanol = 12.8 H, and water =
23.4 H. As the proportion of ethanol increases, the solubility parameter of the solvent mixture decreases, and at low ethanol concentrations, the solubility of sulfamethoxazole increases. The rate of
change in solubility is slow at first, but increases to an approximately constant rate, represented by the rectilinear portion AB of
Fig. 10.5, and then slows down as the solubility parameter of the
solvent mixture approaches that of the solute. The solubility of sulfamethoxazole then passes through a maximum in the region $\delta_1 =$
16.4 H. Beyond this point, solubility decreases as $(\delta_1 - \delta_2)^2$ increases. Similar profiles were observed with other sulfonamides [28],
and there are numerous other examples of such behavior, of which
[29–33] are a selection.

As a first approximation, solubility parameters of solvent blends
can be assumed to be additive and to follow

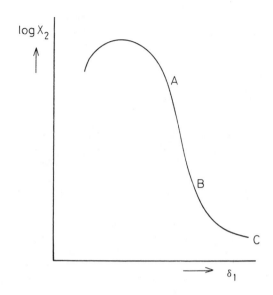

FIGURE 10.5 Variation of solubility of a nonelectrolyte with the solubility parameter of water-cosolvent mixture.

$$\delta_{mixture} = \sum_{\phi=0}^{\phi=1} \phi_i \delta_i \qquad (10.51)$$

where ϕ_i represents volume fraction and δ_i the solubility parameter of each component of the solvent blend. Plots of solubility of solute against solvent composition in binary water-cosolvent mixtures should therefore follow a similar form to the corresponding plots of solubility against solvent blend solubility parameter. Yalkowsky et al. [34] found that the solubilities of a range of alkyl-p-aminobenzoates in propylene glycol-water mixtures increased with increasing propylene glycol concentration. Propylene glycol has a solubility parameter of 15.0 H [35], and calculation using Rheineck and Lin substituent constants [36] gives solubility parameters of the order of 11 H for the alkyl-p-aminobenzoates. The solubility parameter of the solvent mixture will therefore be well removed from that of the solute, even when the volume fraction of propylene glycol is unity, and the plots of solubility against both solvent mixture solubility parameter and volume fraction of water would be expected to take a form similar to the line ABC in Fig. 10.5. This is approximately exponential, and it is therefore not surprising that a rectilinear relationship between log solubility and percentage v/v of propylene glycol in the solvent mixture was found [34]. As a result, the following was proposed:

$$\log M_s = \log M_{s(w)} + \phi_{PG}\sigma \tag{10.52}$$

where M_s and $M_{s(w)}$ represent molar solubilities in solvent blend and water, respectively, ϕ_{PG} is the volume fraction of propylene glycol, and σ is a constant, characteristic of cosolvent and solute.

The equation is useful because the extremes of the line ABC in Fig. 10.5, where predicted results would be expected to deviate from observed, are of limited practical value. Thus in the region of C in Fig. 10.5, the advantage gained by adding cosolvent is too small to be of any use, while at cosolvent concentrations in excess of point A, the aqueous concentration will be too low for most purposes. An estimate of σ can be evaluated by determining solubilities at two cosolvent concentrations, and the region of cosolvent concentration required for the planned concentration of solute determined by substitution in Eq. (10.52).

Equation (10.50) is a binomial relationship between $\log X_2$ and δ_1. The two variables therefore follow a parabolic plot similar to that shown in Fig. 10.5. Solubilities in aqueous systems calculated from Eq. (10.50) are usually greater than experimental values and follow a symmetrical distribution, which is unusual in real situations. Figure 10.6 is an example, and shows the solubilities of caffeine in dioxane-water mixtures. Martin [37] suggested that power series taking the form

$$\frac{\log f_2}{A} = K_1 + K_2\phi_w + K_3\phi_w^2 + K_4\phi_w^3 + K_5\phi_w^4 \tag{10.53}$$

would define the behavior more precisely. f_2 is the activity coefficient of the solute in the saturated solution, ϕ_w is the volume fraction of water in the solvent mixture, and A is defined by

$$A = V_2(2.303RT)\phi_1^2 \tag{10.54}$$

K_1 to K_4 are equation coefficients and are characteristic of the nature of the solute and cosolvent. Multiple regression analysis of experimental solubilities of caffeine in dioxane-water mixtures yielded

$$\frac{\log f_2}{A} = 8.410 - 38.42\phi_w + 109.6\phi_w^2 - 114.4\phi_w^3 \tag{10.55}$$
$$+ 49.38\phi_w^4$$

which provided the line drawn through the experimental points in Fig. 10.6. Similar equations have been obtained with other systems

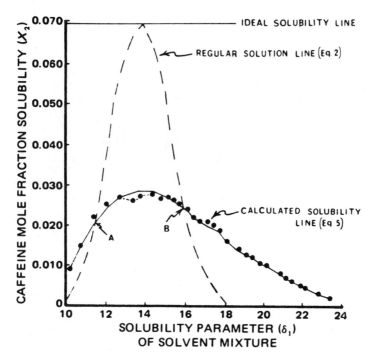

FIGURE 10.6 Variation of solubility of caffeine with the solubility parameters of dioxane-water solvent mixtures. (From Ref. 37.)

[30,31], all requiring fewer power series terms than Eq. (10.55). The procedure may be used to search for solvent compositions capable of attaining a required solubility. Solubility determinations in each of the two pure solvents, and three others in solvent blends spread over the composition range, are sufficient to produce an exploratory series up to the fourth power.

Example

Use the information listed below, together with Eq. (10.55), to predict the solubility of caffeine in a 40% v/v solution of dioxane in water at 25°C. Enthalpy of fusion of caffeine = 5.044 kcal mol^{-1}, molar volume = 114 cm^3 mol^{-1}, and melting point = 239°C. Gas constant = 1.987 cal mol^{-1} deg^{-1}.

Solution:

Ideal solubility is given by Eq. (4.27),

$$-\log X_2^i = \frac{\Delta S^f}{2.303R} \times 2.303 \log \frac{T_m}{T}$$

Therefore, since $\Delta S^f = \Delta H^f / T_m$,

$$-\log X_2^i = \frac{5044}{1.987 \times (273 + 239)} \log \frac{273 + 239}{273 + 25}$$

$$= 1.165$$

From Eq. (10.54), approximating ϕ_1^2 to unity,

$$A = \frac{144}{2.303 \times 1.987 \times 298} = 0.1056$$

From Eq. (10.55),

$$\frac{\log f_2}{A} = 8.410 - 38.42 \times 0.6 + 109.6 \times 0.6^2 - 114.4 \times 0.6^3$$
$$+ 49.38 \times 0.6^4$$
$$= 6.503$$

Therefore,

$$\log f_2 = 6.503 \times 0.1056 = 0.6867$$

Since,

$$X_2^i = f_2 X_2 \qquad \text{or} \qquad \log X_2 = \log X_2^i - \log f_2$$

$$\log X_2 = -1.165 - 0.6867 = -1.852$$

Therefore,

$$X_2 = 0.0140$$

Observed $X_2 = 0.0164$.

A better estimate would be obtained by substituting ϕ_1^2 calculated from $X_2 = 0.0141$ into Eq. (10.55), and repeating the process by successive approximations until a constant value of X_2 is obtained (see p. 203).

Yalkowsky et al. [38] explained the solubilities of the p-aminobenzoates in aqueous solvent mixtures in terms of the two-dimensional approach to solubility (Section III in Chapter 5), and derived

$$\log X_s = \log X_{s(w)} + \frac{CN \, \Delta\gamma\phi_c(HSA)}{2.303RT} \tag{10.56}$$

as a means of predicting solubilities in mixed solvents. X_S and $X_{S(w)}$ are mole fraction solubilities in solvent mixture and water respectively. C is the curvature correction factor [see Eq. (5.49)], which corrects experimental interfacial tensions to those acting across molecular interfaces, N is Avogadro's number, and HSA the hydrophilic surface area of the solute (page 365). $\Delta \gamma$ is the difference between the interfacial tensions of water and pure cosolvent, measured against tetradecane, and ϕ_c is the volume fraction of cosolvent. C was found to have a value around 0.5 for the systems under scrutiny.

Example

The interfacial tensions of water and propylene glycol against tetradecane at 37°C are 51.9 and 28.9 dyn cm^{-1}, respectively. Hexyl-p-aminobenzoate has a hydrophilic surface area (HSA) of 210 A^2 and a mole fraction solubility in water of 1.93×10^{-6} at 37°C. Assuming a curvature correction factor of 0.5, calculate the solubility of hexyl-p-aminobenzoate in 40% v/v aqueous propylene glycol at 37°C. Avogadro's number = 6.024×10^{23} mol^{-1}; gas constant = 8.315×10^7 erg mol^{-1} deg^{-1}.

Solution:

$$1A = 10^{-10} \ m$$

$$210 \ A^2 = 210 \times (10^{-10})^2 \times 100^2 = 2.1 \times 10^{-14} \ cm^2$$

$$\log 1.93 \times 10^{-6} = -5.714$$

Therefore,

$$\log X_S = -5.714 +$$

$$\frac{0.5 \times 6.024 \times 10^{23} \times (51.9 - 28.9) \times 0.4 \times 2.1 \times 10^{-14}}{2.303 \times 8.315 \times 10^7 \times 310}$$

$$= -5.714 + 0.980 = -4.734$$

$$X_S = antilog - 4.734 = 1.8 \times 10^{-5}$$

Observed $X_S = 5.8 \times 10^{-5}$

It is not essential for the cosolvent to be a liquid. Sucrose has been used to increase the solubilities of quinine base, phenobarbital, p-aminobenzoic acid, and sulfanilamide in water, and correlations between solubility and dielectric constant of the medium demonstrated graphically [39]. Dielectric constant is rectilinearly related to solubility parameter [40], so the observed increases in solubility can be interpreted in the same way as above.

The influence of one nonelectrolyte on the aqueous solubility of another cannot always be explained in terms of solubility parameters and/or dielectric constants. Lakshmi and Nandi [41] found that the aqueous solubilities of phenylalanine, tryptophane, tyrosine, and their N-acetylethyl esters decreased, rather than increased, in the presence of glucose, glycerol, propylene glycol, and sucrose. In contrast, 1-butanol increased the solubilities of the ethyl esters. They suggested that the overall behavior could be described by

$$\log f = K'_s c_s \qquad (10.57)$$

which is similar to the Setschenow equation. f represents the activity coefficient of the solute, and K'_s is the value of f when the molar concentration of the added nonelectrolyte (c_s) is unity. Nango et al. [42] observed similar deviations from normal behavior in the solubilities of three aromatic hydrocarbons in sugar solutions. Solubilities increased in the order glucose, fructose, sucrose, but there was also a component in the behavior related to the molecular size of the solute. Thus the solubilities in benzene were reduced and the solubilities of phenanthrene increased in the presence of the sugars, while biphenyl occupied an intermediate position in which solubility was reduced by glucose and fructose, but increased by sucrose. The terms *sugaring-in* and *sugaring-out* were used to describe the behavior.

The aqueous solubilities of nonelectrolytes can be increased by the addition of urea. The process is not associated with solubility parameters, nor is it generally due to solute-urea complexation. Water is considered to consist of two species (see Section VI in Chapter 2); one is ordered and consists of "icebergs" of hydrogen-bonded water molecules, and the other represents the "sea between the icebergs," consisting of unassociated water molecules. The two species are in equilibrium, as shown by

$$\text{associated water} \rightleftharpoons \text{unassociated water} \qquad (10.58)$$

and the molecules are continuously transferring from one species to the other. Finer et al. [43] have presented nuclear magnetic resonance (NMR) evidence which indicates that urea forms short-range, short-lived hydrogen bonds with water but not with itself. The result is the destruction of the long-range order of the "icebergs," thereby moving the equilibrium represented by Eq. (10.58) farther to the right. Urea therefore enhances aqueous solubilities through a process of solvent structure breaking. This peculiar property of urea is attributed to its structure. It resembles water, with which it forms hydrogen bonds, but it has the wrong geometry to take part in the associated species of water. The behavior is not unique to urea; Feldman and Gibaldi [44] have demonstrated similar properties with N-methyl and 1,3-dimethyl urea, both of which enhance the aqueous solubilities of benzoic acid and salicylic acid.

III. AQUEOUS SOLUBILITIES OF ELECTROLYTES

The process of solution of electrolytes follows the same sequence as for nonelectrolytes, involving the three phases outlined previously. In the first stage, individual ions break away from the pure solute. Electrolytes are almost invariably solids, and the energy change involved is analogous to that associated with the formation of ideal solutions of solid nonelectrolytes. However, the forces involved with electrolytes are considerably greater than those of nonelectrolytes. The units forming an electrolyte crystal are intensely charged, and each is held in the crystal lattice by the opposite charges of the ions surrounding it. The resultant attractive energy is termed the lattice energy (ΔU_{lat}), and its magnitude can be judged by the fact that inorganic salts can rarely be melted under normal laboratory conditions. A consequence of this high lattice energy is that electrolytes are rarely soluble in organic solvents, but dissolve only in solvents with high dielectric constants. Water is usually the only suitable solvent in this class, but other, less convenient fluids such as liquid ammonia, hydrogen fluoride, and anhydrous acetic acid are capable of dissolving electrolytes. These solvents find most use in nonaqueous titrations and as solvents for reactions in which hydrolysis is to be avoided. Sometimes they are better solvents than water; silver iodide, for example, is soluble in only one part of ammonia at $0°C$, in comparison with about 10^9 parts of water.

Lattice energy is defined as the energy of the reaction that occurs when gaseous ions are brought together from infinite separation to their equilibrium positions in the solid. Thus for a uni-uni electrolyte AB, the lattice energy is the energy of the reaction

$$A^+_{gas} + B^-_{gas} = A^+B^-_{solid} \qquad\qquad (10.59)$$

Since it depends on the electrostatic interaction between ions, lattice energy increases with the magnitude of the charges on the ions and is, in fact, proportional to the squares of these charges. Thus an electrolyte $A^{2+}B^{2-}$ will have four times the lattice energy of a molecule A^+B^-, provided that they occupy structures with the same geometry. Lattice energy is also dependent on interionic spacing, which is, in turn, dependent on the structure of the lattice and the radii

of the ions. Thus for a given structure, lattice energy will decrease as the atoms taking part come from positions lower in the
periodic table. This is illustrated in Table 10.7. The dependence
of lattice energy on the spatial arrangement of the ions is expressed
as the Madelung constant, a proportionality factor that is characteristic for each type of configuration. They differ only slightly from
one configuration to another, so that their influence is considerably
less than that arising from ionic charge and radius.

The second stage of solution involves the separation of water
molecules to make space for the incoming solute molecules. Energy
is required to overcome attraction between the dipoles of adjacent
water molecules, and this is an important factor in the consideration
of solubilities of nonelectrolytes. It is, however, negligible in comparison with the energy involved in the dissolution and hydration of
ions, and can therefore be ignored when electrolyte solutions are
considered.

When the solute ions are released into the aqueous environment,
they attract the dipoles of the water molecules. Each solute cation
becomes surrounded by water molecules with their oxygen atoms
oriented toward the cation, and each anion acquires a similar shell
with the aqueous hydrogen atoms directed inward. These electrostatic interactions are dependent on the same factors as is lattice
energy, namely ionic charge and ionic radius, and show up thermo-
dynamically as the enthalpy of hydration, which becomes increasingly
more negative as the intensity of the ionic charge is increased and
as the ionic radius is decreased. These trends are illustrated in
Table 10.8.

TABLE 10.7 Observed and Calculated Lattice Energies for Silver
and Potassium Halides

	Lattice energy ($kJ\ mol^{-1}$)			
	Ag^+		K^+	
Halide ion	Observed	Calculated	Observed	Calculated
F	954	920	801	805
Cl	904	833	698	703
Br	895	816	672	675
I	883	778	632	638

Source: Ref. 45.

TABLE 10.8 Enthalpies and Entropies of
Hydration of Some Inorganic Ions

Ion	$-\Delta H$ (kJ mol^{-1})	$-\Delta S$ (J deg^{-1} mol^{-1})
Li$^+$	543	106
Na$^+$	433	73.1
K$^+$	349	39.4
Rb$^+$	324	27.6
Cs$^+$	291	24.7
Mg^{2+}	1980	267
Al^{3+}	4748	480
F$^-$	409	116
Cl$^-$	336	58.6
Br$^-$	302	41.8
I$^-$	259	20.9

Source: Ref. 46.

    If entropy effects are ignored, solubilities can be compared in
terms of enthalpies of solution, which have been shown to represent
the balance between lattice energy put into the system to separate
the solute ions and hydration energy released when the ions are
solvated. Enthalpy of solution is therefore a small difference between two large quantities; for example, for KCl,

$$\text{enthalpy of solution} = \Delta H_s = 698 - 349 - 336 = +13 \text{ kJ mol}^{-1}$$

Small, normally acceptable errors in the large thermodynamic properties will thus give rise to large, unacceptable errors in the heats
of solution, so that the procedure gives only a rough guide to the
anticipated solubilities of electrolytes.

    In view of the known large positive entropies of solution of non-
electrolytes, ignoring the entropy of hydration of electrolytes would
seem to be an ill-founded approximation. However, the anticipated
increase in disorder resulting from the transfer of ions from a crystal lattice to a liquid system is compensated by increased order in
the solvent resulting from orientation of its molecules around the

solute ions, resulting in a negative entropy of hydration. Justification for ignoring entropy is supported by the entropies of hydration quoted in Table 10.8. Thus the mean entropy of hydration is only 114 J mol^{-1} K^{-1}, which takes only 3.9% from the mean free energy of hydration of 872,600 J mol^{-1}.

Despite its failure to provide a quantitative basis for comparing electrolyte solubilities in water, some generalizations can be derived from this approach. Thus ionic charge has a greater influence on lattice energy than enthalpy of hydration, so that an increase in the valency of the ions will result in a decrease in the solubility of the salt, provided that the form of the solid state does not change too drastically. Examples of this can be seen in Table 10.9, which shows that the solubilities of group II salts are lower than those of group I. Another interesting feature is that whereas solubilities of salts vary considerably on a weight in weight basis, molal solubilities are usually reasonably constant within periodic table groups.

When the cation of a salt is small and highly charged and the anion is large with a diffuse electron cloud, the cation can induce a dipole on the anion. The result is the formation of an ion-dipole component to the lattice energy, additional to the ion-ion component. The resultant lattice energy is therefore higher than anticipated. This ability to induce a dipole is called the polarizing power and is greatest in small atoms with large positive charges relative to ionic volume, such as Li^+ and Al^{3+}. The effect is so great with beryllium and boron that they do not form monoatomic ions. The observed lattice energies of silver salts are larger than the anticipated values for this reason, and decrease progressively from the fluoride to the iodide, as shown in Table 10.7. In comparison, the differences for the potassium halides are small, and the calculated values are greater than observed. The enhanced polarizing power of the silver ion is attributed to its full d ring, and the phenomenon is probably the reason for the low solubilities of silver and cuprous salts compared with those of the alkali metals, as demonstrated in Table 10.9.

An interesting consequence of the polarizing power of the silver ion concerns the use of soaps as emulgents. The Harkins theory of emulsification suggests that because the charged head of a monovalent soap, located on the aqueous side of an oil-water interface, is broader er than the alkyl chain on the nonaqueous side, it will act as a wedge, causing the interface to form a concave surface on the lipid side. Formation of oil globules is thereby promoted and the emulgent is said to be oil in water inducing. The fact that silver stearate is a monovalent soap but is not oil-in-water inducing, has been used as evidence against the wedge theory, but the objectors have overlooked the probability that the salt is not ionized, or at best, weakly ionized.

In large molecules, the attractive forces in the solid are greater than the hydration energies, so that solubility decreases with

TABLE 10.9 Solubilities at Ambient Temperature

Ion	Formate		Acetate		Benzoate		Salicylate	
	Molal	% w/w	Molal	% w/w	Molal	% w/w	Molal	% w/w
Li^+	6.1	31	—	—	2.5	32	—	—
Na^+	7.2	49	3.4	33	2.4	35	3.3	52
K^+	9.4	79	6.4	73	2.7	42	3.1	54
Rb^+	6.5	85	5.3	85	2.8	57	3.1	69
Cs^+	4.6	82	4.4	92	3.0	75	—	—
Ag^+	—	—	0.2	1.1	0.01	0.26	0.002	0.095
Ca^{2+}	1.1	14	1.6	26	0.10	2.8	0.06	2.3
Sr^{2+}	0.7	12	1.4	29	0.14	5.0	0.07	3.0
Ba^{2+}	1.0	24	1.7	44	0.12	5.0	—	—

Source: Abstracted from Ref. 50.

increasing size, eventually becoming insignificant. This also applies to large ions. Large ions with reasonable aqueous solubilities can be precipitated by ions of equal and opposite charge, and the process is most efficient when the ions are of similar size. Classical examples of this behavior occur when a large cation such as cetyltrimethylammonium is added to an emulsion stabilized with an anionic surfactant, such as sodium lauryl sulfate, and breaks the emulsion. Similarly, a large anion, as is found for example in an alkaloidal salt, will cause separation of an emulsion stabilized with a cationic emulgent.

Johnson [47] has shown that salts in which the sizes of anion and cation are markedly different are more soluble than those with evenly matched ions, and give lithium fluoride and tetramethylammonium fluoride as examples. The reason was advanced that the "mismatch" caused difficulties in the packing of the solid, with resultant decrease in lattice energy. The same factor in reverse is the probable reason that large ions are more readily precipitated by ions of equal size (and opposite charge). Johnson [47] also included inorganic salts, which were freely soluble in organic solvents, due to imbalance between ionic sizes.

A common belief often assumed in the formulation of electrolyte solutions is that potassium salts tend to be more soluble than sodium salts. This is often true when the salt concentration is measured by weight, but is seldom so when molarities are considered. The observed higher solubilities are usually due to the difference between the atomic weights of the two cations, and when the object of the exercise is to get as much anion into solution as possible, there is no advantage in using the salt with the larger molecular weight.

IV. EFFECT OF ADDITIVES ON AQUEOUS SOLUBILITIES OF ELECTROLYTES

A. Electrolytes

1. With a Common Ion. The equilibrium operating in a saturated aqueous solution of a strong electrolyte is given by

$$A^+B^-_{solid} \rightleftharpoons A^+_{aq} + B^-_{aq} \tag{10.60}$$

Application of the law of mass action gives

$$K = \frac{[A^+_{aq}][B^-_{aq}]}{[A^+B^-_{solid}]} \times f_{A^+} f_{B^-} \tag{10.61}$$

where K is the equilibrium constant of Eq. (10.60) and f represents activity coefficient. K is another way of expressing solubility, since the greater its value, the greater will be the solubility.

If another electrolyte, having B^- for its anion, is dissolved in the solution, B_{aq}^- in Eq. (10.61) will increase, with the result that some A^+ and B^- ions will combine and precipitate in order to reduce the numerator in Eq. (10.61), thereby keeping K constant. This effect of a common ion, in this case B^-, on the solubility of an electrolyte is called the common-ion effect. The classical example occurs when HCl gas is bubbled through a saturated solution of sodium chloride. The gas, which is very soluble in water, puts more chloride ions into solution and some of the sodium chloride is precipitated out. Since Eq. (10.61) is used here to express a qualitative effect, the extra accuracy derived by the activity coefficients is not required and is usually ignored.

Sodium chloride in very soluble in water, so that $[Na_{aq}^+][Cl_{aq}^-]$ is large, comparible in size to $[NaCl_{solid}]$. With sparingly soluble electrolytes, such as silver chloride, $[Ag_{aq}^+][Cl_{aq}^-]$ is very small and normally insignificant compared with $[AgCl_{solid}]$, as expressed in

$$K_{AgCl} = \frac{[Ag_{aq}^+][Cl_{aq}^-]}{[AgCl_{solid}]} \qquad (10.62)$$

$[AgCl_{solid}]$ can therefore be considered to be constant, which leads to

$$K_{AgCl}[AgCl_{solid}] = [Ag_{aq}^+][Cl_{aq}^-] = K_{sp} \qquad (10.63)$$

K_{sp} is the solubility product. It is constant at constant temperature and characteristic of the electrolyte it represents. Solubility products are usually calculated using molar concentrations. However, for accurate work, activities should be used; that is,

$$K_{sp}' = [Ag_{aq}^+][Cl_{aq}^-] \times f_{Ag^+} f_{Cl^-} \qquad (10.64)$$

K_{sp}' is the thermodynamic solubility product. Activity coefficients may be calculated using the Debye-Hückel equations (Section III.A of Chapter 1) or by the experimental methods described in Chapter 1. Many activity coefficients can be found in the literature (e.g., [23,48]).

For an electrolyte A_aB_b, the equilibrium is represented by

$$A_aB_b = aA^{b+} + bB^{a-} \tag{10.65}$$

and the solubility product is therefore given by

$$K_{sp} = [A^{b+}]^a [B^{a-}]^b \tag{10.66}$$

Example

The molar solubility product of calcium sulfate is 6.56×10^{-5} mol^2 dm^{-6} at 25°C. Calculate the thermodynamic solubility product.

Solution:

$$[Ca^{2+}][SO_4^{2-}] = 6.56 \times 10^{-5}$$

Therefore,

$$\text{molar concentration} = \sqrt{6.56 \times 10^{-5}} = 8.099 \times 10^{-3}$$

$$\text{ionic strength} = I = 0.5(c_{Ca^{2+}}z_{Ca^{2+}}^2 + c_{SO_4^{2-}}z_{SO_4^{2-}}^2$$

$$= 0.5(2 \times 8.099 \times 10^{-3} \times 2^2) = 3.240 \times 10^{-2}$$

This figure is greater than $I = 0.01$ and less than $I = 0.25$; therefore, Eq. (1.12) must be used to calculate the activity coefficient; that is,

$$\log f = \frac{-0.51 \times 2 \times 2 \sqrt{3.240 \times 10^{-2}}}{1 + \sqrt{3.240 \times 10^{-2}}}$$

$$= -0.3111$$

Therefore,

$$f = \text{antilog} -0.3111 = 0.488$$

$$K'_{sp} = [Ca^{2+}][SO_4^{2-}] \times f_{Ca^{2+}} \times f_{SO_4^{2-}}$$

$$= K_{sp} \times f_{Ca^{2+}} \times f_{SO_4^{2-}}$$

$$= 6.56 \times 10^{-5} \times 0.488^2$$

$$= 1.55 \times 10^{-5}$$

Example

The solubility of procaine penicillin in water is 1 in 200 at 25°C. Calculate its molar solubility product at this temperature, assuming complete dissociation into procaine and penicillin ions. What would be the equilibrium percentage w/v of procaine penicillin in solution if an excess of procaine penicillin is suspended in a 1.0% w/v solution of procaine hydrochloride in water at 25°C? Molecular weights: procaine penicillin, 589; procaine hydrochloride, 273.

Solution:

Molar solubility of procaine penicillin in water $= \dfrac{1 \times 1000}{200 \times 589}$

$$= 8.49 \times 10^{-3} \text{ mol dm}^{-3}$$

Solubility product $= K_{sp} = [\text{procaine-H}^+][\text{penicillin}^-]$

$$= (8.49 \times 10^{-3})^2 = 7.21 \times 10^{-5}$$

Molar concentration of procaine hydrochloride $= \dfrac{1 \times 1000}{100 \times 273}$

$$= 3.66 \times 10^{-2} \text{ mol dm}^{-3}$$

Ignoring the procaine ion concentration coming from the procaine penicillin yields

$$[\text{Penicillin}^-] = \frac{7.21 \times 10^{-5}}{3.66 \times 10^{-2}} = 1.97 \times 10^{-3} \text{ mol dm}^{-3}$$

Taking the procaine ions coming from the procaine penicillin into consideration gives

$$[\text{Penicillin}^-] = \frac{7.21 \times 10^{-5}}{3.66 \times 10^{-2} + 1.97 \times 10^{-3}} = 1.87 \times 10^{-3} \text{ mol dm}^{-3}$$

Substitution of 1.87×10^{-3} for 1.97×10^{-3} in the equation above gives no significant reduction in the result; therefore, the concentration of procaine penicillin dissolved in the aqueous phase is

$$\frac{1.87 \times 10^{-3} \times 589}{10} = 0.11 \% \text{ w/v}$$

Miyazaki et al. [27,49] used the Setschenow equation (10.39) to study the common-ion effect of sodium chloride on a selection of organic hydrochlorides. They were able to use the equation to quantify the common-ion effect for moderately soluble combinations of ions. This work is described in more detail elsewhere (page 381).

2. Without a Common Ion. In a solution containing two electrolyte solutes, A^+B^- and C^+D^-, the following four equilibria will operate:

$$AB_{solid} \rightleftharpoons A^+ + B^- \tag{10.67}$$

$$CD_{solid} \rightleftharpoons C^+ + D^- \tag{10.68}$$

$$CB_{solid} \rightleftharpoons C^+ + B^- \tag{10.69}$$

$$AD_{solid} \rightleftharpoons A^+ + D^- \tag{10.70}$$

As a first approximation, precipitation will occur when the aqueous solubility of the pair of ions having the lowest equilibrium constant is exceeded.

The other ions will influence the solubility of the pair of ions with the lowest equilibrium constant, through their mean activity coefficient, by increasing ionic strength (page 10). Thus if in the foregoing example involving the solubility product of calcium sulfate, a mixture of sodium sulfate and calcium chloride were under consideration, the ionic strength expression would become

$$I = 0.5(c_{Ca^{2+}}z_{Ca^{2+}}^2 + c_{SO_4^{2-}}z_{SO_4^{2-}}^2 + c_{Na^+}z_{Na^+}^2 + c_{Cl^-}z_{Cl^-}^2) \tag{10.71}$$

which would reduce the activity coefficient of calcium sulfate, together with the value of the solubility product operating under the given conditions.

If the concentrations of the ions are too great to employ one of the Debye-Hückel limiting equations (Section III.A of Chapter 1),

activity coefficients corresponding to the calculated ionic strength
can often be obtained from tables of activity coefficients (e.g., in
[23] and [48]).

B. Strong Acids and Bases

As explained in Chapter 3, salts of organic acids and bases are
usually very soluble in water because they are completely ionized
in this medium and because the resulting charged group is highly
hydrophilic and capable of bringing large hydrophobic groups into
solution.   On the other hand, the undissociated weak acid or base
is a weak electrolyte and therefore only feebly ionized in water.
The resulting uncharged group is only weakly hydrophilic, so that
only those acids and bases with small hydrophobic groups are able
to dissolve in water to any great extent.   Another property of weak
acids and bases is that their aqueous solubilities are sensitive to
pH, so that an uncharged, water-insoluble molecule can be changed
to a charged, water-soluble species simply by changing the hydrogen ion concentration.   As an example, sodium salicylate is considerably more soluble in water than salicylic acid, due to the different hydrophilic powers of COO^- and $COOH$, so that if a strong acid
is added to an aqueous solution of sodium salicylate, there will be
a drastic fall in solubility and salicylic acid will be precipitated.   A
strong base has the same effect on weak bases.

A weak acid, HA, will dissociate in aqueous solution according to

$$HA + H_2O \rightleftharpoons H_3O^+ + A^- \tag{10.72}$$

but the equilibrium will be primarily to the left.   Application of the
law of mass action, and ignoring activity coefficients, gives

$$K = \frac{[H_3O^+][A^-]}{[HA][H_2O]} \tag{10.73}$$

and since $[H_2O]$ is much greater than the other terms, then

$$K[H_2O] = K_a = \frac{[H_3O^+][A^-]}{[HA]} \tag{10.74}$$

and

$$[A^-] = \frac{K_a[HA]}{[H_3O^+]} \tag{10.75}$$

K_a is the acid dissociation constant of HA. The total molar solubility (M_S) of the dissociated and undissociated acid is given by

$$M_S = [HA] + [A^-] \tag{10.76}$$

[HA] is the solubility of the undissociated acid and is independent of pH. If [HA] is given the symbol S_O and $[A^-]$ is substituted from Eq. (10.75), then

$$M_S = S_O + K_a \frac{S_O}{[H_3O^+]} \tag{10.77}$$

Rearranging yields

$$\frac{M_S - S_O}{S_O} = \frac{K_a}{[H_3O^+]} \tag{10.78}$$

Taking logs and substituting for $pK_a = -\log K_a$ and $pH = -\log H_3O^+$ gives

$$pH_p = pK_a + \log \frac{M_S - S_O}{S_O} \tag{10.79}$$

pH_p is the pH of precipitation, that is, the pH below which the solute will be precipitated as the undissociated acid from a solution of molar concentration M_S.

If S_O is considered to be negligible in comparison with M_S, rearrangement of Eq. (10.79) will give

$$\log M_S = pH - pK_a + \log S_O \tag{10.80}$$

Example

Phenobarbital is a weak monobasic acid with a pK_a value of 7.41 and an aqueous solubility of 1 in 830 at 25°C. Calculate its percentage solubility in an aqueous solution having a pH value of 8.2. Molecular weight of phenobarbital = 232.

Solution:

$$\text{Molarity of a saturated solution} = \frac{1000}{830 \times 232} = 5.19 \times 10^{-3} \text{ mol dm}^{-3}$$

$$\log S = pH - pK_a + \log S_o$$

$$= 8.2 - 7.41 + \log (5.19 \times 10^{-3})$$

$$= -1.49$$

Therefore,

$$S = \text{antilog} (-1.49) = 3.24 \times 10^{-2} \text{ mol dm}^{-3}$$

$$= \frac{3.24 \times 10^{-2} \times 232}{10} = 0.752\% \text{ (expressed as the acid)}$$

A similar argument can be applied to weak bases; for example,

$$B + H_2O = BH^+ + OH^- \qquad\qquad (10.81)$$

is the equilibrium for a base B, which can be substituted into the mass action equation,

$$K_b = \frac{[BH^+][OH^-]}{[B]} \qquad\qquad (10.82)$$

which defines the basic dissociation constant K_b. $[H_2O]$ is assumed to be constant and in large excess and is incorporated into the dissociation constant. The ionic product for water, K_w, is defined by

$$K_w = [H_3O^+][OH^-] \qquad\qquad (10.83)$$

and substitution for $[OH^-]$ from this into Eq. (10.82), leads to

$$[BH^+] = \frac{K_b[B][H_3O^+]}{K_w} \qquad\qquad (10.84)$$

As before, the total solubility (S) is the sum of the solubilities of the protonated base and the free base, that is,

$$S = [BH^+] + [B] \qquad\qquad (10.85)$$

or calling [B], S_o,

$$S = [BH^+] + S_o \qquad\qquad (10.86)$$

Substitution for [BH$^+$] and [B] in Eq. (10.84) gives

$$\frac{S - S_o}{S_o} = \frac{K_b}{K_w} [H_3O^+] \tag{10.87}$$

which on conversion to logs gives

$$pH_p = pK_w - pK_b - \log \frac{S - S_o}{S_o} \tag{10.88}$$

or in terms of the dissociation constant of the conjugate acid of the base (pK_a) $(= pK_w - pK_b)$, to

$$pH_p = pK_a - \log \frac{S - S_o}{S_o} \tag{10.89}$$

For weak bases, pH_p is the pH value *above* which the solute will be precipitated from a molar solution.

If S_o is considered to be negligible in comparison with S, rearrangement of Eq. (10.89) will give

$$\log S = pK_a - pH + \log S_o \tag{10.90}$$

analogous to Eq. (10.80) for weak acids.

Example

The molar solubility of cocaine in water is 5.60×10^{-3} at 25°C, and the molecular weight of its hydrochloride is 340. What is the highest pH permissible for complete solubility of a 0.5% solution of the hydrochloride at the same temperature? pK_a for cocaine = 8.41.

Solution:

The molarity of a 0.5% solution of cocaine hydrochloride is

$$\frac{0.5 \times 1000}{100 \times 340} = 1.47 \times 10^{-2}$$

Therefore,

$$pH_p = 8.41 - \log \frac{1.47 \times 10^{-2} - 5.60 \times 10^{-3}}{5.60 \times 10^{-3}} = 8.20$$

C. Nonelectrolytes

The Setschenow equation [Eq. (10.39)] is a well-established device for predicting the influence of electrolytes on the solubilities of non-electrolytes in water. McGowan [51] suggested that a similar equation should be applicable to the influence of nonelectrolytes on the aqueous solubilities of electrolytes, and proposed

$$\log M_s = \log M_{s(w)} - k'_s V^* C_{NE} \qquad (10.91)$$

taking the same form as that of Setschenow, but dependent on the molar volume of the nonelectrolyte. $M_{s(w)}$ and M_s are the solubilities in mol m^{-3} of the salt in water and water-nonelectrolyte mixture, respectively. k'_s is a constant, characteristic of the salt, but independent of the nature of the nonelectrolyte, and C_{NE} is the concentration of the nonelectrolyte in mol m^{-3}. V^* is described as the characteristic volume of the nonelectrolyte, equal to the parachor in cgs units, multiplied by 10^{-6}.

The solubilities of silver bromate (AgBrO$_3$) in methanol-water mixtures will be given as an example. The parachor for methanol can be calculated from Table 9.20 as follows:

$$[P] = 4 \times 24.7 + 46.35 + 35.25 - 5 \times 18.6 = 87.4$$

$$V^* = 8.74 \times 10^{-5} \; m^3 \; mol^{-1}$$

For a 10% w/w solution of methanol (molecular weight = 32.04) in water, a mixture having a density of 980.2 kg m^{-3},

$$C_{NE} = \frac{10 \times 980.2 \times 1000^2}{32.04 \times 1000 \times 100} = 3.06 \times 10^3 \; mol \; m^{-3}$$

k'_s for AgBrO$_3$ is 0.6, and the aqueous solubility of silver bromate is 8.12 mol m^{-3} [52]; therefore, substituting in Eq. (10.91),

$$\log M_s = \log 8.12 - 0.6 \times 8.74 \times 10^{-5} \times 3.06 \times 10^3$$

$$= 0.910 - 0.161 = 0.750$$

$$M_s = \text{antilog } 0.750 = 5.62 \; mol \; m^{-3}$$

Observed value [52] = 5.51 mol m^{-3}.

Observed and predicted value for other methanol-water mixtures are given in Table 10.10 and indicate the usefulness of Eq. (10.91). Factors for other electrolytes are given in Table 10.11.

TABLE 10.10 Observed and Predicted Solubilities of Silver Bromate in Methanol-Water Mixtures at 25°C

% w/w methanol	Density of solvent $(kg\ m^{-3})$	Solubility $(mol\ m^{-3})$	
		Predicted	Observed
0	998.7	—	—
10	980.2	5.62	5.51
20	965.0	3.93	3.79
30	949.2	2.78	2.65
40	931.8	2.00	1.82
50	912.3	1.46	1.24
60	890.8	1.08	0.83

The concept appears to be very useful in that the factor k_S' is independent of the nonelectrolyte mixed with the water, and that the cosolvent dependent term is readily calculated. The range of values of k_S' given by McGowan is restricted, but given solubilities in one solvent system, k_S' for a particular electrolyte can be calculated and used to calculate solubilities of that electrolyte in other solvent mixtures. Equation (10.91) fails if the electrolyte is soluble in the nonelectrolyte.

The equation is also a useful device for detecting interaction between the electrolyte and the nonelectrolyte, which is characterized by a significant difference between observed and predicted solubilities. Thus, by substituting observed solubilities (M_S) of silver sulfate in various water-cosolvent systems in Eq. (10.91) to predict aqueous solubilities, McGowan found that six of the cosolvents, comprising one ester, one ketone, and four alcohols, gave a mean value of 27.1 ± 1 (p' = 0.01) mol m^{-3}, compared with an

TABLE 10.11 k_S' Values for Calculation of Solubilities of Electrolytes in Water-Cosolvent Mixtures

Electrolyte:	$KBrO_3$	K_2SO_4	$AgBrO_3$	Ag_2SO_4	Li_2CO_3	$PbSO_4$
k_S':	0.8	1.0	0.6	1.1	10.5	1.6

observed value of 26.7, while acetonitrile and phenol gave 60.7 and 50.1 mol m^{-3}, respectively. It was therefore concluded that silver salts complex with acetonitrile and with phenol.

REFERENCES

1. C. McAuliffe, Solubility in water of paraffin, cycloparaffin, olefin, acetylene, cycloolefin and aromatic hydrocarbons, *J. Phys. Chem.*, *70*, 1267–1275 (1966).
2. S. S. Davis, T. Higuchi, and J. H. Rytting, Determination of thermodynamics of the methylene group in solutions of drug molecules, *J. Pharm. Pharmacol.*, *24* (Suppl.), 30P–46P (1972).
3. N. A. Armstrong, K. C. James, and C. K. Wong, Inter-relationships between solubilities, distribution coefficients and melting points of some substituted benzoic and phenylacetic acids, *J. Pharm. Pharmacol.*, *31*, 627–631 (1979).
4. K. C. James, Free energies of solution in water of some androstanolone, nandrolone and testosterone esters, *J. Pharm. Pharmacol.*, *28*, 929–931 (1976).
5. S. H. Yalkowsky, G. L. Flynn, and T. G. Slunick, Free energies of solution of alkyl-p-aminobenzoates, *J. Pharm. Sci.*, *61*, 852–857 (1972).
6. J. C. McGowan, The physical toxicity of chemicals: I. Vapours, *J. Appl. Chem.*, S120–S126 (1951).
7. J.C. McGowan, Molecular volumes and the periodic table, *Chem. Ind.*, 495–496 (1952).
8. J. C. McGowan, Molecular volumes and structural chemistry, *Recl. Trav. Chim. Pays-Bas Belg.*, *75*, 193–208 (1956).
9. S. Sugden, A relation between surface tension, density and chemical composition, *J. Chem. Soc.*, 1177–1189 (1924).
10. A. I. Vogel, W. T. Cresswell, G. J. Jeffery, and J. Leicester, Bond refractions and bond parachors, *Chem. Ind.*, 358 (1950).
11. J. C. McGowan, The physical toxicity of chemicals: II. Factors affecting physical toxicity in aqueous solutions, *J. Appl. Chem.*, *2*, 323–328 (1952).
12. J. C. McGowan, The physical toxicity of chemicals: IV. Solubilities, partition coefficients and physical toxicities, *J. Appl. Chem.*, *4*, 41–47 (1954).
13. J. A. V. Butler, C. N. Ramchandani, and D. W. Thomson, The solubility of non-electrolytes: Part 1. The free energy of hydration of some aliphatic alcohols, *J. Chem. Soc.*, 280–285 (1935).
14. J. A. V. Butler and C. N. Ramchandani, The solubility of non-electrolytes: Part II. The influence of the polar group on the free energy of hydration of aliphatic compounds, *J. Chem. Soc.*, 952–955 (1935).

15. G. L. Amidon, S. H. Yalkowsky, and S. Leung, Solubility of nonelectrolytes in polar solvents: II. Solubility of aliphatic alcohols in water, *J. Pharm. Sci. 63*, 1858—1866 (1974).

16. R. B. Herman, Theory of hydrophobic bonding: II. The correlation of hydrocarbon solubility in water with solvent cavity surface area, *J. Phys. Chem.*, *76*, 2754—2759 (1972).

17. G. L. Amidon, S. H. Yalkowsky, S. T. Anik, and S. C. Valvani, Solubility of nonelectrolytes in polar solvents: V. Estimation of the solubility of aliphatic monofunctional compounds in water using a molecular sufrace area approach, *J Phys. Chem.*, *79*, 2239—2246 (1975).

18. S. C. Valvani, S. H. Yalkowksy, and G. L. Amidon, Solubility of nonelectrolytes in polar solvents: VI. Refinements in molecular surface area computations, *J. Phys. Chem.*, *80*, 829—835 (1976).

19. S. H. Yalkowsky and S. C. Valvani, Solubility and partitioning: I. Solubility of nonelectrolytes in water, *J. Pharm. Sci.*, *69*, 912—922 (1980).

20. S. C. Valvani, S. H. Yalkowsky, and T. J. Roseman, Solubility and partitioning: IV. Aqueous solubility and octanol-water partition coefficients of nonelectrolytes, *J. Pharm. Sci.*, *70*, 502—507 (1981).

21. G. L. Amidon and N. A. Williams, A solubility equation for nonelectrolytes in water, *Int. J. Pharm.*, *11*, 249—256 (1982).

22. S. Glasstone and A. Pound. Solubility influences: Part I. The effect of some salts, sugars and temperature on the solubility of ethyl acetate in water, *J. Chem. Soc.*, 2660—2667 (1925).

23. H. S. Harned and B. B. Owen, *The Physical Chemistry of Electrolytic Solutions*, Rheinhold, New York, 1964.

24. W. Herz and F. Hiebenthal, Über Loslichkeitbesinfluesungen (About solubility), *Z. Anorg, Chem.*, *177*, 363—380 (1929).

25. F. A. Lang and W. F. McDevit, Activity coefficients of nonelectrolyte solutions in aqueous salt solutions, *Chem. Rev.*, *51*, 119—169 (1952).

26. P. Dedye and J. McAuley, Das elektrische Feld der Ionen und die Neutralsalzwirkung (The electric field of ions and the action of neutral salts), *Phys. Z.*, *26*, 22—29 (1925).

27. S. Miyazaki, M. Oshiba, and T. Nadai, Precaution on use of hydrochloride salts in pharmaceutical formulation, *J. Pharm. Sci.*, *70*, 594—596 (1981).

28. C. Sunwoo and H. Eisen, Solubility parameters of selected sulfonamides, *J. Pharm. Sci.*, *60*, 238—244 (1971).

29. M. J. Chertkoff and A. N. Martin, The solubility of benzoic acid in mixed solvents, *J. Pharm. Sci.*, *49*, 444—447 (1960).

30. A. Martin, P. L. Wu, A. Adjei, R. E. Lindstrom, and P. H. Elworthy, Extended Hildebrand solubility approach and log linear solubility equation, *J. Pharm. Sci.*, *71*, 849–856 (1982).

31. A. Martin, J. Newburger, and A. Adjei, Extended Hildebrand solubility approach: II. Solubility of theophylline in polar binary solvents, *J. Pharm. Sci.*, *69*, 487–491 (1980).

32. A. N. Paruta and J. W. Manger, Solubility of sodium salicylate in mixed solvent systems, *J. Pharm. Sci.*, *60*, 432–437 (1971).

33. N. G. Lordi, B. J. Sciarrone, T. J. Ambrosio, and A. N. Paruta, Dielectric constants and solubility, *J. Pharm. Sci.*, *53*, 463–464 (1964).

34. S. H. Yalkowsky, G. L. Flynn, and G. L. Amidon, Solubility of nonelectrolytes in polar solvents, *J. Pharm. Sci.*, *61*, 983–984 (1972).

35. K. L. Hoy, New values of the solubility parameters from vapor pressure data, *J. Paint Technol.*, *42*, 76–118 (1970).

36. A. E. Rheineck and K. F. Lin, Solubility parameter calculations based on group contributions, *J. Paint Technol.*, *40*, 611–616 (1968).

37. A. Adjei, J. Newburger, and A. Martin, Extended Hildebrand approach III. Solubility of Caffeine in dioxane-water mixtures, *J. Pharm. Sci.*, *69*, 659–661 (1980).

38. S. H. Yalkowsky, S. C. Valvani, and G. L. Amidon, Solubility of non-electrolytes in polar solvents: IV. Non-polar drugs in mixed solvents, *J. Pharm. Sci.*, *65*, 1488–1494 (1976).

39. A. N. Paruta, Solubility of several solutes as a function of the dielectric constant of sugar solutions, *J. Pharm. Sci.*, *53*, 1252–1254 (1964).

40. A. N. Paruta, B. J. Sciarrone, and N. G. Lordi, Correlation between solubility parameters and dielectric constants, *J. Pharm. Sci.*, *51*, 704–705 (1962).

41. T. S. Lakshmi and P. K. Nandi, Effects of sugar solutions on the activity coefficients of aromatic amino acids and their N-acetyl ethyl esters, *J. Phys. Chem.*, *80*, 249–252 (1976).

42. M. Nango, H. Yamamoto, K. Joukou, M. Ueda, A. Katayama, and N. Kuroki, Solubility of aromatic hydrocarbons in water and aqueous solutions of sugars, *Chem. Commun.*, 105–106 (1980).

43. E. G. Finer, F. Franks, and M. J. Tait, Nuclear magnetic resonance studies of aqueous urea solutions, *J. Am. Chem. Soc.*, *94*, 4424–4429 (1972).

44. S. Feldman and M. Gibaldi, Effect of urea on solubility, *J. Pharm. Sci.*, *56*, 370–375 (1967).

45. K. M. Mackay and R. A. Mackay, *Introduction to Modern Inorganic Chemistry*, 3rd ed., International Textbook Company, London, 1981.

46. R. M. Noyes, Thermodynamics of ion hydration as a measure of effective dielectric properties of water, *J. Am. Chem. Soc.*, *84*, 513–522 (1962).

47. D. A. Johnson, The standard free energies of solution of anhydrous salts in water, *J. Chem. Educ.*, *45*, 236–240 (1968).

48. R. A. Robinson and R. H. Stokes, *Electrolyte Solutions*, Butterworths, London, 1970.

49. S. Miyazaki, M. Oshiba, and T Nadai, Unusual solubility and dissolution behaviour of pharmaceutical hydrochloride salts in chloride-containing media, *Int. J. Pharm.*, *6*, 77–85 (1980).

50. W. F. Linke, *Solubility*, Van Nostrand, New York, Vol. 1, 1958, Vol. 2, 1965.

51. J C. McGowan, Effects of nonelectrolytes on the solubilities of salts in water, *Nature*, *252*, 296–297 (1974).

52. B. B. Owen, The medium effect of various solvents upon silver bromate at 25°, *J. Am. Chem. Soc.*, *55*, 1922–1928 (1933).

Index